Techniques in Diagnostic Radiology

Where is the wisdom we have lost in knowledge?
Where is the knowledge we have lost in information?
T. S. Eliot, *The Rock*.

Techniques in Diagnostic Radiology

Edited by

G. H. WHITEHOUSE, MB, BS, MRCP, MRCS, LRCP, FRCR, DMRD
Professor of Diagnostic Radiology
University of Liverpool

B. S. WORTHINGTON, BSC, LIMA, MB, BS, LRCP, MRCS, FRCR, DMRD
Professor of Diagnostic Radiology
University of Nottingham

BLACKWELL SCIENTIFIC PUBLICATIONS
OXFORD LONDON EDINBURGH BOSTON MELBOURNE

© 1983 by
Blackwell Scientific Publications
Editorial offiecs:
Osney Mead, Oxford, OX2 0EL
8 John Street, London, WC1N 2ES
9 Forrest Road, Edinburgh, EH1 2QH
52 Beacon Street, Boston
    Massachusetts 02108, USA
99 Barry Street, Carlton
    Victoria 3053, Australia

First published 1983

Typeset by CCC, printed and bound in Great Britain by
William Clowes Limited Beccles and London

DISTRIBUTORS

USA
    Blackwell Mosby Book Distributors
    11830 Westline Industrial Drive
    St Louis, Missouri 63141

Canada
    Blackwell Mosby Book Distributors
    120 Melford Drive, Scarborough
    Ontario, M1B 2X4

Australia   Blackwell Scientific Book Distributors
    31 Advantage Road, Highett
    Victoria 3190

British Library
Cataloguing in Publication Data

Techniques in diagnostic radiology.
    1. RM
    I. Whitehouse, G. H.   II Worthington, B. S.
    616.07′57   R895

ISBN 0-632-00874-1

Contents

SECTION 6. MISCELLANEOUS

List of Contributors

C. I. BARTRAM, *MB, BS(Lond), MRCP, FRCR, DMRD*, Consultant Radiologist; St. Bartholomew's Hospital and St. Marks Hospital for Diseases of the Rectum and Colon, London.

T. A. S. BUIST, *MB, ChB(Edin), FRCR, FRCP(Ed), FRCS(Ed), DObst, RCOG*, Consultant Radiologist; Edinburgh Royal Infirmary.

R. DICK, *MB, BS(Sydney), FRCR, MRACR*, Consultant Radiologist; Royal Free Hospital, London.

A. F. EVANS, *MB, ChB(L'pool), FRCR, DMRD*, Consultant Radiologist, Whiston Hospital, Merseyside.

C. D. R. FLOWER, *MA(Cantab), MB, BChir, FRCP Canada, FRCR*, Consultant Radiologist; Addenbrooke's Hospital, Cambridge.

R. W. GALLOWAY, *MD(L'pool), FRCR, DMRD, DObst, RCOG*, Consultant Radiologist; Royal Liverpool Hospital.

R. G. GRAINGER, *MD(Leeds), FRCP, FRCR, DMRD, Hon FACR, Hon FRACR*, Consultant Radiologist; Royal Hallamshire Hospital and Northern General Hospital, Sheffield.

R. K. LEVICK, *TD, MB, ChB(Wales), FRCP, FRCR, DMRD*, Consultant Radiologist; Sheffield Children's Hospital.

G. A. S. LLOYD, *MA, DM(Oxon), FRCR, DMRD*, Consultant Radiologist; Royal National Throat, Nose and Ear Hospital and Moorfields Eye Hospital, London.

J. S. MACDONALD, *MB, ChB(Edin), FRCP(Ed), FRCR, DMRD*, Consultant Radiologist; Royal Marsden Hospital, London.

D. J. NOLAN, *MD, MB, BCh, BAO(NUI), MRCP, FRCR, DMRD*, Consultant Radiologist, John Radcliffe Hospital, Oxford.

J. P. OWEN, *MB, BS(Newc), FRCR, DMRD*, Senior Lecturer in Diagnostic Radiology, University of Newcastle.

E. J. ROEBUCK, *MBBS(Lond), FRCR, DMRD*, Consultant Radiologist; University Hospital, Queens Medical Centre, Nottingham.

N. S. RUSSELL, *BMedSci, BM, BS*, University Hospital and Medical School, Queens Medical Centre, Nottingham.

N. J. D. SMITH, *MPhil, MSc, BDS*, Professor of Dental Radiology; Kings College Hospital Dental School, London.

S. L. SNOWDON, *MB, ChB(L'pool), FFARCS*, Senior Lecturer; Department of Anaesthesia, University of Liverpool.

H. L. WALTERS, *MBChB(Wales), FRCR, DMRD*, Consultant Radiologist; Kings College Hospital, London.

G. H. WHITEHOUSE, *MB, BS(Lond), MRCP, MRCS, LRCP, FRCR, DMRD*, Professor of Diagnostic Radiology, University of Liverpool.

B. S. WORTHINGTON, *BSc, MB, BS(Lond), FRCR, DMRD*, Professor of Diagnostic Radiology, University of Nottingham.

Preface

The scope and complexity of diagnostic imaging has greatly increased in recent years; with the development of interventional radiology, ultrasonography, radionuclide imaging, computed tomography and nuclear magnetic resonance. All these modalities have increased the knowledge demanded of trainee radiologists. It is necessary, however, for the trainee radiologist to be well versed in the practical radiological procedures which still have an important role in the day to day practice of diagnostic radiology. The common investigations, such as barium studies and intravenous urography, are performed by all general radiologists and should be carried out with the same scrupulous care as the esoteric angiograms performed by the experienced few.

It is intended that this book should fill a void in the radiological literature by providing a comprehensive and up-to-date compendium of practical radiological procedures. The increasing importance of an economical and rational approach to diagnostic imaging is reflected by the systematic elaboration of the indications and contra-indications of each technique, and its relationship to other modalities. The risks of the procedure have to be weighed against the need for information and the patient's best interests. Modifications to the basic method are necessary in specific instances. This format has been followed for each body system, pathological considerations being raised only for the understanding of a particular technique. In some instances, as in the orbits and the breast, it has been deemed relevent to extend the description to cover plain radiography. The physical properties and chemical nature of contrast media, pertaining to their application, have been given detailed description. The role of the anaesthetist is the X-ray Department, including the use of his skills in clinical measurement, have also merited consideration.

In essence, it is hoped that this book will be a useful guide to all radiologists, especially those in training, and will provide a convenient encapsulation of many facts which are otherwise disseminated throughout the radiological literature. We would envisage that it will also be a helpful reference source to radiographers as well as to radiologists.

We are indebted to the many contributors who have devoted time and effort to writing their sections, despite their many other commitments. Our gratitude is due to Miss Joan Doyle for preparing the manuscript. It is also a pleasure to acknowledge the consistent help and encouragement of Richard Zorab and the work of Bridget Cook of Blackwell Scientific Publications.

Graham Whitehouse, Brian Worthington, July 1983

SECTION 1
THE GASTROINTESTINAL TRACT

The Salivary Glands

1

N. J. D. SMITH

The term 'Sialography' appears to have been coined by the anatomist Antonio Nuck in 1690 to describe the casts he made of the salivary glands by injecting wax into the ducts. It is now used to describe the radiographic demonstration of the major salivary glands after the injection of contrast medium into the duct system.

The first recorded sialogram was made by Arcelin (1912) using a contrast medium containing bismuth. Further development was delayed because of the inadequacy of this and other available contrast media. Following the development of iodized oil as a contrast medium, Uslenghi (1925) and Carlsten (1926) independently pioneered the routine clinical use of sialography. Subsequently, sialography has become a firmly established technique in the investigation of salivary gland disease (Ollerenshaw & Rose, 1951).

Indications

The presenting symptoms of disorders affecting the salivary glands are relatively few and include pain, swelling, which may be recurrent, xerostomia, bad taste and, rarely, sialorrhoea (Mason & Chisholm, 1975).

Sialography should only be performed when the information derived from the examination may be of assistance in reaching a diagnosis or in the subsequent management of the patient.

The indications for sialography include the following.

Suspected calculi

A sialogram is indicated in the presence of a salivary calculus in order to ascertain whether or not there is normal salivary gland tissue beyond it, when this information will alter the subsequent management of the case. Sialography also demonstrates whether or not a calcific opacity lies within the gland system.

Swelling Sialography is indicated when there is unilateral or bilateral enlargement of the glands for which the cause is unknown, or when there are recurrent episodes of swelling, and in the presence of a suspected tumour mass.

Xerostomia There are many causes of dry mouth resulting from conditions extrinsic to the glands and which exert their effect either through the salivary centre or the nervous pathways to the glands. When there is doubt, sialography is indicated to distinguish these conditions from intrinsic causes of xerostomia, which include Sjogren's syndrome.

Contra-indications

The examination must not be performed in the presence of acute infection in the salivary glands. It is contra-indicated in cases of known iodine allergy, but these are rare.

Basic technique

The basic requirements are relatively few and should be readily to hand on a trolley during the examination (Fig. 1.1).

Probes

A set of graded probes is needed to explore and dilate the orifice of the salivary duct. The preference is for Liebreich's double-ended lacrimal probes which usually come in sets of four, graded 00/0, 1/2, 3/4 and 5/6. Only the two finer probes, 00/0 and 1/2 are required for sialography.

Directional control of the probe is easily achieved by holding the flat portion at the centre of the instrument lightly between fore-finger and thumb.

Cannula

It is best to introduce the contrast medium through a flexible cannula. A 30 cm Portex intravenous cannula with an outside diameter of 1.02 mm and a pink Luer connection is most suitable. The distal end of the cannula should then be drawn out to a fine diameter tip. This is achieved by grasping the end of the cannula in a pair of Spencer-Wells forceps, at the same time holding the main part of the cannula firmly between finger and thumb near to the forceps and drawing out the intervening segment to a smaller diameter by giving a sharp tug on the forceps. The

3

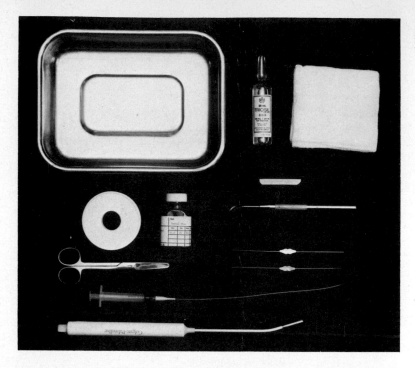

narrow part of the cannula is now cut with a sharp scalpel to produce a fine tip for insertion into the orifice after minimal dilatation. The thicker portion gives sufficient rigidity for the operator to handle the cannula and control the direction of movement (Fig. 1.2).

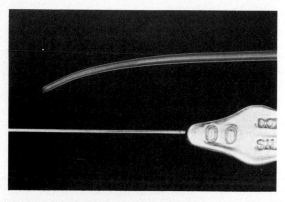

Fig. 1.2 The finely drawn out tip of a Portex cannula shown alongside a size 00 Liebreich's lacrimal probe.

A variety of metal cannulae have been used in sialography, varying from blunted hypodermic needles to metal tipped-catheters. The danger of inadvertently piercing the duct wall, with subsequent extravasation of the contrast medium, is greater with a metal cannula than with a flexible cannula.

Syringe

A 2 ml disposable syringe is suitable since it is rare to use more than this volume of contrast medium.

Dental mirror

There should always be a good external light source. It is sometimes difficult to illuminate directly the orifices of the sub-mandibular ducts because of their position behind the lower incisor teeth, and a dental mirror may be found useful to reflect light on to the floor of the mouth. The back of the mirror also prevents the tip of the tongue moving forward to cover the orifice.

Flexible examination light

As well as external illumination, an additional light source such as the *Hoyt*(TM)* flexible examination light which has a small bulb at the end of a flexible stalk, may be helpful when held close to the orifice of the duct by an assistant.

Gauze

Identification of the orifice of the salivary ducts is facilitated by a dry mucosa, particularly in the case of the sub-mandibular duct where saliva pools in the

* Colgate-Palmolive

floor of the mouth. Excess saliva can be easily removed by sterile gauze squares.

Stainless steel dish

As a result of reflex stimulation of the salivary glands, patients sometimes produce excessive saliva which may be collected in a suitable dish. During the later clearing stages, when contrast medium mixed with saliva is being passed into the mouth, the patient should be able to spit into a dish.

Plaster tape

A roll of sticking plaster and scissors should be available to tape the syringe to the forehead at the end of the injection of contrast medium.

Lemon or ascorbic acid tablets

A slice of fresh lemon is the ideal way to produce reflex stimulation of saliva before taking 'clearing' radiographs, although ascorbic acid tablets make an acceptable substitute.

Contrast medium

Either a water-soluble contrast medium such as Triosil 440 or the oil-based medium Lipiodol Ultra Fluide are used in sialography, the subject having been reviewed by Trester (1968). The oil-based media have the disadvantages of being more viscous and remaining *in situ* for many years should they be accidentally injected into the tissues surrounding the duct. For these reasons, many prefer to use water-soluble contrast agents.

Preliminary radiographs

Plain radiographs should be taken before embarking on sialography because a considerable proportion of salivary gland pathology is associated with opaque calculi within the glands themselves or their ducts, particularly in the submandibular gland (Fig. 1.3).

The projections used for these preliminary radiographs are the same as those described later for sialography. In addition a dental film, placed in the buccal sulcus *outside* the upper molar teeth, will be found useful if a calculus is suspected near the orifice of the parotid duct.

Procedure

It is usual to carry out the procedure with the patient lying on an X-ray couch in the supine position.

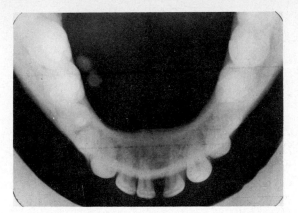

Fig. 1.3 A mandibular occlusal film showing two calculi in the right sub-mandibular duct.

Parotid gland

The orifice of the parotid duct (Stenson's duct) opens on to a small papilla on the inner surface of the cheek, approximately opposite the crown of the upper second molar tooth. The orifice itself cannot usually be identified by inspection alone. The inner surface of the cheek should first be dried with a gauze square and then the gland itself should be gently massaged by means of external pressure applied by the fingers just behind the posterior border of the ascending ramus of the mandible. This usually results in a bead of saliva becoming visible on the inner surface of the cheek where the duct opens into the mouth. In many cases, the opening of the orifice itself becomes visible at the same time. Gentle exploration with the finest probe should now follow and, once the orifice has been located, the probe should be inserted into it. Resistance will be met after the probe has passed about one centimetre into the duct, because of the sharp bend where it penetrates the buccinator muscle in its passage across the anterior border of the masseter. On no account should any attempt be made to force the probe further along the duct.

The probe should be left in the duct for a minute or two in order to dilate the orifice. This probe should then be withdrawn and immediately replaced with the next largest size. The orifice is almost invariably visible for a few seconds after the probe has been withdrawn. Ideally, this procedure should be repeated until a size 2 Liebreich's probe is inserted into the duct. Sometimes this cannot be achieved, especially when a stricture is present, and in these cases an attempt must be made to cannulate the duct through a smaller opening.

It is a great help when changing probes to be able to pass the probe which has just been withdrawn to an

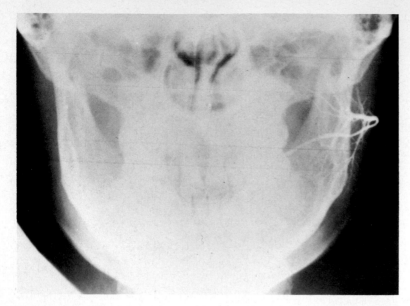

Fig. 1.4 A postero–anterior projection of a normal parotid sialogram.

assistant, who then replaces it with one of the next size. Constant observation of the orifice may therefore be maintained by the operator.

Once the orifice has been dilated sufficiently, the fine end of the cannula, which has been filled with contrast medium, is inserted into the duct and advanced until resistance is felt at the point where the duct turns to pierce the buccinator. The orifice usually closes around the wider portion of the cannula, forming an effective seal, which prevents reflux of contrast medium into the mouth. The contrast medium should now be injected *tediously* slowly at a rate of approximately 0.2 ml/min. Between 0.5 and 0.75 ml of contrast medium should be sufficient to outline the duct system within a healthy gland, but more may be needed where there is gross dilation of the duct or an abscess cavity. The injection is terminated when either 1 ml of contrast medium has been injected or as soon as the patient indicates discomfort by a pre-arranged signal. With the cannula still within the duct, the syringe barrel is taped to the contra-lateral side of the forehead, rather than in the mid-line where it may interfere with radiography. This produces a slight hydrostatic pressure of contrast medium and prevents premature emptying of the gland.

An oblique lateral radiograph should be taken at this time. If there is satisfactory filling of the gland, then radiography should be completed as soon as possible. A small 'top up' of contrast medium is made just before each exposure. Where filling is inadequate, further contrast medium should be injected before taking a radiograph.

Postero–anterior (P–A) and lateral radiographs

should be taken, and may be complemented by an axial projection to show that portion of the gland which lies medial to the mandible. The best P–A view is an offset occipito–frontal projection, centring through the gland with the lower border of the ala of the ear making a good surface marking (Fig. 1.4). The traditional lateral projection is the 15° oblique lateral (Fig. 1.5), while an excellent alternative lateral view may be obtained with dental panoramic equipment (Fig. 1.6). If the patient is positioned about 2 cm further forward than is the case for a dental examination, then the region behind the posterior border of the mandible which contains the parotid gland will be in the tomographic cut (Pappas & Wallace, 1970; Azouz, 1978).

Sub-mandibular gland

The orifices of each sub-mandibular duct (Wharton's duct) is considerably more difficult to identify and cannulate than a parotid duct. The duct orifices open on to very flaccid papillae which lie on either side of the mid-line, in the lax tissues of the floor of the mouth behind the central incisor teeth. In some patients, tongue thrusting is an almost involuntary reaction and can make sialography very difficult. A dental mirror, as well as reflecting light, is invaluable in holding the tongue out of the way.

After drying the floor of the mouth with gauze squares, the position of the sub-mandibular orifice is often identified by the expression of a few drops of saliva after external massage of the gland. This is achieved by forward pressure from the fingers just

Fig. 1.5 The oblique lateral projection. This is the lateral view of the sialogram shown in Fig. 1.4.

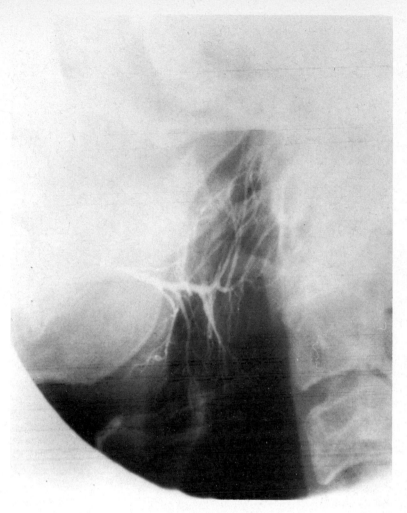

behind the angle of the mandible. Sometimes the orifice itself can be identified as it opens momentarily, but in other cases the position is only indicated by the formation of beads of saliva. Very gentle exploration by the finest lacrimal probe should identify the orifice. The probe should be steadied above the papilla, applying only slightly more pressure than is available from its own weight. Too much pressure merely depresses the mucosa in the floor of the mouth, making it harder to find the orifice. Once the orifice has been located, the probe may usually be inserted further than in the parotid duct. Thereafter, the procedure is the same as that described for the parotid duct except that the cannula should be inserted further along the duct, since tongue movement can all too easily displace the cannula.

The usual projections are an oblique lateral (Fig. 1.7) and a true lateral, supplemented by a mandibular occlusal radiograph to show the course of the duct in the floor of the mouth. As in the case of the parotid

gland, an excellent lateral view is obtained by using dental panoramic equipment.

The sub-mandibular gland is awkwardly placed for P–A radiography and, in an attempt to overcome the superimpositions resulting from the anatomical position of the gland, Park & Bahn (1968) have recommended a sub-mento-vertical projection while an oblique antero–posterior projection was described by Hollender & Lindvall (1977).

Pain

Patients vary considerably in their assessment of the degree of discomfort experienced during sialography. The exploration that is sometimes necessary to discover the orifice of the gland, especially in the case of the sub-mandibular gland, together with the slow injection may be tedious and uncomfortable. The procedure, however, should not cause acute pain or distress.

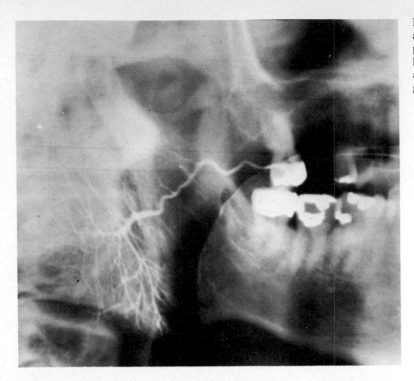

Fig. 1.6 The illustration shows part of a dental panoramic tomogram (ortho-pantomograph). This view gives excellent visualization of both the parotid and the sub-mandibular salivary glands.

The too rapid injection of contrast medium often results in pain within the healthy gland. When the gland is diseased, especially when much glandular tissue has been destroyed, it often becomes relatively insensitive and for this reason it is unwise to place too much reliance on the onset of pain as the end-point for injection.

Pain appears to occur more readily with a water-soluble contrast medium than an oil-based agent.

Clearing films

After the routine radiographs have been taken, it is possible to obtain a crude indication of the functional status of the gland after stimulating secretory activity. The cannula should be removed and the patient asked to suck a piece of lemon or an ascorbic acid tablet.

After an interval of approximately five minutes, one further radiograph is taken and, if normal secretory activity is present, no contrast medium will be seen.

Variations on basic technique

Hydrostatic sialography (Gullmo & Böök Henderström, 1958; Park & Mason, 1966), replaces the imprecise hand injection technique by gravity feed of the contrast medium through the cannula. Mason and

Chisholm (1975) have shown that the secreting pressure of stimulated salivary gland lies between 54 and 76 cm of water. By raising an open reservoir of contrast medium to a height of between 70 and 90 cm above the orifice, the hydrostatic pressure from the contrast medium exceeds that exerted by the secreting gland and then runs into the gland.

Another attempt to avoid excessive intra-glandular pressure during sialography is the method of Ferguson *et al.* (1977) who use a constant flow rate infusion pump connected to a pressure transducer in order to monitor the injection pressures.

Subtraction sialography

The use of subtraction radiography in sialography is described by Liliequist and Welander (1969) and Buchignani and Shimkin (1971). It is unlikely to have any significant advantage over routine radiographs and the difficulty in obtaining accurate masks effectively limits this technique to a single projection which is taken just before the injection of contrast medium.

Xeroradiography

The use of xeroradiography in sialography has been described by Glassman *et al.* (1974) and Ferguson *et al.* (1976). It is claimed that the edge enhancement effect reveals more detail of the opacified ducts, particularly where they are overlaid by bone.

Fig. 1.7 A lateral oblique projection of a normal sub-mandibular sialogram.

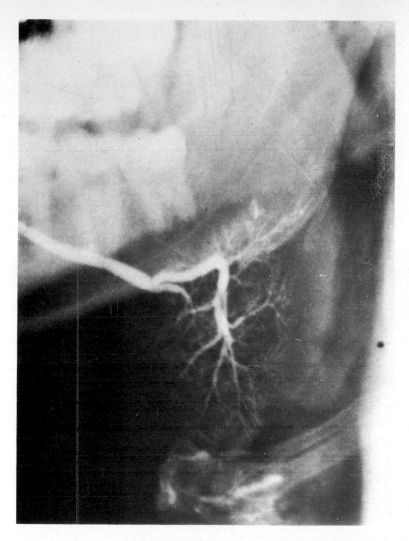

Complications

Serious complications are rare during sialography (Ansell, 1968). Glottic oedema in one case followed as an allergic reaction to iodine. The accidental injection of contrast medium into the tissues of the floor of the mouth is more of a hazard with oil-based media. Extravasated oil-based contrast media are not readily absorbed and may persist in the extrasalivary tissues for several years.

Relationship to other imaging modalities

Radioisotope scanning

Isotope scanning of the salivary glands with Tc^{99m} pertechnetate has been in use for some years (Schmitt *et al.*, 1966; Gates & Work, 1967; Harden *et al.*, 1967).

This isotope has very similar biological properties to the iodide ion, being taken from the bloodstream and concentrated by the salivary glands. Its uptake following intravenous injection gives an indication of salivary gland function but does not materially assist in the evaluation of salivary gland disease.

The lack of consistency in the results coupled with the limited resolution detract from the routine use of radioisotope scanning as an adjunct to sialography. The rare case of congenital absence of some or all of the major salivary glands may, however, be confirmed using this technique (Smith & Smith, 1977).

Computed tomography

Sialographic examination has been combined with computed tomography to distinguish between lesions within the deep lobe of the parotid and those extrinsic parapharyngeal masses which tend to compress and laterally displace the gland (Som & Biller, 1979; Rice et al., 1980).

REFERENCES

Ansell G. (1968) A national survey of radiological complications: interim report. *Clin. Radiol.*, **19**, 175–91.

Arcelin (1921) Radiographie d'un calcul salivaire de la glande sub-linguale. *Lyon Medecine*, **118**, 769–73.

Azouz E. M. (1978) The panoramic view of sialography. *Radiology*, **127** (1), 267–8.

Carlsten D. B. (1926) Lipiodolinjecktion in den Ausführungsgang der Speicheldrusen. *Acta Radiol.*, **6**, 221–3.

Ferguson M. M., Evans A. & Mason W. N. (1977) Continuous infusion pressure-monitored sialography. *Internat. J. Oral Surg.*, **6**, 84–9.

Ferguson M. M., Davidson M., Evans A. & Mason W. N. (1976) Application of xeroradiography in sialography. *Internat. J. Oral Surg.*, **5**, 176–9.

Gates G. A. & Work W. P. (1967) Radioisotope scanning of the salivary glands. *Laryngoscope*, **77**, 861.

Glassman L. M., O'Hara A. E. & Cregar D. (1974) Xerosialography. *Arch. Otolaryng.*, **100**, 341–3.

Gullmo A. & Böök-Henderström E. (1958) A method of sialography. *Acta Radiol.*, **49**, 17–24.

Harden R. McG., Hilditch T. E., Kennedy I., Mason D. K., Papadopoulos S. & Alexander W. D. (1967) Uptake and scanning of the salivary glands in man using pertechnetate 99mTC. *Clin. Sci.*, **32**, 49.

Hollender L. & Lindvall A. M. (1977) Sialographic technique. *Dentomaxillofacial Radiol.*, **6**, 34–40.

Liliequist B. & Welander U. (1969). Sialography—new application of the subtraction technique. *Acta Radiol. Diagn.*, **8**, 228–34.

Mason D. K. & Chisholm D. M. (1975) *Salivary Glands in Health and Disease*. London. W. B. Saunders Co. Ltd.

Nuck A. (1690) Sialographia.

Ollerenshaw R. & Rose S. (1951) Radiological diagnosis of salivary gland disease. *Brit. J. Radiol.*, **24**, 538–48.

Pappas G. C. & Wallace W. R. (1970) Panoramic sialography. *Dental Radiog. Photog.*, **43**, 17–33.

Park W. M. & Bahn S. L. (1968) Sialography simplified. *Oral Surg.*, **26** (5), 728–35.

Reid J. M. (1969) Sialography. *Australas. Radiol.*, **13** (2), 148–60.

Rice D. H., Mancuso A. A. & Hanaffee W. N. (1980) Computerized tomography with simultaneous sialography in evaluating parotid tumours. *Arch. Otolaryngol.*, **106**, 472–3.

Schmitt G., Lehmann G., Strotges M. W., Wehmer W., Reinecke V., Teske H. J. & Rottinger E. M. (1976) The diagnostic value of sialography and scintigraphy in salivary gland disease. *Brit. J. Radiol.*, **49**, 326–9.

Smith N. J. D. & Smith P. B. (1977) Congenital absence of major salivary glands. *Brit. Dent. J.*, **142**, 259–60.

Som P. M. & Biller H. F. (1979) The combined computerised tomography sialogram. A technique to differentiate deep lobe parotid tumours from extraparotid pharyngomaxillary space tumours. *Ann. Otol. Rhinol. Laryngol.*, **88**, 590–5.

Trester P. H. (1968) The development and use of contrast media in sialography. *J. Canad. dent. Ass.*, **34**, 210–13.

Uslenghi J. P. (1925) Nueva technica papa la investigacion radiologica de las glandulas salivarires. *Rev. Soc. Argent Radiol. Electrol.*, **1**, 4–16.

The Upper Gastrointestinal Tract

D. J. NOLAN

PLAIN ABDOMINAL RADIOGRAPHS

Plain radiographs are important in patients who present with symptoms or signs of an acute abdomen. The essential views are an upright chest, supine abdomen and left lateral decubitus of the abdomen. If properly taken they can show as little as 1 ml of gas from a ruptured viscus and should demonstrate fluid levels in abcess cavities, in the peritoneal cavity, or in distended intestine (Miller & Nelson, 1971; Miller, 1973).

A left lateral decubitus view of the abdomen should be taken first (Miller & Nelson, 1971). The patient needs to be in this position for 5–10 min before the radiograph is taken in order to allow adequate time for free gas to collect between the lateral abdominal wall and the highest point of the peritoneal cavity. This may be the only view to show a small volume of intraperitoneal gas and the exposure should be less than is normally employed in abdominal radiography. There are two sites in the peritoneal cavity where gas is likely to collect—the peritoneal cavity between the liver edge and the right wall of the abdomen, and over the right ilium. If perforation of the stomach, duodenum or proximal small intestine is suspected and there is doubt about the presence of free gas on the left decubitus view, 50–100 ml of air may be injected into the stomach via a nasogastric tube (Miller, 1973).

Upright radiographs of the chest and abdomen are taken next in those patients who are able to sit or stand. The patient should be in the upright position for 5–10 min before taking the radiograph. The view of the erect abdomen should include the pelvis. Finally, a supine view of the abdomen is taken.

The indications for plain radiographs are suspected perforation or rupture of an abdominal organ, intestinal obstruction or ileus, volvulus, acute colitis or toxic megacolon, acute conditions of the gall-bladder and biliary tract, acute pancreatitis, urinary calculi or other acute conditions of the urinary tract, abscess, foreign body, appendix calculi or an abdominal aneurysm.

THE DOUBLE CONTRAST BARIUM MEAL

The double contrast barium meal is now widely used and is the method of choice for the barium examination of the upper gastrointestinal tract, having largely replaced the single contrast technique. The use of the double contrast method owes much to Japanese radiologists who refined the technique and have been routinely performing successful double contrast studies of the stomach for almost 30 years. The aim of the double contrast method is to distend the stomach and duodenum with gas after coating the mucosa with a thin even layer of barium. The lesions are shown en face and details of the size, shape and margin are clearly shown. Compression radiography and the filling method are incorporated in the examination.

Indications

Indications for the double contrast barium meal include patients who present with dyspepsia, unexplained weight loss, anaemia, gastrointestinal bleeding or a palpable mass in the upper abdomen. A single contrast barium examination without the use of hypotonic or effervescent agents is indicated in patients who present with vomiting due to a suspected obstructive lesion of the gastric antrum or duodenum.

Contra-indications

Barium should not be given to patients with suspected perforation of the upper gastrointestinal tract. The presence of barium in the gastrointestinal tract may make it impossible to carry out satisfactory angiography and it should, therefore, not be used in patients who present with bleeding until the question of performing angiography has been fully considered.

The barium suspension

Many advocate that barium suspensions for double contrast examinations should be of medium density and low viscosity, arguing that they give good mucosal coating, the barium suspension is stable and the density is suitable for obtaining compresssion views. Suitable concentrations range from 82.5 w/v % (Op den Orth & Ploem, 1977) to 120 w/v %. Others prefer higher density barium suspensions which are prepared shortly before use by adding water to barium sulphate. The local water supply has an effect upon the performance of these suspensions (Miller & Skucas, 1977). If the type of water used is unsatisfactory, artefacts, such as foam and bubble formation, may cause problems. As a result some barium sulphate preparations perform satisfactorily in one Radiology Department but not in another.

Gas

There are numerous ways of introducing gas into the stomach and duodenum for double contrast examinations. Initially, naso-gastric intubation was used (Shirakabe, 1971) but it is unsuitable for routine use and has been superseded by effervescent agents in the form of powder, granules, tablets and aerated liquids. James *et al.* (1976), in a study comparing the different methods, found effervescent tablets to be the best. Bubble formation remains a problem, even with tablets, and it is necessary to add a little antifoam to the barium suspension. Some of the more recently introduced granules appear to rapidly effervesce without the problem of bubble formation. The 'bubbly barium' method (Pochaczevsky, 1973; Op den Orth & Ploem, 1977; Dainty *et al.*, 1980) is another satisfactory technique for introducing gas. Refrigerated barium is put in a soda-making dispenser and carbon dioxide cartridges are attached to the syphon resulting in a slow release of gas into the barium.

Hypotonic agents

The best double contrast studies are obtained by using smooth muscle relaxants so that the stomach and duodenum are examined in a state of hypotonia. Glucagon and hyoscine butylbromide (Buscopan) are widely used for this purpose, generally being safe and effective agents (Barrowman, 1975).

Glucagon, a straight-chain polypeptide derived from the islets of Langerhans, produces gastric and duodenal hypotonia. Nausea and vomiting may occur, but are rare with the dose used for double contrast studies. Glucagon may produce severe hypertension in patients with phaeochromocytoma and is also contra-indicated in insulinoma. Sensitization reactions occur although they are rare. A dose of 0.15 mg given intravenously at the beginning of the examination is adequate for the double contrast examination. There may be a slight delay before the barium and gas pass through the pylorus with the use of glucagon. This has an advantage in that views of the stomach can normally be obtained before barium passes into the distal part of the duodenum and partially obscures the lower half of the stomach.

Buscopan is a quaternary ammonium synthesized from scopolamine (Ayre-Smith, 1976). It is a ganglion-blocking agent but, unlike scopolamine, has no central action. It causes only minor atropine-like side-effects unless used in doses over 40 mg. Massive gastric dilatation is a rare complication. Contra-indications to its use are cardiac failure, angina pectoris, prostatism and glaucoma. The dose normally used for the double contrast examination—20 mg intravenously— is unlikely to aggravate heart failure or angina or cause urinary retention. Buscopan produces transient loss of accommodation but vision should have returned to normal within an hour of the injection.

Examination technique

The aim of the examination is to obtain views of all parts of the stomach distended with gas. The mucosal surface should be outlined with an even coating of barium to show details of the mucosal pattern. Enough gas is used to put the gastric mucosa under slight tension so that lesions that lack distensibility such as ulcers, ulcer scars and carcinomas, produce a clearly visible series of converging folds (Gelfand, 1975), making it possible to identify small lesions and slight irregularity of the mucosa. Views of the oesophagus and duodenum are also taken. It is essential that the method adopted is quick to perform and reproducible. The technique described here is similar to the methods of Shirakabe (1971) and Kreel *et al.* (1973).

The patient arrives in the department after fasting for at least six hours. A short history is taken and the patient is given an intravenous injection of 0.15 mg of glucagon or 20 mg of Buscopan. Effervescent granules or tablets, enough to produce 300–400 ml of gas, are taken by the patient and washed down with 50 ml of barium suspension. With the table horizontal, the patient lies in the prone position and a radiograph is taken (Fig. 2.1). The patient drinks a further 150 ml of barium suspension and turns once, or preferably twice, on to the right side and then on to the left side before lying supine. A radiograph is taken of the whole stomach in this position (Fig. 2.2) and shows the mucosal pattern of the body and antrum. The mucosa of the antrum and body is again washed with barium by rotating the patient as before and a view is obtained in the right anterior oblique position to show the mucosal pattern of the antrum (Fig. 2.3). A left anterior oblique radiograph is taken to show the mucosal pattern of the fundus and upper body of the stomach (Fig. 2.4). If the patient turns from the left anterior oblique to the supine position, about half the barium remains in the antrum while the remainder passes to the fundus and a spot mucosal view of the

Fig. 2.1 Prone view showing anterior wall of the stomach.

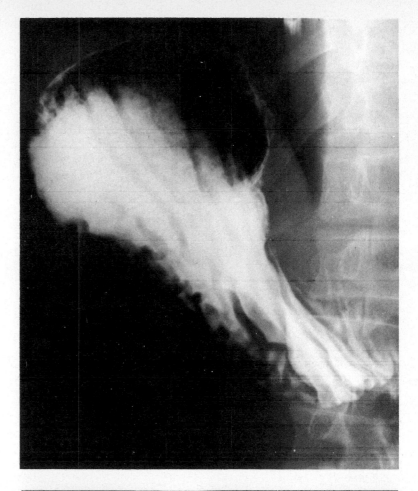

Fig. 2.2 Supine double contrast view of the lower body and proximal antrum of the stomach.

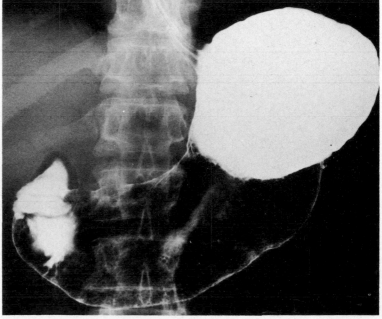

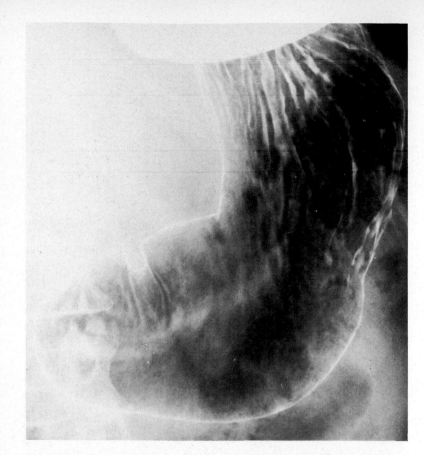

Fig. 2.3 Supine right anterior oblique view of the antrum and body of the stomach.

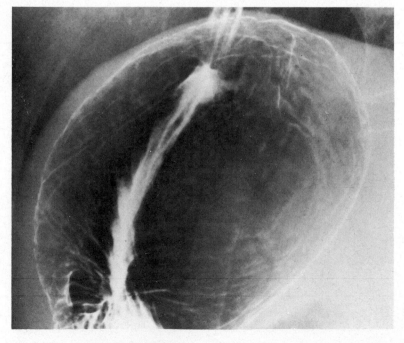

Fig. 2.4 Double contrast view of the upper body and fundus of the stomach taken with the table horizontal and the left side raised.

upper body of the stomach is obtained in this way (Fig. 2.5).

A mucosal view of the fundus of the stomach is taken with the patient in the supine left anterior oblique (Fig. 2.6) or the prone left posterior oblique position with the head of the table elevated to an angle of 45°. The table is then brought to the upright position and compression is applied to the barium-filled body and antrum of the stomach. Radiographs are taken only if an abnormal feature is recognized on fluoroscopy. Protuberant lesions are often shown best with compression. Finally, a single contrast view of the stomach is taken with the patient standing straight or rotated slightly into the right anterior oblique position.

Anterior wall lesions are uncommon (Goldsmith *et al.*, 1976) and, when present, are normally detected during the standard double contrast examination. The prone view and the compression parts of the technique are important in this respect. A double contrast examination of the anterior wall of the stomach is occasionally indicated. Such a technique was described by Goldsmith *et al.* (1976) and involves the use of a small amount of barium suspension and gas. The patient is turned from side to side in the prone position. Radiographs are taken with the patient prone in a 15° head down position with the right side elevated and a pad under the left side, in the prone horizontal position, and prone with the head of the table raised.

Radiographs of the duodenum are normally obtained when the table is horizontal after the left anterior oblique view or the supine view showing the upper body of the stomach. Double contrast views of the duodenal cap are taken with the patient in the right anterior oblique position. It may be necessary to elevate the head of the table slightly from the horizontal position in order to drain the barium from the apex of the cap into the second part of the duodenum. The patient is turned on the left side and then prone, sometimes with the left side raised a little, to obtain a double contrast anterior wall view of the duodenal cap and the duodenal loop. Further spot views of the duodenal cap may be taken with the patient standing.

Another method for obtaining good views of the duodenum is described by Stevenson *et al.* (1980). The patient is first turned on to the right side so that barium fills the duodenum. This occurs more quickly and reliably with Buscopan than with glucagon, since Buscopan relaxes the pylorus. The patient is then rotated to lie on the left, a pad is placed under the upper abdomen, and the patient is rolled forward to lie semi-prone on the pad. The pad compresses the proximal antrum against the spine, and the patient's respiration helps drive air from the distal antrum around the duodenal loop. A film is taken either prone oblique, with the second part of the duodenum seen through the air-filled antrum, or prone with the second part of the duodenum clear of the stomach. The patient is turned supine and a supine right anterior oblique view is taken (Fig. 2.7).

Patients who are not fit to stand while undergoing double contrast studies may be examined in the horizontal position with relatively good results. A smaller amount of barium and effervescent agent is used in immobile elderly patients.

Views of the oesophagus may be taken at the beginning of the examination. However, double contrast views of the oesophagus are best obtained after the examination of the stomach and duodenum (Nolan, 1980). Good double contrast views of the whole oesophagus can be obtained by getting the patient to drink the barium suspension while standing and holding his nose, so that large amounts of air are swallowed with the barium. The swallowed air distends the oesophagus and the barium forms a coating on the walls. Views of the pharynx and full length of the oesophagus should be taken in patients with oesophageal symptoms such as dysphagia. Antero–posterior and lateral views of the pharynx and upper oesophagus are obtained on full-size radiographs by careful timing or by using rapid serial or cine radiography. Cine radiography is necessary to evaluate neuromuscular disorders of swallowing. It is important to obtain views of oesophageal strictures with the patient swallowing the barium in the head-down position, the upper and lower margins of the narrowed segment being clearly identified by this method. Patients with suspected oesophageal varices should be examined in the supine right anterior oblique position, with the oesophagus in a relaxed state and with a good residual coating of barium. Buscopan and the Valsalva manoeuvre are useful for detecting small varices.

Some modifications to the double contrast technique are necessary in patients who have had previous gastric surgery. A smaller quantity of barium is required initially in patients with a previous Billroth I partial gastrectomy, although further quantities of barium and effervescent agent may be necessary as barium and gas escape through the anastomosis into the small intestine. It is important to outline the afferent loop in patients with a Polya or Billroth II type partial gastrectomy. This is normally achieved by getting the patient to drink the barium suspension while lying on his right side with the head of the table slightly elevated (Op den Orth, 1977). In this way barium should pass into the afferent loop. When the

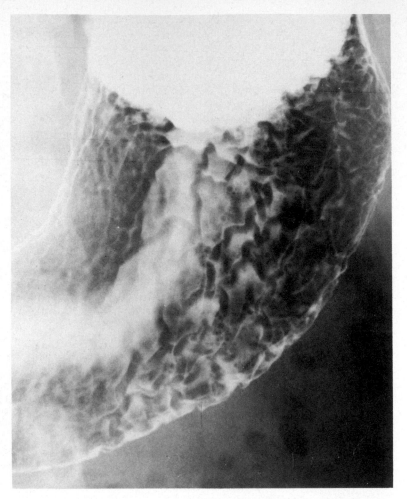

Fig. 2.5 Supine double contrast view of the upper body of the stomach.

barium has outlined the afferent loop, the table is returned to the horizontal position. Normally, the gas passes into the afferent loop if the patient turns into the right anterior oblique position. Radiographs of the afferent loop are obtained in the supine right anterior oblique and prone positions.

VARIATIONS ON BASIC TECHNIQUE

Hypotonic duodenography

The duodenum as far as the ligament of Treitz should be shown on at least one view during a routine double contrast examination of the upper gastrointestinal tract. If the prime interest is the duodenal loop, hypotonic duodenography should be carried out as a separate study. Although it is possible to obtain good views of the duodenum in some cases by the tubeless method, intubation gives consistently better results,

particularly in the investigation of a suspected pancreatic lesion. The amount of barium and air insufflation can be controlled and there is no overlying barium in the gastric antrum or jejunal loops (Eaton & Ferrucci, 1978).

The duodenal intubation technique is described in the next chapter. The tip of the catheter is placed in the lower part of the descending duodenum and about 40 ml of barium suspension is injected through it. As this fills the second part of the duodenum, a smooth muscle relaxant such as 20 mg Buscopan or 0.25 mg glucagon, is injected into a vein. Air is then injected through the catheter. The best projections for showing the duodenal loop are judged on fluoroscopy and are normally a supine right anterior oblique and a prone view with a pad under the right side. The proximal duodenum is often shown best with the head of the table elevated about 45–60°. Narrowed segments of duodenum are demonstrated better by the single contrast barium column.

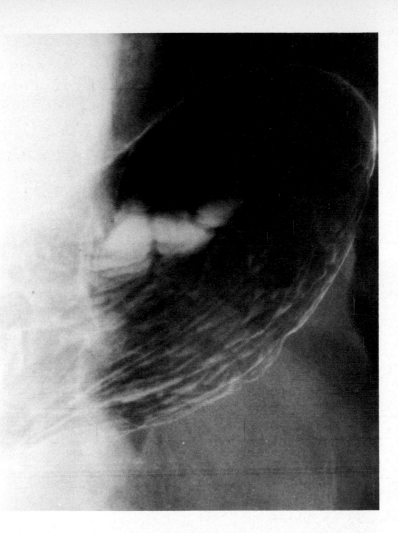

Fig. 2.6 Double contrast view of the fundus of the stomach taken with the patient in the supine right anterior oblique position and with the head of the table elevated to an angle of 45°.

Hypotonic duodenography is indicated if routine studies have resulted in equivocal findings, or if there is a suspicion of a primary lesion of the duodenum or pancreas. Patients admitted to hospital with obstructive jaundice due to suspected pancreatic or duodenal disease are best examined by fine needle percutaneous transhepatic cholangiography and hypotonic duodenography performed as a combined procedure (Gourtsoyiannis & Nolan, 1979).

Tubeless hypotonic duodenography is similar to the duodenal part of the double contrast examination. A smaller amount of barium is used and the hypotonic agent is injected after the barium outlines the duodenum.

Relationship to other diagnostic techniques

Barium studies versus endoscopy

Modern fibreoptic endoscopes are now widely used and make it possible to visualize, photograph and obtain aimed biopsy and cytology specimens from lesions in the upper gastrointestinal tract. The proper detection and diagnosis of lesions in the upper gastrointestinal tract is best achieved by close cooperation between the radiologist performing the double contrast studies and the endoscopist (Scobie, 1970; Fevre *et al.*, 1976; Dekker & Op den Orth, 1977).

When fibreoptic endoscopy was first introduced, many studies showed that it was superior to the single contrast barium meal. Studies comparing the accuracy of the double contrast examination and endoscopy however, show that the double contrast examination of the stomach is an accurate investigation (Laufer, 1976; Salter, 1977). The accuracy of both double contrast barium studies and endoscopy depends on the experience and skill of the person performing the examination.

It is not unusual for an endoscopist to miss a lesion that is subsequently demonstrated on a double contrast

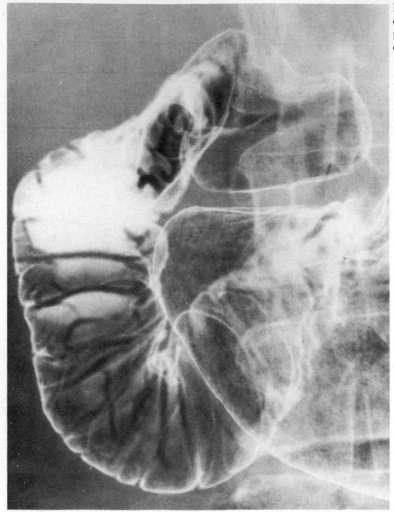

Fig. 2.7 A double contrast view of the duodenal cap and loop taken with the patient in the supine right anterior oblique position.

barium meal. This is most likely to occur if the lesion lies in one of the 'blind' areas, such as the upper lesser curve of the stomach or the base of the duodenal cap, or just distal to the anastomosis in patients who have had a previous partial gastrectomy (Nolan, 1980). In the latter group it is important to perform both a double contrast barium study and endoscopy to fully evaluate the anastomosis site.

The double contrast barium meal has a number of advantages over endoscopy; it is quick to perform and is safer and more comfortable for the patient. Each radiograph obtained provides an image of a large area of gastric and duodenal mucosa which may be retained as a permanent record available at any time for detailed review.

Radionuclide studies

Gastro-oesophageal reflux, is safely, rapidly and reliably demonstrated, using a gamma camera, following the ingestion of 300 µCi Tc^{99m} sulphur colloid (Malmud & Fisher, 1980). Protagonists of this technique claim it to be more sensitive than any other diagnostic test of gastro-oesophageal reflux and that it permits quantitation of the reflux.

Radionuclide studies are also used to evaluate the rate of gastric emptying, following the ingestion of a solid meal which is mixed with a radionuclide (Griffiths *et al.*, 1966; Scheiner, 1977). Enterogastric reflux has also been assessed, using radionuclides, after gastric surgery (Tolin *et al.*, 1979).

The administration of Tc^{99m}-pertechnetate has been used to delineate heterotopic gastric mucosa in the oesophagus (Berquist *et al.*, 1975).

Angiography

Selective visceral angiography may be invaluable in certain patients who present with acute bleeding from the upper gastrointestinal tract. There are two reasons for performing angiography in patients who present with acute bleeding: to locate the site of bleeding and to stop the bleeding by selective infusion of drugs or embolic material into the bleeding territory (Allison, 1980). Both applications apply in some cases, therapeutic embolization being particularly indicated when the patient is a poor operative or anaesthetic risk. The technique for performing selective visceral angiography is described elsewhere (Chapter 8).

A bleeding site with a blood loss of 0.5–0.6 ml/min or more should be shown on a technically satisfactory angiogram (Frey *et al.,* 1970). Coeliac axis and superior mesenteric angiography should be performed for acute upper gastrointestinal bleeding. When the bleeding point has been found, the haemorrhage may be controlled by the selective infusion of vasopressin (Athanasoulis *et al.,* 1974) or by the deliberate injection of embolic material (Allison, 1980) such as sterile absorbable gelatine sponge (Sterispon), lyophilized human dura mater (Lyodura), steel coils, acrylic polymers or detachable balloons.

Selective coeliac and superior mesenteric angiography is a useful diagnostic procedure in patients with intermittent acute bleeding. The angiogram should be performed during an episode of active bleeding to demonstrate the site of leakage of contrast medium (Allison, 1980). Angiography should not be performed if the bleeding has stopped; endoscopy or barium studies should be performed instead. Barium studies should not, however, be performed if there is a strong possibility of another acute bleed within two days as the presence of residual barium in the intestine may obscure the field for angiography. Angiography is indicated when endoscopy and barium studies fail to find the lesion and if there is recurrence of the bleeding.

Water-soluble contrast examinations

Plain abdominal radiographs are the initial diagnostic procedure in patients with suspected perforation of the stomach or duodenum. Water-soluble contrast agents should be used when perforation is still suspected but the plain radiographs fail to show the presence of free gas. The water-soluble contrast medium is injected through a naso-gastric tube directly into the stomach. The examination is either conducted completely under fluoroscopic control or the contrast medium may be injected with the patient lying on the right side with a right decubitus radiograph being taken after a short interval. About 50 ml of contrast medium is usually adequate. If perforation of the lower oesophagus is suspected, the nasogastric tube is withdrawn slowly through the lower oesophagus during injection of the contrast medium.

The water-soluble contrast agents are hyperosmolar and draw fluid into the intestinal lumen. Their use may cause shock and possible death, particularly in infants, children, the aged and the very ill (Margulis, 1977). It is therefore, important to monitor the fluid and electrolyte balance of those patients at risk. Water-soluble contrast medium should not be used if there is any danger of it being inhaled or passing into the lungs through an oesophagobronchial fistula. In difficult cases when there is a danger of both inhalation and extravasation, particularly when there is a new anastomosis high in the oesophagus, aqueous Dionosil is an appropriate contrast medium.

Studies using diatrizoate in the form Gastrografin are frequently requested by clinicians. Gastrografin is more likely to produce local tissue reaction than other water-soluble contrast agents (Margulis, 1977). Therefore, Gastrografin should only be used for suspected perforation or an anastomotic leak in the stomach and duodenum when the patient takes the contrast medium by mouth. It is recommended that the term 'water-soluble contrast examination' should be adopted in place of the 'Gastrografin examination' so often requested by clinicians.

REFERENCES

Allison D. J. (1980) Gastrointestinal bleeding. Radiological diagnosis. *Brit. J. Hosp. Med.,* **23**, 358–64.
Athanasoulis C. A., Baum S., Waltman A. C., Ring E. J., Imembo A. & Vander Salm J. T. (1974) Control of acute gastric mucosal haemorrhage. Intra-arterial infusion of posterior pituitary extract. *New Engl. J. Med.,* **290**, 597–603.
Ayre-Smith G. (1976) Hyoscine-N-butylbromide (Buscopan) as a duodenal relaxant in tubeless duodenography. *Acta Radiol. Diagn.,* **17**, 701–13.
Barrowman J. (1975) Anti-cholinergics/glucagon in barium meal examinations. In the Double Contrast Barium Meal, Proceedings of a Seminar, pp. 27–33. Rickmansworth, Concept Pharmaceuticals.
Berquist T. H., Nolan N. G., Stephens D. H. & Carloon H. C. (1975) Radioisotope scintigraphy in diagnosis of Barretts oesophagus. *Amer. J. Roentgenol.,* **123**, 401–11.
Dekker W. & Op den Orth J. O. (1977) Early gastric cancer. *Radiol. clin.* (Basel), **46**, 115–29.
Eaton S. B. & Ferrucci J. T. (1978) Commentary. *Gastrointestinal Radiol.,* **3**, 233–4.

Fevre D. I., Green P. H. R., Barratt P. J. & Nagy G. S. (1976) Review of five cases of early gastric cancer. *Gut*, **17**, 41–7.

Frey C. F., Reuter S. R. & Bookstein J. J. (1970) Localization of gastrointestinal haemorrhage by selective angiography. *Surgery*, **67**, 548–55.

Gelfand D. W. (1975) The double contrast upper gastrointestinal examination in the Japanese style. *Amer. J. Gastroenterol.*, **63**, 216–20.

Goldsmith M. R., Paul R. E. Jr., Poplack W. E., Moore J. P., Matsue H. & Bloom S. (1976) Evaluation of routine double contrast views of the anterior wall of the stomach. *Amer. J. Roentgenol.*, **126**, 1159–63.

Gourtsoyiannis N. C. & Nolan D. J. (1979) Combined fine needle percutaneous transhepatic cholangiography and hypotonic duodenography in obstructive jaundice. *Clin. Radiol.*, **30**, 507–12.

Griffiths G. H., Owen G. M., Kirkman S. & Shields R. (1966) Measurement of rate of gastric emptying using the scintillation camera and ^{129}Cs. *Lancet*, **i**, 1244–5.

James W. B., McCreath G., Sutherland G. R. & McDonald M. (1976) Double contrast barium examination—a comparison of techniques for introducing gas. *Clin. Radiol.*, **27**, 99–101.

Kreel L., Herlinger H. & Glanville J. (1973) Technique of the double contrast barium meal with examples of correlation with endoscopy. *Clin. Radiol.*, **24**, 307–14.

Laufer I. (1976) Assessment of the accuracy of double contrast gastroduodenal radiology. *Gastroenterology*, **71**, 874–8.

Lunderquist A. & Vang J. (1974) Transhepatic catheterization and obliteration of the coronary vein in patients with portal hypertension and oesophageal varices. *New Engl. J. Med.*, **291**, 646–9.

Malmud L. S. & Fisher R. S. (1980) Gastro-eosophageal scintigraphy. *Gastrointestinal Radiol.*, **5**, 195–204.

Margulis A. R. (1977) Water-soluble radiographic contrast agents in the gastrointestinal tract. In *Radiographic Contrast Agents* (Eds. Miller R. E. & Skucas J.), pp. 169–88. University Park Press, Baltimore.

Miller R. E. (1973) The technical approach to the acute abdomen. *Seminars in Roentgenology*, **8**, 267–79.

Miller R. E. & Nelson S. W. (1971) The roentgenologic demonstration of tiny amounts of free intraperitoneal air: experimental and clinical studies. *Amer. J. Roentgenol.*, **112**, 574–85.

Miller R. E. & Skucas J. (1977) *Radiographic Contrast Agents*. University Park Press, Baltimore.

Nolan D. J. (1980) *The Double Contrast Barium Meal. A Radiological Atlas.* HM + M Publishers, Aylesbury.

Op den Orth J. O. (1977) Tubeless hypotonic examination of the afferent loop of the Billroth II stomach. *Gastrointestinal Radiol.*, **2**, 1–5.

Op den Orth O. & Ploem S. (1977) The standard biphasic—contrast gastric series. *Radiology*, **122**, 530–2.

Pochaczevsky R. (1973) 'Bubbly barium'. A carbonated cocktail for double contrast examination of the stomach. *Radiology*, **107**, 461–2.

Salter R. H. (1977) X-ray negative dyspepsia. *Brit. med. J.*, **ii**, 235–6.

Scheiner H. J. (1975) Gastric emptying tests in man. *Gut*, **16**, 235–47.

Scobie B. A. (1970) Early gastric carcinoma. *Australasian Radiology*, **14**, 181–2.

Shirakabe H. (1971) *Double Contrast Studies of the Stomach*. Bunkodo Company, Tokyo.

Stevenson G. W., Somers S. & Virjee J. (1980) Routine double-contrast barium meal: appearances of the normal duodenal papillae. *Diagnostic Imaging*, **49**, 6–14.

Tolin R. D., Malmud L. S., Stelzer F., Menin R., Makler P. T., Applegate G. & Fisher R. S. (1977) Enterogastric reflux in normal subjects and patients with Billroth II gastroenterostomy. *Gastroenterology.*, **77**, 1027–33.

The Small Intestine

3

D. J. NOLAN

There are a number of radiological techniques available for investigating the small intestine. Plain abdominal radiographs may be helpful in patients who present with acute symptoms. The barium examination is the method of choice for examining the small intestine in patients whose symptoms present less acutely and it is well-established in the diagnosis and management of diseases of the small intestine. Water-soluble contrast agents are of little practical value for investigating the small intestine.

Plain abdominal radiographs

The technique used for obtaining plain radiographs in patients with an acute abdomen has been described in Chapter 2. Plain abdominal radiographs are indicated in patients with suspected obstruction or perforation of the small intestine.

Barium studies

The barium follow-through is the most widely used method of examining the small intestine with contrast medium. The follow-through is not an accurate technique for detecting and demonstrating diseases which cause morphological changes in the small intestine, duodenal intubation techniques having replaced the follow-through in many centres (Nolan, 1981). Excellent visualization of the small intestine is achieved when the barium is introduced directly through a tube into the small intestine. Reports from centres using intubation techniques indicate that these give much more accurate information than the follow-through. The single contrast dilute barium infusion method described by Sellink is very satisfactory and is regarded as being the method of choice for examining the small intestine with barium.

In some centres, intestinal tubes are used for decompressing the distended intestine in patients with small intestinal obstruction. Useful diagnostic information is obtainable by injecting barium suspension through these intestinal tubes when they are no longer advancing and have reached the site of obstruction (Herlinger, 1978). The small intestine is also evaluated by refluxing barium through the ileocaecal valve during barium enema examinations, while the terminal ileum is shown by a per oral pneumocolon examination of the ileocaecal region (Kellett et al., 1977).

BARIUM FOLLOW-THROUGH

The barium follow-through examination is indicated in elderly patients with suspected jejunal diverticulosis who present with malabsorption. It is also necessary to use the follow-through in patients who are unwilling to have intubation performed and in those for whom it is impossible for some reason to pass the catheter to the duodenum.

A barium meal to examine the oseophagus, stomach and duodenum is normally carried out before proceeding to examine the small intestine.

A total volume of 500–600 ml of barium suspension, diluted by the addition of an equal volume of water is used for the follow-through examination. Large radiographs of the abdomen (43 cm × 35 cm) are taken at half-hourly intervals as the barium progresses along the small intestine. The first radiograph to show the proximal jejunum is taken supine at the end of the barium meal or about 15 min later (Marshak & Lindner, 1976). The remainder of the radiographs are taken with the patient in the prone position. A pad is placed under the right iliac fossa when the barium has reached the distal ileum in order to separate the loops of ileum. Spot compression views of the terminal ileum are also obtained at this time.

The head of the barium column normally takes between two and six hours to reach the terminal ileum and caecum. A number of suggestions have been made for increasing the speed of barium through the small intestine. Metoclopramide 20 mg, intravenously after the barium meal part of the examination (James & Hume, 1968) or orally beforehand (Kreel, 1970), promotes gastric emptying and accelerates the transit of barium along the small intestine. Adding Gastrografin to the barium also reduces the time taken for barium to pass through the small intestine (Rosenquist, 1975). Other pharmacological agents which have been used include neostigmine (Marshak & Lindner, 1976), glucagon (Kreel, 1975), cholecystokinin (Parker & Beneventano, 1970) and ceruletide

(Novak, 1980; Robins *et al*., 1980). Preliminary cleansing of the colon, combined with the use of 10 oz or more of oral barium suspension, and placing the patient in the right lateral recumbent position has been suggested by Nice (1963). However, the advantage of decreasing the transit time is offset by diminished anatomical detail, particularly in the terminal ileum (Robbins *et al*., 1980).

The action of the pyloric sphincter, combined with the tone and peristaltic activity of the small intestine, prevent the small intestine from being distended with the barium contrast medium. Most of the loops of the small intestine are shown in a collapsed state and, for this reason, the barium follow-through is not as accurate as the duodenal intubation techniques.

BARIUM INFUSION

There has been renewed interest during the last decade in duodenal intubation techniques for examining the small intestine, mainly due to the work of Sellink. Sellink developed an infusion technique, using a modification of the Bilbao-Dotter tube for duodenal intubation and a barium suspension of particular specific gravity, which saved considerable time and yielded information which was far superior to that achieved with the barium follow-through. He suggested that the oral administration of contrast medium should be abandoned and replaced by the infusion as a routine technique (Sellink, 1974).

Indications

A barium infusion examination is indicated when diseases causing morphological changes in the small intestine are suspected; such as Crohn's disease, tuberculosis, tumours, radiation damage and ischaemia. Unexplained abdominal pain, diarrhoea and weight loss are the most common presenting features of these conditions. Sometimes they present as unexplained anaemia or as an 'acute abdomen'. The barium infusion examination is useful in detecting recurrent Crohn's disease in patients who have previously had a resection of small intestine performed for the disease. It is also indicated in patients with recurrent bleeding from the gastrointestinal tract when full investigation of the upper gastrointestinal tract and colon is negative.

The barium infusion has proved very useful in patients where the clinical findings are suggestive of small intestinal obstruction and the plain radiographs are either negative or do not give sufficient information about the site or cause of obstruction. There is sometimes a reluctance to use barium for contrast studies of an obstructed small intestine for fear of converting a partial to a complete obstruction by impaction of barium. This is unlikely because the small intestine secretes fluid which dilutes the barium. In a restrospective review of 172 patients with proven small intestinal obstruction, Miller and Brahme (1969) found no record of impaction of barium in the small or large intestine. Their findings confirmed the results of earlier studies on the effects of barium in experimental small intestinal obstruction in animals (Donato *et al*., 1954; Nelson *et al*., 1963). Barium suspension was shown to be superior to water-soluble iodinated compounds because of the greater density of barium. It also has fewer side-effects, barium producing less vomiting and crampy abdominal pain. In addition, water-soluble compounds can cause dehydration and electrolyte imbalance.

Malabsorption is often quoted as an indication for performing a barium study of the small intestine. Coeliac disease is one of the more common conditions causing malabsorption and a jejunal biopsy is diagnostic in the vast majority of cases. A jejunal biopsy should therefore be the initial diagnostic procedure in patients with suspected coeliac disease presenting with malabsorption. The barium infusion study should be reserved for those patients with malabsorption in whom the jejunal biopsy is normal, or for patients with a suspected complication of coeliac disease such as lymphoma of the small intestine.

Contra-indications

Barium is contra-indicated in suspected perforation of the small intestine. In practice, gross disruption is usually recognized on clinical grounds and contrast studies are unnecessary. In difficult cases, the better quality barium infusion study may demonstrate a small leak, outweighing the theoretical consideration of toxicity due to leakage of barium (Freeark *et al*., 1968).

Technique

The barium infusion examination of the small intestine described below is similar to Sellink's method (Sellink, 1976; Miller & Sellink, 1979).

Preparation of the patient

A clean colon is necessary for the barium column to flow freely through the distal ileum into the caecum.

It has been shown that a full caecum or distal ileum causes the flow of intestinal contents to be seriously retarded in the ileum (Nice, 1963). A low residue diet and aperients are prescribed, and fluids are encouraged on the day before the examination. The usual aperient is twelve ounces of magnesium sulphate, but it is not given to patients with known Crohn's disease or severe diarrhoea. Cleansing enemas are not performed because the cleansing fluid and faecal material may be washed into, and retained in, the distal ileum.

The patient fasts overnight prior to the barium examination.

Duodenal intubation

The catheter is made of radio-opaque polyvinyl chloride and is size 12 French, measuring 135 cm in length with six holes at the distal closed end (Fig. 3.1).* It is a modification of the Bilbao–Dotter tube (Bilbao *et al.*, 1967) differing in that the latter is a size 14 French and 115 cm long. The catheter was modified to make it easier to pass through the nose and more flexible in its passage through the duodenum (Nolan, 1979). It bends at acute angles and, as a result, passes with ease through the apex of the duodenal cap and the junction of the second and third parts of the duodenum. A Teflon-coated guide wire, 1.65 mm in diameter and 135 cm long, acts as a stiffener inside the catheter as it passes through the stomach (Fig. 3.1).

Local anaesthetic (lignocaine) is applied in the form of a spray or gel to the patient's nostril and a thin coating of the lignocaine gel is applied to the catheter. The patient sits in a chair while the tip of the catheter is passed through his nostril and is swallowed by him. It is passed by mouth in patients who express a preference for the oral route. The tip of the catheter should be swallowed by the patient with his neck flexed in order to prevent the catheter from passing into the trachea. It may be necessary to give the patient a small mouthful of water to facilitate swallowing. Some patients, particularly those with previous experience of having had a nasogastric tube passed, find it easier to coordinate the swallowing by passing the catheter themselves.

The patient is placed supine on the fluoroscopic table when the tip of the catheter is presumed to have reached the gastric antrum. The guide wire is introduced into the catheter and is passed to within 3 cm of the distal end. The catheter is then advanced to the pylorus and is gently eased forward through the

* William Cook Europe ApS.

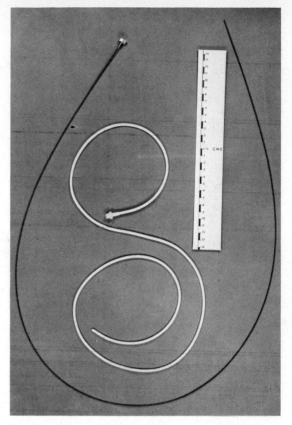

Fig. 3.1. The catheter and guide wire used for duodenal intubation.

pyloric sphincter into the duodenal cap under fluoroscopic control. This part of the procedure is best performed with the patient on his left side. In this position the prepyloric gastric antrum and the duodenal cap fill with air, facilitating the passage of the catheter tip through the pyloric sphincter. The acute angle between the first and second portions of the duodenum also diminishes in this position and makes it easier for the catheter to pass into the second part of the duodenum. If there is doubt about the anatomical arrangement of the antrum or duodenum, an injection of 50 ml of air through the catheter provides information and also excites peristalsis (Herlinger, 1978).

The catheter is then advanced through the duodenum, while the guide wire is slowly withdrawn so that its tip lies in the catheter proximal to the pylorus (Fig. 3.2). Thus, the catheter in the stomach remains stiff, while the part passing through the duodenum is flexible. The catheter is advanced until it reaches the ligament of Treitz. Ideally, the tip of the catheter should be positioned about 10 cm into the jejunum

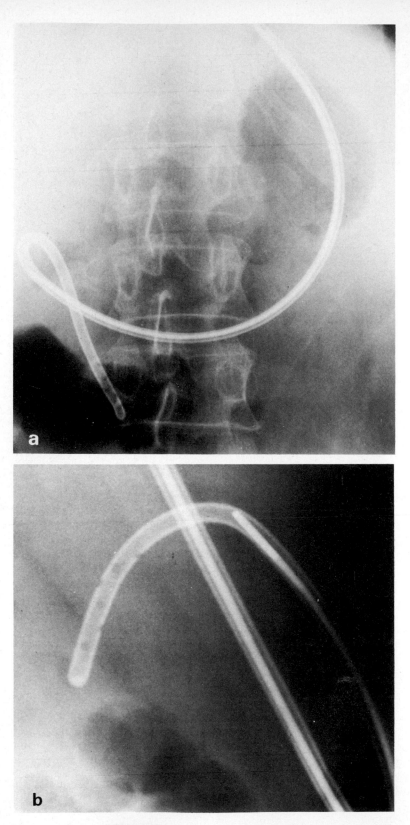

Fig. 3.2. (a) An antero–posterior view showing the tip of the catheter being passed through the duodenum. The guide wire is slowly withdrawn so that its tip lies in the catheter just proximal to the pylorus. (b) A lateral spot view.

Fig. 3.3. The catheter in position with the tip in the jejunum about 10 cm distal to the ligament of Treitz.

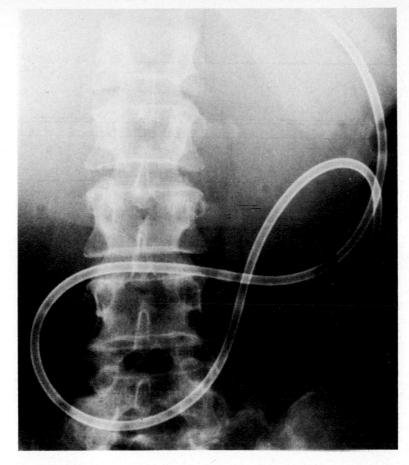

(Fig. 3.3), as this considerably reduces the chance of barium refluxing through the pylorus into the stomach.

Difficulty arises if the catheter coils in the fundus of the stomach. This is less likely to occur if the catheter is passed through the stomach with the patient standing. If coiling of the catheter does occur, it should be withdrawn until only 3 cm of the distal end remains pointing towards the fundus. The guide wire should be introduced and passed to within 3 cm of the distal end of the catheter (Fig. 3.4). It is possible to twist the distal end of the catheter and direct it downwards before advancing it to the antrum by rotating the catheter and applying torque. A guide wire with a curved or angled tip may be introduced and, by rotating the knurled handle of the guide wire, it is often possible to turn the tip of the catheter out of the fundus and direct it towards the antrum (Shipps *et al.*, 1979).

One can also tilt the fluoroscopic table upright and withdraw the catheter a little to uncoil the loop in the fundus. The guide wire is introduced and passed to the distal end of the catheter. The catheter is then advanced under intermittent fluoroscopic control with the patient erect. The weight of the guide wire helps to carry the tip of the catheter downwards under gravity to the antrum. Sometimes it is easier to get the tip of the catheter, with the guide wire inside, to pass to the gastric antrum if the patient is lying on the right side. In patients with a transverse stomach, it is sometimes impossible to pass the tip of the catheter downwards and out of the fundus. In such cases, it is best to let the catheter follow the curve of the fundus and pass it along the lesser curve to the antrum (Fig. 3.5).

The catheter may form a coil in the antrum and fail to pass easily into the duodenum. If this occurs, the catheter should be withdrawn a little so as to uncoil it. It is then advanced slowly while the radiologist's right hand, in a lead glove, exerts upward pressure on the distal part of the greater curve aspect of the gastric antrum. This manoeuvre usually works but, in a small number of cases, it may be necessary to inject a little barium to show the position of the pylorus. The injection of barium may also stimulate peristalsis and

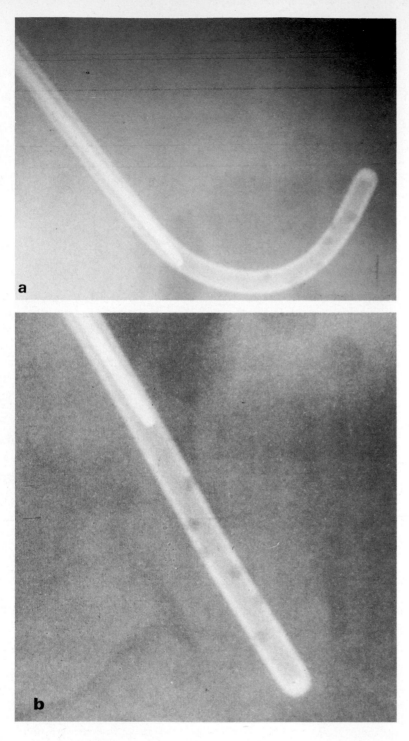

Fig. 3.4 Turning the tip of the catheter out of the fundus. The catheter coiled in the fundus of the stomach. It was then withdrawn and the guide wire introduced. (a) A spot view shows the distal end of the catheter directed towards the fundus. (b) After rotating the catheter the distal end is pointing downwards.

aid the passage of the catheter into the duodenum. Sometimes turning the patient prone enables the catheter to pass through the pyloric sphincter.

The tip of the catheter may be arrested during its passage through the duodenum by passing into a duodenal diverticulum. In cases where the catheter fails to advance through the duodenum, the guide wire should be withdrawn and a small amount of barium

Fig. 3.5 The catheter has passed along the greater curve of the fundus before passing to the gastric antrum.

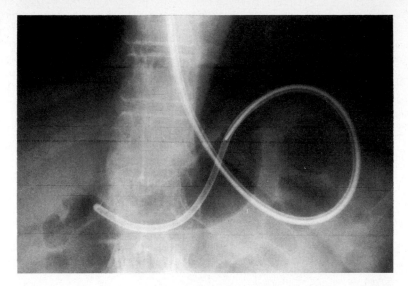

injected. If a diverticulum is outlined, the catheter is withdrawn a little and then advanced past the diverticulum under fluoroscopic control.

Great care should be taken with the guide wire in the distal end of the catheter, as it is possible for the guide wire to pass out through one of the side-holes and damage the wall of the stomach. Passing the guide wire through the distal 3 cm of the catheter should always be conducted under fluoroscopic control.

During fluoroscopy the X-ray beam should be coned down so that only the distal end of the catheter is seen. A low tube current, 0.5 mA or less, is normally sufficient to show the catheter on the television monitor. However, it may be necessary to increase the mA when the patient is in the lateral position. Fluoroscopy should be intermittent in order to keep the total screening time to a minimum. The radiation dose received by the patient during the intubation procedure is small, provided attention is paid to careful collimation, a low mA and short periods of intermittent fluoroscopy.

With practice, the whole intubation procedure is performed in 4–7 min in the majority of patients.

The infusion

Sellink realized that the specific gravity of the contrast fluid was a very important factor which had hitherto received insufficient attention. Following experiments, Sellink decided that a barium suspension diluted to a specific gravity of 1.25–1.32 was most suitable for examining the small intestine (Sellink, 1971).

Barium suspension, diluted to a specific gravity of 1.27 for adult patients and more dilute for younger

patients, is used for the infusion. A barium hydrometer* is necessary to obtain the correct specific gravity. Barium is infused into the jejunum at a rate of about 75 ml per minute. A total volume of 1200 ml of contrast medium is prepared and is put into a transparent plastic enema bag.

The tubing of the bag is connected by a Portex connector† to the catheter. The barium is infused into the jejunum at a rate of about 75 ml per minute. Occasionally, the barium column only reaches the terminal ileum after 1200 ml of barium has been infused and it is then necessary to add water to the infusion to maintain the flow of contrast medium. If water is required, it should be added before the bag becomes empty as any interruption may cause delay in the passage of barium. (Fig. 3.6)

A radiograph (30 cm × 24 cm) is taken of the jejunum after infusion of about 300 ml of barium. A large-sized radiograph (35 cm × 35 cm) is taken when 600 ml of contrast medium is in the small intestine. A further large radiograph (35 cm × 35 cm) is taken after contrast medium reaches the terminal ileum. Spot films are taken, often with compression, of the pelvic loops of ileum, the terminal ileum and any other segment of interest. Finally, another large radiograph (43 cm × 35 cm) of the abdomen is taken when the right-half of the colon, as well as the small intestine, is outlined with contrast medium. All radiographs are taken at high kilovoltage (115–120 kV).

The radiographs should be developed immediately and reviewed so that spot views may be taken of any abnormal segments not seen at fluoroscopy. Patients should be warned that an episode of diarrhoea often develops after the examination.

* Phillips Medical Systems   † Portex Ltd.

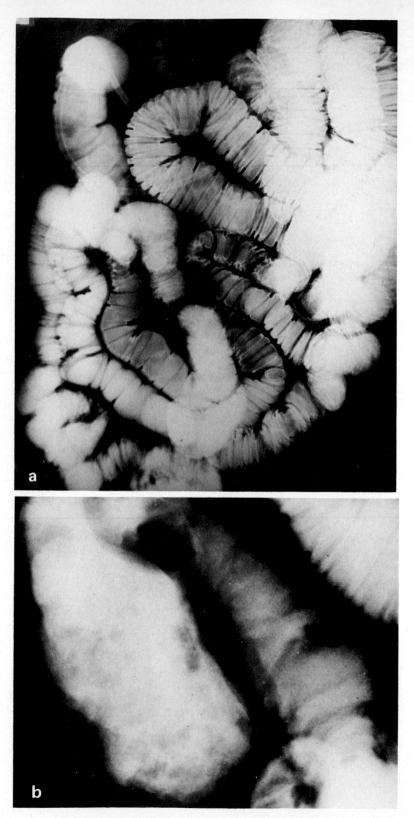

Fig. 3.6 Normal barium infusion examination of the small intestine. (a) A radiograph showing the small intestine outlined with dilute barium. (b) A spot view of the terminal ileum.

Modifications of basic technique

A modification of the Sellink method has been advocated by Herlinger (1978) and Vallance (1980), who inject 200 ml of moderate density barium suspension (85% w/v) through the catheter by means of 20 ml syringes at a rate of about 100 ml/min. A total of 1–2 litres of an 0.5% aqueous suspension of methylcellulose is then injected, using 50 ml syringes at an approximate rate of 100 ml/min. The barium column is pushed forward leaving a thin coating of barium to give a double contrast outline to the small intestine. Excellent mucosal detail of the normal intestine is obtained but diseased segments are demonstrated much better by the barium at the head of the column than by the double contrast produced by the combined barium and aqueous suspension of methylcellulose. It may be that the increased secretions of the abnormal mucosa make it difficult for the thin layer of barium to remain adherent to the wall of the diseased segment as the aqueous solution flows past. The dilute barium, used in the Sellink method, distends the diseased segment and need not adhere to the mucosa to produce good visualization. The infusion technique is also easier and quicker to perform.

Ekberg (1977) prefers a double-contrast method using barium and air. Barium suspension (600 ml) is injected into the duodenum. When the column of barium has reached the caecum, air is injected to obtain a double-contrast outline of the small intestine and radiographs are then taken. Dilute barium is considered to give much better distension of the intestine than air which passes through very quickly and fails adequately to distend narrowed segments. Severe stenosis may be overlooked on the double contrast views because overlapping ring shadows are not as clearly and diagnostically shown as a loop well-filled with barium (Miller & Sellink, 1979). The air-contrast method is unlikely to demonstrate sinuses and fistulae as well as the dilute barium technique.

Small intestinal intubation

A number of tubes are used for decompressing the distended intestine in patients with small intestinal obstruction. The Miller–Abbott type tube (Miller & Abbott, 1934) is a double lumen tube with a balloon at the tip. The balloon is inflated with air when it reaches the duodenum and the peristaltic activity carries the tube along the small intestine until it stops at the site of obstruction. Other tubes have a mercury-filled bag at the tip which is taken to the site of obstruction by peristalsis. When the tube is arrested at the site of obstruction, barium suspension may be injected to outline the obstructing lesion. The barium suspension needs to be of low viscosity because of the length and narrowness of the lumen of the Miller–Abbott tube (Herlinger, 1978).

REFLUX EXAMINATION

The terminal ileum may be examined by refluxing barium through the ileocaecal valve during a barium enema examination (Fig. 3.7), a method which has been advocated as the technique of choice for radiologically demonstrating the terminal ileum (Figiel & Figiel, 1964; Spiro, 1977). The terminal ileum is often involved with Crohn's disease and its delineation by partial reflux is very helpful in patients with inflammatory bowel disease. Evidence of recurrent disease is obtainable by partial reflux during a barium enema examination in patients who have previously had a right hemicolectomy and ileocolic anastomosis for Crohn's disease. Other abnormalities are also detectable on careful observation of the distal ileum when performing barium enemas. In ileostomy patients, barium may be injected directly into the small intestine in a retrograde manner.

It is possible to demonstrate all the small intestine by refluxing barium from the colon into the terminal ileum using a technique described by Miller (1965). The patient is prepared as for a double contrast barium enema with a low residue diet, increased fluid intake, laxatives and a cleansing enema. Preparation is omitted in patients with suspected intestinal obstruction. Normally, a single contrast study of the colon is performed first, using a dilute barium suspension. With the patient supine the barium is allowed to flow under fluoroscopic control through the terminal ileum in a retrograde direction to initially fill the ileum and then the jejunum. The flow is stopped when the barium column reaches the duodenum or when 4500 ml of barium suspension has been infused. The presence of small intestinal obstruction should be clearly shown, whereupon spot films are taken. When the barium reaches the duodenum, a single large radiograph (43 cm × 35 cm) is exposed with the patient turned into the prone position. The barium is then drained off with the patient in the supine position and a further large radiograph is exposed in this position. Fluoroscopy is performed in order to detect any lesion of the small intestine. The patient is then sent to the toilet to void as much barium as possible, further prone and supine radiographs being taken immediately after his return.

A large volume of barium suspension (2000–

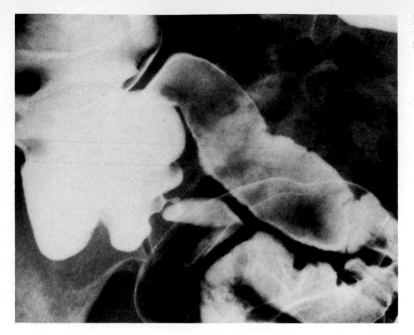

Fig. 3.7 Normal terminal ileum. A view obtained during a double contrast barium enema examination.

4500 ml) is required for this examination. Discomfort from the procedure may require analgesia. The ileocaecal valve is competent in some patients and a smooth muscle relaxant such as 0.5 mg of glucagon of 20 mg hyoscine butylbromide (Buscopan) should then be given intravenously to relax the valve and allow barium to flow into the terminal ileum. Failure to reflux barium through the ileocaecal valve occurred in only 3 out of 75 patients examined by Miller (1965).

The main indication for the complete reflux examination is the diagnosis and assessment of distal small intestinal obstruction. The technique is of particular value in marked distal small intestinal obstruction when it is necessary to establish the diagnosis or to obtain further information about the cause or site of hold-up. The excess fluid proximal to the site of obstruction is likely to cause considerable delay in the passage of barium if it is introduced into the proximal jejunum in these patients. The complete reflux examination should not be attempted in patients in whom there is a risk of perforation of the colon.

Per oral pneumocolon examination of the ileocaecal region

Excellent visualization of the ileocaecal region is obtainable by giving barium by mouth and introducing air per rectum when the barium is in the region of the terminal ileum and caecum (Kellett *et al.*, 1977). The patient is prepared as for a double-contrast enema with a low residue diet, increased fluid intake, laxatives and a cleansing enema. The progress of the barium is observed and air is introduced when the head of the column reaches the transverse colon. This air distends the caecum and terminal ileum, radiographs then being taken (Fig. 3.8). Crohn's disease of the terminal ileum and carcinoma of the caecum are particularly well demonstrated by this technique.

RELATION OF BARIUM STUDIES TO OTHER DIAGNOSTIC TECHNIQUES

Angiography

The main indication for selective visceral angiography of the small intestine is to determine the cause of obscure gastrointestinal bleeding when barium studies of the upper gastrointestinal tract, small intestine and colon, as well as fibre-optic endoscopy, are negative. The small intestine may be the site of angiomatous malformations, small tumours and Meckel's diverticulum, all of which may present as persistent or recurrent iron deficiency anaemia or recurrent acute bleeding. Selective catheterization of the coeliac axis, superior mesenteric artery and inferior mesenteric artery may be necessary when angiography is performed in the investigation of gastrointestinal bleeding (Allison, 1980).

Fig. 3.8 Normal terminal ileum shown on a per oral pneumocolon examination of the ileocaecal region.

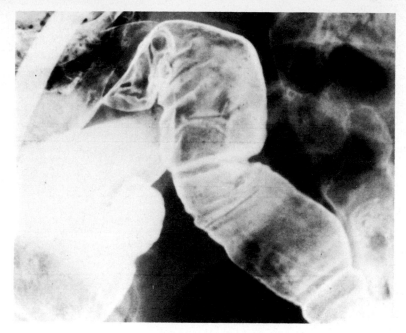

Radionuclide studies

Bleeding sites in the small intestine and colon may be detected with radionuclides (Alavi, 1980). The general anatomical location of bleeding is identified in the majority of patients and further investigations, such as barium studies or angiography, can then be performed to define the precise bleeding site. ^{51}Cr-tagged red cells (Ebaugh et al., 1958), ^{99}Technetium^{m} labelled albumin (Miskowiak et al., 1977) and in vivo and ex vivo labelling of red cells with pyrophosphate have all been used in the detection of bleeding. Alavi (1980), however, recommends the use of freshly prepared ^{99}Technetium^{m} sulphur colloid in patients with clinical evidence of lower gastrointestinal tract bleeding, 10 mCi (370 Bq) ^{99}Tc^{m} sulphur colloid are injected by the intravenous route. Serial images of the abdomen and pelvis are taken at two minute intervals. If extravasation is demonstrated, further images are taken to define the site of bleeding. If no bleeding is detected, images are taken of the upper abdomen to include the liver and spleen. If no bleeding site is demonstrated, a left anterior oblique projection is used to scan the splenic flexure and proximal small intestine in the left upper quadrant. The examination is extended for an additional 30–45 minutes if the bleeding site is not identified on the early scans. Alavi (1980) claims that bleeding rates of as low as 0.05–0.1 ml/min are detected by this method.

Meckel's diverticulum is detectable by radionuclide imaging using ^{99}Technetium^{m} pertechnetate, a technique which should precede other radiological studies where there is suspicion of this condition (Conway, 1980). A dose of 100 µCi of ^{99}TC^{m} pertechnetate per pound (3.7 mBq/kg) is injected intravenously and images are taken at 5–10 min intervals for 45 min. The area of ectopic uptake is identified as an area of increased radionuclide activity in the lower abdomen, usually on the right side, within the first 5–10 minutes of injection and becoming more intense with time.

Ultrasonography and CT scanning have at present no practical application in the investigation of the small intestine. Fibre-optic endoscopy has not developed to the point where it may be considered a normal technique for investigating the small intestine.

REFERENCES

Alavi A. (1980) Scintigraphic demonstration of acute gastrointestinal bleeding. *Gastrointestinal Radiol.*, **5**, 205–8.

Allison D. J. (1980) Gastrointestinal bleeding. Radiological diagnosis. *Brit. J. Hosp. Med.*, **23**, 358–65.

Bilbao M K., Frische L H., Dotter C. T. & Rosch J. (1967) Hypotonic duodenography. *Radiology*, **89**, 438–43.

Conway J. J. (1980) Radionuclide diagnosis of Meckel's diverticulum. *Gastrointestinal Radiol.*, **5**, 209–13.

Donato H., Mayo H. W. & Barr L. H. (1954) The effect of peroral barium in partial obstruction of the small bowel. *Surgery*, **35**, 719–23.

Ebaugh F. G. Jr., Clemens T. J., Rodnan G. & Peterson R. E. (1958) Quantitative measurement of gastrointestinal blood loss. The use of radioactive ^{51}Cr in patients with gastrointestinal haemorrhage. *Amer. J. Med.*, **25**, 169–81.

Ekberg O. (1977) Double contrast examination of the small bowel. *Gastrointestinal Radiol.*, **1**, 349–53.

Figiel L. S. & Figiel S. J. (1964) Tumours of the terminal ileum. Diagnosis by retrograde filling during the barium enema study. *Amer. J. Roentgenol.*, **91**, 816–18.

Freeark R. J., Love L. & Baker R. J. (1968) An active diagnostic approach to blunt abdominal trauma. *Surg. clin. N. Amer.*, **48**, 97–109.

Herlinger H. (1978) A modified technique for the double contrast small bowel enema. *Gastrointestinal Radiol.*, **3**, 201–7.

James W. B. & Hume R. (1968) Action of metoclopramide on gastric emptying and small bowel transit time. *Gut*, **9**, 203–5.

Kellett M. J., Zboralske F. F. & Margulis A. R. (1977) Per oral pneumocolon examination of the ileocaecal region. *Gastrointestinal Radiol.*, **1**, 361–5.

Kreel L. (1970) The use of oral metoclopramide in the barium meal and follow-through examination. *Brit. J. Radiol.*, **43**, 31–5.

Kreel L. (1975) Pharmaco-radiology in barium examination with special reference to glucagon. *Brit. J. Radiol.*, **48**, 691–703.

Marshak R. H. & Lindner A. E. (1976) *Radiology of the Small Intestine*, 2e, W. B. Saunders Company, Philadelphia.

Miller R. E. (1965) Complete reflux small bowel examination. *Radiology*, **84**, 457–63.

Miller R. E. & Brahme F. (1969) Large amounts of orally administered barium for obstruction of the small intestine. *Surg., Gynec. Obstet.*, **129**, 1185–8.

Miller R. E. & Sellink J. L. (1979) Enteroclysis: the small bowel enema. How to succeed and how to fail. *Gastrointestinal Radiol.*, **4**, 269–83.

Miller T. G. & Abbott W. O. (1934) Intestinal intubation: a practical technique. *Amer. J. med. Sci.*, **187**, 595–9.

Miskowiak J., Nielsen S. L., Munk O. & Anderson B. (1977) Abdominal scintiphotography with 99 m technetium labelled albumin in acute gastrointestinal bleeding. *Lancet*, **ii**, 852–4.

Nelson S. W., Christoforidis A. J. & Roenick W. J. (1963) Barium suspension vs. water soluble iodine compounds in the study of obstruction of the small bowel. An experimental study of physiologic characteristics and radiographic value. *Radiology*, **80**, 252–4.

Nice C. M. Jr. (1963) Roentgenographic pattern and motility in small bowel studies. *Radiology*, **80**, 39–45.

Nolan D. J. (1979) Rapid duodenal and jejunal intubation. *Clin. Radiol.*, **30**, 183–5.

Nolan D. J. (1981) The barium examination of the small intestine. Progress report. *Gut*, **22**, 682–94.

Novak D. (1980) Acceleration of the small intestine contrast study by ceruletide. *Gastrointestinal Radiol.*, **5**, 61–5.

Parker J. G. & Beneventano T. C. (1970) Acceleration of small bowel contrast study by cholecystokinin. *Gastroenterology*, **58**, 679–84.

Robbins A. H., Wetzner S. M. & Landy M. D. (1980) Ceruletide-assisted examination of the small bowel. *Amer. J. Roentgenol.*, **134**, 343–7.

Rosenquist C. J. (1975) Methods of acceleration of small intestinal radiographic examination. *West. J. Med.*, **122**, 320.

Sellink J. L. (1971) *Examination of the Small Intestine by means of Duodenal Intubation*. H. E. Stenfert Kroese B.V., Leiden.

Sellink J. L. (1974) Radiologic examination of the small intestine by duodenal intubation. *Acta Radiol., Diagn.*, **15**, 318—32.

Sellink J. L. (1976) *Radiological Atlas of Common Diseases of the Small Bowel*. H. E. Stenfert Kroese, B. V., Leiden.

Shipps F. C., Sayler C. B., Egan J. F., Green G. S., Weinstein C. J. & Jones J. M. (1979) Fluoroscopic placement of intestinal tubes. *Radiology*, **132**, 226–7.

Spiro H. M. (1977) *Clinical Gastroenterology*, 2e, p. 697. Macmillan Publishing Company, New York.

Vallance R. (1980) An evaluation of the small bowel enema based on an analysis of 350 consecutive examinations. *Clin. Radiol.*, **31**, 227–32.

The Colon

C. I. BARTRAM

THE DOUBLE CONTRAST BARIUM ENEMA

The double contrast barium enema (DCBE) is now established as the definitive and routine radiological method for the examination of the large bowel. The radiologist must take responsibility for all aspects of the examination.

Technique

Bowel preparation

Poor bowel preparation is the commonest cause of error in barium enemas, since the presence of excess faecal residue invalidates the examination. Most methods of cleansing the large bowel involve a combination of dietary restriction, purgation, and water enemas. (Table 4.1).

Table 4.1 Standard bowel preparation

Day before barium enema	Day of barium enema
Clear fluids only	Clear fluids only
30 ml castor oil *or* 71 ml X-prep* at 2 pm	2 cleansing water enemas

* X-prep—142 mg sennosides A and B in 71 ml.
Napp Laboratories Ltd, Hill Farm Avenue, Watford WD2 7RA

Dietary restriction   A low residue diet for several days before the barium enema reduces the faecal content, but is often difficult to implement as a routine. In practice, it is simplest to instruct the patient to take only clear fluids once purgation has begun. This also prevents dehydration from the resultant intestinal fluid loss. The patient should be told to drink a certain volume every hour for a given period.

Purgatives   Recent investigations suggest that all laxatives have a similar effect on the intestinal tract, causing secretion of water and electrolytes instead of the normal absorption. Whether this change is due to active electrolyte secretion, decreased electrolyte absorption, increased intraluminal osmolarity, or increased hydrostatic pressure, is uncertain. The net

effect is an increase in the faecal excretion of water, which is the mechanism by which laxatives cause diarrhoea. The additional role of altered bowel motility and the site at which laxatives act is not clear. The following purgatives are in common use:

1. *Castor oil* is broken down in the small intestine which is when the active ingredient, rinoleic acid, is absorbed. There is an increased secretion of water and electrolytes in the small intestine and colon, but the exact site of action is unknown.
2. *Bisacodyl* inhibits water reabsorption in the intestine and has been shown to increase ileostomy output by 15%. Five per cent of the oral dose is absorbed.
3. *X-Prep** is a standardized preparation of senna fruit extract. It contains some alcohol and is therefore contra-indicated in patients taking disulfiram.
4. *Magnesium salts* including citrate, hydroxide and sulphate, probably work through their osmotic effect, although cholecystokinin release may be partly responsible.
5. *Oxyphenisatan* induces a mass peristalsis when instilled into the colon. Its oral use has declined following reports of the development of hepatitis, which is probably a rare sensitivity reaction.

Non-washout regimes are derived from Brown's original method of bowel preparation which involved a complex low-residue diet combined with an osmotic irritant laxative to purge the bowel. A modern equivalent is given in Table 4.2.

Cleansing water enemas   Miller has recommended that a cleansing water enema should consist of 2 litres of warm tap water. This amount is usually sufficient to reach the caecum and distend the colon. The water should be run in slowly with the patient first on their left side, then prone, and finally turning on to the right side to fill the caecum. If fluid is introduced too fast, the rectum is over-distended, and the patient will complain of discomfort and may be incontinent. The reservoir should be only 2–3 ft above the patient but is lowered if the patient experiences discomfort. When

* X-Prep. 142 mg sennosides A and B in 71 ml Napp Laboratories Ltd, Hill Farm Ave, Watford WD2 7RA

Table 4.2   Non-washout bowel preparation

Day before barium enema	Day of barium enema
Clear fluids only	Clear fluids only
7–8 a.m. one sachet of Picolax† dissolved in water and drunk	
3–4 p.m. one sachet of Picolax dissolved in water and drunk	

N.B. When Picolax is added to water an exothermic reaction occurs. Patients should be warned of this. Only a small quantity of water should be used initially and the solution diluted to 150 ml after 5 minutes.
† Picolax—each sachet contains 16.3 g of powder which is composed of 10 mg of sodium picosulphate with magnesium citrate.
Ferring Pharmaceuticals Ltd. Feltham, Middlesex TW13 6JG.

the colon has been filled, the patient is sent immediately to the toilet with instructions to evacuate as completely as possible. Providing the colon has been filled well, this usually results in rapid emptying of the bowel. A repeat enema ensures that the bowel is completely clean. Three grams of oxyphenistan may be added to the second water enema and has no ill effect, but a marginal benefit on colonic evacuation. A 15–30 minute interval should be allowed between complete evacuation of the water enema and the commencement of the barium enema to allow for reabsorption of residual water in the colon. Standard regimens for bowel preparation are shown in Tables 4.1 and 4.2. An alternative approach is saline lavage. The patient drinks, or is given via a naso-gastric tube, a large quantity of saline to flush the bowel through. Although effective, it is uncomfortable for the patient and leaves the colon full of fluid which is unsatisfactory for double contrast barium enemas.

The value of a preliminary radiograph

A plain abdominal radiograph prior to the administration of barium is not essential, but may be useful to show any abnormal calcification or a skeletal lesion that might otherwise be obscured by the barium. If the plain radiograph shows there is still obvious faecal residue, the patient may require further cleansing enemas. Residue may be present, however, although the colon appears clear on the plain radiograph. It is very difficult to clear the colon proximal to a tumour which is almost obstructing the lumen. If plain radiography shows extensive residue in a patient who could have an obstructing lesion, some barium may be given per rectum to exclude an obstruction before repeating the bowel preparation. Intestinal obstruction, toxic megacolon or perforation are excluded by

a plain radiograph. The plain radiograph is an integral part of the instant enema. In the interests of economy and reduced radiation it may be omitted from the routine DCBE.

Administration of the barium suspension and air insufflation

The barium suspension must be sufficiently viscose to ensure that the mucosal layer has a radiographic density which is clearly visible en face. If the barium suspension is too thick, it will not flow easily and the coating will be uneven. Small clumps of barium produce artefacts and should not be present. (Fig. 4.1). The colon will reabsorb some water from the suspension, but this should not cause any loss of elasticity with flaking of barium. (Fig. 4.2). Persistant bubble formation during the administration of air should not occur, (Fig. 4.3).

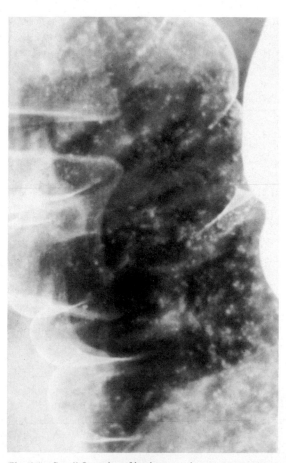

Fig. 4.1   Small floccules of barium causing numerous dense particles on the mucosal surface.

Fig. 4.2 Flaking of the barium coating due to loss of elasticity in the barium suspension.

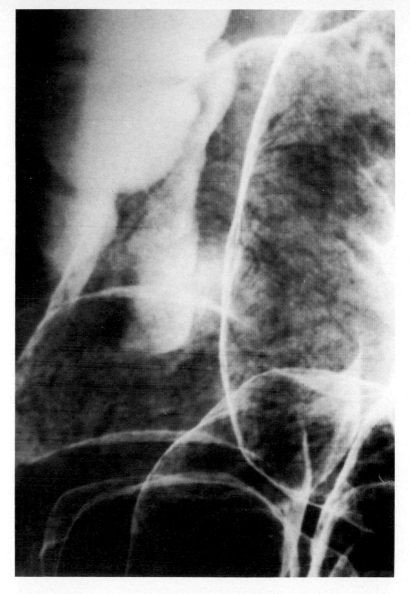

A higher viscosity barium suspension is needed to obtain good coating after a cleansing water enema than after non-washout preparation techniques. This has the advantage that a smaller volume of barium may be used, with less pooling so that more of the bowel is seen in double contrast. Visualization of the innominate grooves is usually only possible if a low viscosity suspension is used without any water cleansing enema.

Most apparatus now available for barium enemas is disposable (Fig. 4.4). The barium is administered from a large container via a tube and disposable enema tip (Fig. 4.5). With the patient in the prone position, the enema tip is covered with a lubricating jelly and inserted so that the end is lodged just inside the anal canal. In the few instances where it is necessary to use a balloon catheter, the balloon should be of small volume and symmetrical when inflated so that it does not impale the enema tip on the rectal wall. The balloon should form a seal against the anal sphincter and yet not occlude the rectum. Over-inflation of the balloon is dangerous, while distension of the rectum reflexly lowers sphincteric tone and paradoxically forces the patient to be incontinent.

A balloon catheter may be used, with caution, to overcome incontinence. Prior to doing so the patient should be given an i.v. smooth muscle relaxant and the head of the table lowered. Both these measures

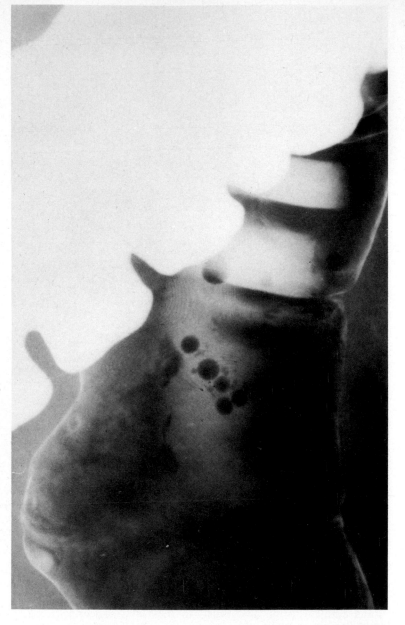

Fig. 4.3 Small air bubbles trapped in
the surface coating of barium.

facilitate rectal drainage into the colon, thus reducing
the pressure in the rectum and the risk of incontinence.

The rate at which barium flows into the colon
depends on its viscosity, the diameter of the tubing
and the height of the reservoir. Too rapid filling may
induce colonic contraction, while overdistension of
the rectum will lead to pain and incontinence.

The requisite volume of barium varies with the
configuration of the colon. Most colons require 350–
650 ml to reach the splenic flexure. The objective is to
fill the colon with a sufficient volume of barium to
achieve uniformly good coating without large segments becoming obscured by being completely filled
with barium. In practice this is achieved by running
barium as far as the transverse colon, and in most
cases 300–500 ml is sufficient.

As much barium as possible should be drained from
the rectum to obtain optimum double contrast views
of the recto-sigmoid. Barium may be drained into a
kidney dish, or back into the bag of a closed system.
Drainage is facilitated by elevating the head of the
table and the use of wide-bore tubing. The simplest

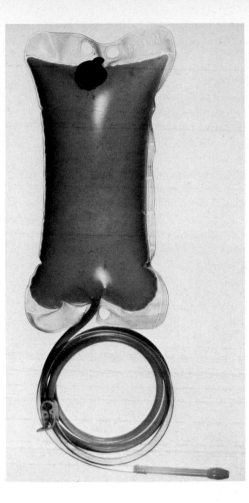

Fig. 4.4 Self-contained disposable barium enema giving set. Sufficient barium for a normal DCBE is in the bag (520 bag from E–Z–EM), which has been inflated with air and may be used to insufflate the colon without the need for further apparatus. (E–Z–EM: Henley Medical Supplies Ltd., London N8 ODL.)

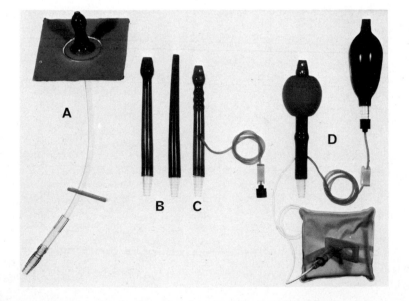

Fig. 4.5 Selection of disposable enema tips (E–Z–EM).
(a) Colostomy enema tip. The square flange is adhesive and holds the tip in position.
(b) Two standard enema tips with different ends.
(c) Enema tip with air line.
(d) Enema tip with air line and bulb inflator attached. This is a self retaining catheter. Note the small balloon and square plastic inflator, which distends the balloon to a measured volume to prevent over-inflation.

method, particularly when a closed system is used, is to distend the rectum with air in the prone position, and then to let it drain out. The force of the rectum collapsing aids evacuation of the barium.

Air insufflation

Air may be insufflated with a Higginson's syringe, a bulb inflator, or from the bag of a closed system. For the latter, the bag must be blown up and clamped prior to running in the barium. The tube is best cleared of barium by placing the bag on the table and leaning on it with both hands, making sure that one hand covers the seal which will otherwise be forced open. Once the tube is empty of barium, air will rush in and it is then necessary to reduce the pressure. It is best to insufflate gently but constantly, rather than intermittently with large volumes.

The principle of air insufflation is to drive the barium around the colon as a column (Fig. 4.6). Air pushes the barium into the transverse colon when the patient is prone. The barium must travel uphill to enter the hepatic flexure. Continued air insufflation in the prone position results in distension of the transverse colon, following which the caecum will be distended by air. The barium remains in the transverse colon, unless the patient is turned on to the right side, whereupon the hepatic flexure becomes dependent and fills with barium (Fig. 4.7). There is often a critical angle of obliquity at which barium enters the ascending colon, best observed on screening whilst turning the patient. When barium is seen to enter the ascending colon, several large puffs of air help the forward propulsion of the barium column. Barium may not fill the caecum in this position but, as the patient is turned prone again, the caecum becomes dependent and barium cascades into it (Fig. 4.7).

The minimum manoeuvring of the patient required during air insufflation is prone–right lateral–prone. Turning the patient prone–right lateral–supine–left lateral–prone–right lateral–prone, aids emptying of the left colon with more of the barium reaching the proximal colon. The more the patient is turned, the better is the coating; but placing the patient in the supine position increases the chance of refluxing barium through the ileo-caecal valve. This is not a problem in the prone position as the ileo-caecal valve is uppermost, so that only air should reflux through it. Intermittent screening is essential to check progress.

Mass contractions or persistent physiological ring contractions are the commonest indication for giving intravenous smooth muscle relaxants. An i.v. smooth muscle relaxant should be given when more than one colonic contraction occurs during filling, otherwise

parts of the colon may be in spasm during radiographic exposure. A dose of 0.25 mg of glucagon or 20 mg of Buscopan are used and will render the entire colon more distensible, with the disadvantage that ileo-caecal reflux is more frequent due to reduced tone in the valve. The indications for i.v. smooth muscle relaxants during barium enema are: generalized or localized spasm, where the distinction from an organic stricture may be difficult; in diverticular disease where improved distension of the sigmoid segment aids the detection of polyps; the differentiation between benign and malignant strictures; and in elderly patients with poor anal tone who have difficulty in retaining the enema. Relaxation of the colon facilitates rectal drainage and lowers the pressure in the rectum.

Radiographic views

Radiographs are taken immediately after the examiner is satisfied that the colon has been adequately filled with barium and properly distended with air. The recommended radiographic sequence and positioning is given in Table 4.3 (Fig. 4.8). The angled

Table 4.3 Film sequence and positioning DCBE

View	Film size (cm)	Positioning
Prone (angled)	35 × 43	Centre level iliac crests in midline. Tube angled 30° caudally.
Left lateral	30 × 40	Centre 3″ below iliac crests in midline with patient lateral.
Right posterior oblique	35 × 43	Patient turned 30° to the right. Centre 1½″ to left midline at level iliac crests.
Left posterior-oblique	35 × 43	Patient turned 30° to the left. Centre 1½″ to right of midline at level of iliac crests.
A–P decubitus with horizontal beam	30 × 40	Patient left lateral. Centre 1″ below iliac crests in midline of parallel grid.
P–A decubitus with horizontal beam	30 × 40	Patient right lateral. Centre 1″ below iliac crests to midline of parallel grid.
A–P erect	35 × 43	Centre in midline 1″ above iliac crests.
or two erect spot views of the flexures		

Fig. 4.6 Diagramatic illustration of the principles of air insufflation during DCBE.

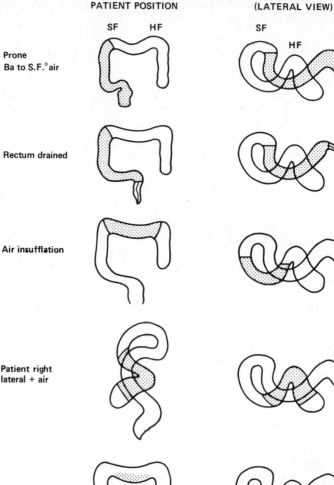

PATIENT POSITION

EQUIVALENT (LATERAL VIEW)

SF   HF

SF

HF

Prone
Ba to S.F.°air

Rectum drained

Air insufflation

Patient right
lateral + air

Patient prone + air

Ba pools in dependant parts

Table 4.4 Optimum views for segments of large bowel

Rectum	P–A with perpendicular tube
	Right lateral
	Decubitus views
Sigmoid	15° RAO with 35° caudal tube angulation, 45° LPO
Descending colon	RPO
	Decubitus views
Transverse colon	Erect
	LPO
Ascending colon and caecum	LPO
	Decubitus views

Modified from Peterson & Miller 1978.

prone view is preferable to the perpendicular projection because it prevents overlapping of the sigmoid loop and proximal rectum, but does not provide an overall view of the colon. The straight prone projection is often the only view which shows the entire large bowel on one radiograph. The optimum projections for various parts of the large bowel, as described by Peterson and Miller (1978), are summarized in Table 4.4. The area of colon visualized by angled and oblique views is less than with a vertical X-ray tube and more radiographs are needed to give coverage of the entire bowel.

The sigmoid segment is undoubtedly the most

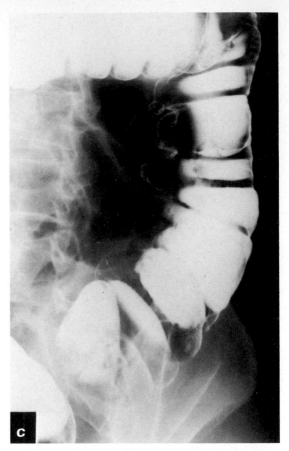

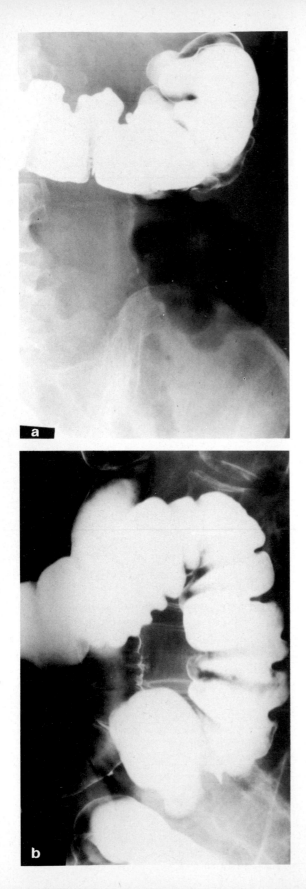

Fig. 4.7 Technique for filling the proximal colon.

(a) Patient prone. The barium has reached the hepatic flexure, but air is in the caecum. Further air insufflation in this position will only distend the caecum with more air, but not barium.

(b) When the patient is turned on to the right side, barium flows into the ascending colon but may not fill the caecum.

(c) With the patient turned back into the prone position, the caecum is dependant and fills with barium.

difficult part of the large bowel to visualize. Special views help to prevent obscuration of lesions due to superimposition of loops, but if the loops are filled with barium the diagnostic accuracy will be downgraded to that of single contrast. Careful air insufflation, rotation of the patient and drainage of the rectum ensures that most of the sigmoid is shown by double contrast. This gives an accurate investigation and allows overlapping loops to be 'seen through', thus reducing the need for specialized views.

The lateral pelvic view is the only other projection, apart from the angled prone view, which demonstrates the rectosigmoid segment. Either a left or a right lateral pelvic view may be used in this situation. Oblique views give an overall coverage of the colon with useful visualization of the sigmoid and transverse segments. The decubitus views are very important and should include the rectum. A common error is to allow the film and grid to tilt, resulting in grid line cut-off. A film holder should be used to maintain the film in a vertical position. The erect views may be taken with the undercouch tube, when it is customary to take two oblique views of the flexures. If a single overcouch projection is taken, it is essential to check that the splenic flexure has been included on the film, as this may be the only view on which this segment is shown. Part of the hepatic flexure may be hidden and spot radiographs are invaluable to show any part of the proximal colon that has not been seen adequately on the standard projections.

VARIATIONS ON BASIC TECHNIQUE

Colostomy enema

Recurrent neoplasia may develop some years after the initial cancer in up to 10% of patients. Follow-up examinations are therefore required, sometimes in patients who have a colostomy.

Cleansing water enemas are very difficult to perform with a colostomy, so that a standard non-washout regimen is a definite advantage in these patients.

The barium suspension should be the same as that used in a regular double contrast enema. The main problem of administering the barium is to prevent leakage without damaging the colostomy. Catheters are available with a flange (Fig. 4.5a), which is held by the patient against the colostomy opening. A Foley catheter, with the balloon inflated, may be used in the same way. The most effective seal however, is obtained by inserting a Foley catheter into the colostomy and inflating the balloon with 10 ml of air, then gently pulling the balloon back until it impinges against the

cutaneous opening of the colostomy. There should be no danger of perforating the bowel at the site of the colostomy with this small volume of air.

Barium may be given from a syringe. The colon should be filled to the hepatic flexure, which usually requires about 250 ml. An i.v. smooth muscle relaxant must be given, otherwise barium filling induces strong peristalsis which continually empties the colon.

Air insufflation is commenced with the patient on the right side in order to propel the barium into the ascending colon. The patient is then turned further over to fill the caecum, and then supine to distend the transverse colon. The same degree of colonic distension as in normal patients is not possible, and forceful over-distension of the colon should be avoided at all times in the colostomy patient.

An advantage of using an indwelling Foley catheter is that a spigot can be applied to the tube before taking the radiographs. A supine radiograph is substituted for the prone view, otherwise the projections are the same as in Table 4.3. Drainage from the colostomy is invariable when the patient stands, so the catheter should be removed with the patient supine and a disposable bag placed over the colostomy before taking the erect radiograph.

The 'instant' barium enema

The technique was developed by Young to provide a double contrast barium enema in patients with ulcerative colitis, without the need for bowel preparation. The 'instant' enema is used to show the extent and severity of colitis which is known to be present from sigmoidoscopy. It may also be used to demonstrate the level and nature of an obstruction in the large bowel, to show a fistula in the distal part of the large bowel, and to demonstrate the rectum and distal ileum in a patient with an ileo-rectal anastomosis.

The contra-indications to an instant enema are: toxic megacolon, suspected perforation, and the possibility of cancer in ulcerative colitis which demands a full barium enema.

An instant enema is feasible in ulcerative colitis because the disease starts distally and remains in continuity. Where the mucosa is inflamed, the lumen is free of residue and good double contrast views are then obtained in the affected bowel (Fig. 4.9). Crohn's disease, on the other hand, is patchy in distribution and early lesions or lesions in the proximal bowel may become obscured by faecal residue. The 'instant' enema is therefore not recommended in Crohn's disease unless the colitis is very active and there is severe anal disease which would make bowel preparation extremely uncomfortable. A barium enema

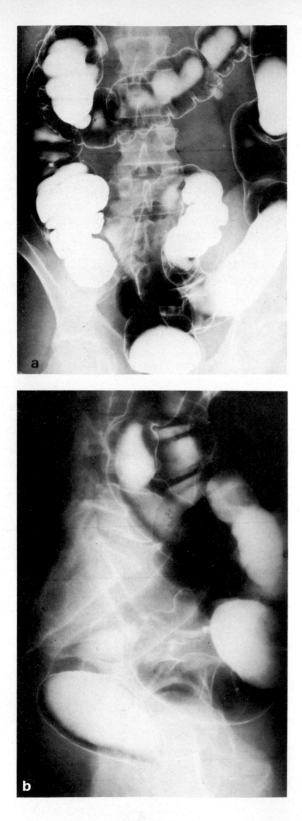

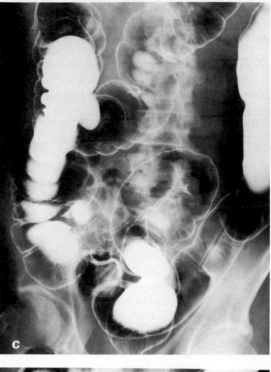

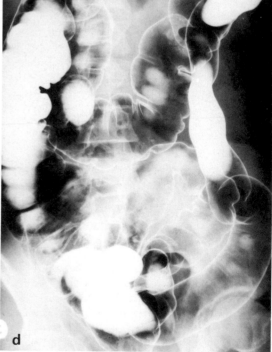

Fig. 4.8 Standard DCBE series.
(a) Prone (X-ray tube vertical).
(b) Left lateral pelvis.
(c) Right posterior oblique.
(d) Left posterior oblique.

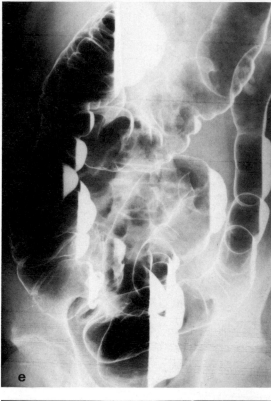

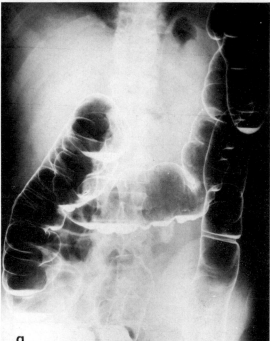

(e) Decubitus, left side down.
(f) Decubitis, right side down.
(g) Erect (overcouch view).

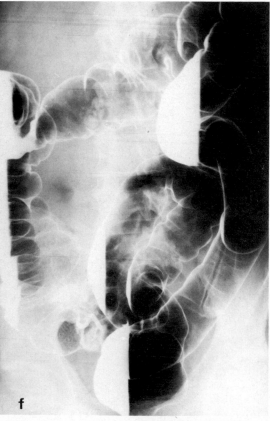

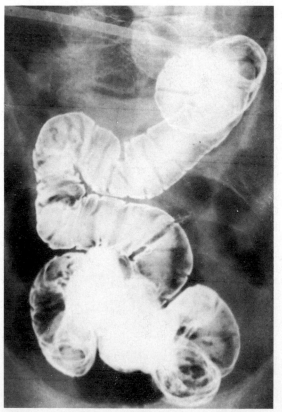

Fig. 4.9 Ileostomy enema—normal distal ileum.

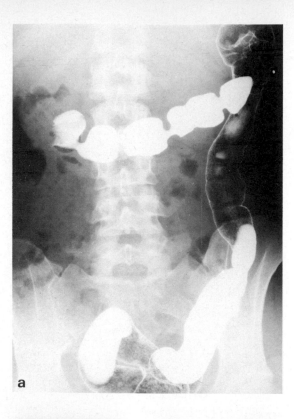

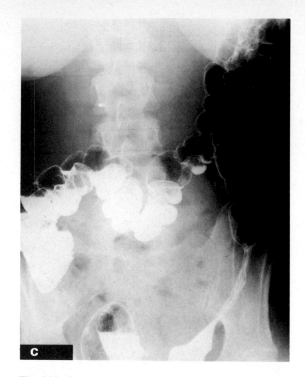

Fig. 4.10 Instant enema.

(a) Prone view—after barium and air. A granular mucosa extends into the transverse colon.

(b) Left lateral pelvic view to show recto-sigmoid.

(c) Erect view—flexures and transverse colon shown in double contrast.

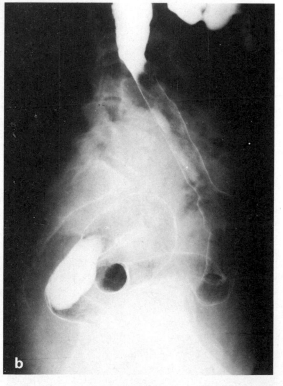

with full bowel preparation is then performed if information from the instant enema is inadequate.

A preliminary radiograph is taken to exclude perforation or toxic megacolon and to show the extent of the faecal residue. The barium suspension is similar to that used for a standard examination. It is run in with the patient prone, until either the splenic flexure is reached, an obstruction is demonstrated, or solid faeces block the flow of barium. Air is then insufflated in a similar fashion to a standard examination. Patients with colitis are intolerant of rectal distension and there is often narrowing of the affected colon. To avoid distressing the patient, only sufficient air should be given to obtain a reasonable double contrast view of the affected colon.

Three radiographs are taken for a complete study (Fig. 4.10) namely the prone, left lateral pelvic, and erect views. Sufficient information is often obtained from the prone radiograph. If the patient is being considered for an ileo-rectal anastomosis, the left lateral view will show the configuration of the rectum. The erect projection gives the best double contrast view of the flexures and transverse colon, and is included if there is doubt as to the extent of the colitis. When the examination is undertaken to show a stricture or fistula, spot radiographs are taken of the lesion, using screening to manouevre the patient into the ideal position.

There is no conclusive evidence that an 'instant' enema causes any deterioration of the colitis. The lack of any bowel preparation is an obvious safety factor. Retention of barium in the proximal colon is common when there is severe active distal disease, but appears to be without clinical effect.

ILEOSTOMY ENEMA

Continent ileostomies, the commonest being the Koch ileostomy, have been developed in an attempt to overcome the disadvantage of a simple terminal ileostomy which necessitates the constant wearing of a drainage appliance. There are differing indications and methods for examining these types of ileostomy.

Terminal ileostomy

It is often difficult to examine the small bowel immediately proximal to an ileostomy by the small bowel follow through. In ileostomy dysfunction, it is important to show the distal small bowel in order to exclude strictures, adhesions, or recurrent disease.

An ileostomy enema is performed by the following technique. The patient's normal appliance is removed and a disposable bag is placed over the ileostomy. A small cut in the bag over the site of the ileostomy enables the examination to be performed through the bag, thus preventing extensive spilling of barium. A Foley catheter is then inserted into the ileostomy, taking care gently to guide the tube into place rather than pushing it. The tube is moved in different directions in order to find the line of the lumen. The balloon is inflated with *10 ml of air only*, the tube then being withdrawn slightly so that the balloon abuts against the inner side of the ileostomy. An i.v. injection of Buscopan 20 mg is then given to arrest peristalsis and allow retrograde filling of the bowel. The injection is repeated if necessary during the examination. The barium suspension (100 wt/vol) is injected slowly with a 60 ml bladder syringe. It is usually only possible to fill the distal 40 cm of bowel, using 120–80 ml of barium. Air is insufflated by a Higginson syringe and spot radiographs are taken in several projections (Fig. 4.10).

Kock's ileostomy

Continence is maintained by the nipple valve, which lies within the reservoir (Fig. 4.11). The reservoir is drained about four to six times a day by inserting a catheter through the valve and into the reservoir. Difficulty in intubation and/or incontinence are common problems, which may be due either to partial retraction or complete eversion of the valve (Fig. 4.12). When examining a Kock's ileostomy, it is essential to show the reservoir, the valve and the position of the valve in relation to the reservoir.

A Foley catheter is inserted just into the valve. Barium is then injected and spot radiographs are taken to show the valve (Fig. 4.13). The catheter is then moved through the valve and into the reservoir. The reservoir is then filled with about 100 ml of barium. The pouch has a capacity of only 100 ml immediately after operation, which increases to 500–800 ml after three months. Air is insufflated and spot radiographs are taken of the pouch, the position of the valve within the pouch, and the small bowel leading into the pouch (Fig. 4.14).

WATER-SOLUBLE CONTRAST ENEMA

A water-soluble contrast medium is indicated where there is a risk of peritoneal contamination, or when the low viscosity of the contrast medium compared to

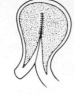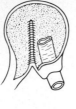

Fig. 4.11 Construction of Kock's ileostomy.

| 30 cm of ileum anastomosed along antimesenteric border | Bowel opened | Efferent limb intussuscepted to form valve 5 cm long | Valve and flap sutured to form reservoir |

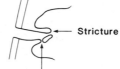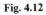

Fig. 4.12

← Stricture

Fistula

Normal   Partial reduction   Complete reduction

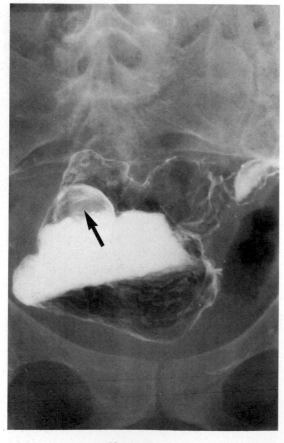

Fig. 4.13 Normal Kock's ileostomy. The valve (arrowed) is seen lying within the reservoir.

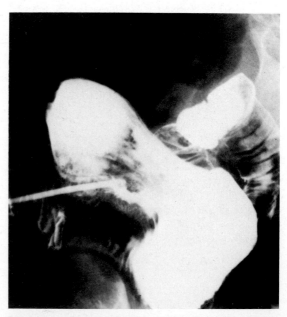

Fig. 4.14 Complete reduction of valve. The Foley catheter is in the valve, which is outside the reservoir.

barium may be an advantage. Specifically, a water-soluble contrast enema is used to demonstrate the site of, or exclude, a colonic perforation; to delineate an anastomosis in the immediate post-operative period; and to outline the rectum and distal colon in patients thought to have megacolon or Hirschsprung's disease.

The water-soluble contrast agent is diluted with either two or three parts of water, depending on its original concentration. Quantities in excess of 500 ml should be avoided. Even small volumes may cause diarrhoea, due to the hypertonicity of the contrast medium. A 1 in 5 dilution of Gastrografin is isotonic, but the density is too low for use in adult studies. Standard enema tips should not be used in patients with low anastomoses.

Anastomoses are examined on about the tenth post-operative day to exclude any leakage. A Foley catheter is inserted carefully into the rectum. It is easiest to introduce contrast medium with the patient in the left lateral position. Supine and lateral views of the distended anastomic area are taken (Fig. 4.15), a small track or pouch indicating a leak at the anastomosis into a small sealed cavity (Fig. 4.16). Free peritoneal spread of contrast is a rare occurrence, the volume of contrast escaping into the peritoneum being kept to a minimum because it may produce a severe ileus. (Fig. 4.17).

The plain abdominal radiograph in patients with megacolon will show gross faecal retention. In order to demonstrate a distal transitional zone in Hirschsprung's disease, it is better not to prepare the bowel but simply to delineate the configuration of the distal large bowel by contrast medium on lateral and prone radiographs.

COMPLICATIONS

Perforation is the commonest serious complication of the barium enema. The incidence is less than 1 in 12 000 examinations. The bowel may be perforated by trauma from an enema tip lacerating the rectum; by overdistention of a balloon tearing or rupturing the rectal wall; because of a weakness of the bowel wall, such as a diverticular abscess which predisposes to perforation even when the colon is subjected to normal pressures; and by hydrostatic bursting due to overdistension of the colon with fluid and/or air.

The damage that results from a perforation depends on its level and degree. A mucosal tear leads to an intramural perforation, whereas complete rupture of the bowel causes either extra-peritoneal or intra-peritoneal perforation depending on whether it occurs below or above the peritoneal reflection. Perforation is not always apparent during the barium enema, and

Fig. 4.15 Water-soluble contrast enema. No leak at the anastomosis (marked by metal clips).

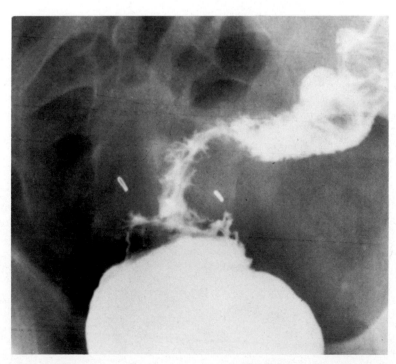

Fig. 4.16 Water-soluble contrast enema. The anastomosis is marked with a metal clip. A small track of contrast medium indicates a leak at the anastomosis, but this is sealed off and the patient was asymptomatic.

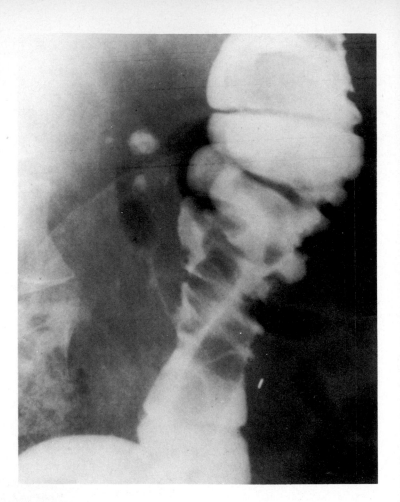

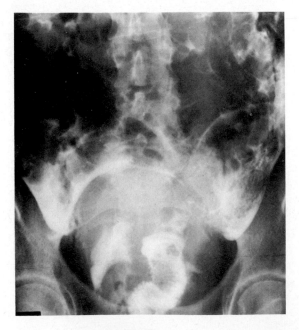

Fig. 4.17 Water-soluble contrast enema. Extensive free spillage of contrast medium throughout the peritoneal cavity was due to a large defect in the colo-anal anastomosis.

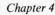

is sometimes not recognized until several hours after the examination.

Intravasation of barium into the wall of the rectum through a mucosal tear results in a barium granuloma. Polypoid granulomatous masses may be mistaken macroscopically for malignant tumours, although their true nature is confirmed histologically by the presence of barium crystals which are anisotrophic in polarized light. The granuloma may ulcerate. Perirectal abscesses may result from small extrusions of barium through the bowel wall.

Intraperitoneal perforation (Fig. 4.18) causes barium peritonitis, the immediate effect being hypovolaemia due to serosal exudation. As the barium is contaminated, this may be compounded by Gram-negative endotoxic shock. There is a high mortality without immediate and intensive treatment. Management consists of intravenous fluids, antibiotics, peri-toneal lavage with resection of the perforated segment, and the formation of a temporary colostomy. The particles of barium sulphate in the peritoneal cavity cause a severe foreign body reaction which leads to extensive fibrosis and adhesions.

Perforation during air insufflation is extremely rare but may lead to retroperitoneal emphysema (Fig. 4.19), pneumoperitoneum or gas in the portal vein.

Venous intravasation is also very rare, but massive pulmonary embolism is lethal. Entry into the portal circulation has resulted in the development of a liver abscess.

The use of non-disposable apparatus involves a risk of cross infection between patients, retrograde flow of barium during a colonic contraction having been shown to contaminate the reservoir of barium several feet above the patient. Disposable apparatus removes

Fig. 4.18 Intraperitoneal perforation of barium during a colostomy enema, due to rupture of a small diverticular abscess. Barium has spread throughout the peritoneal cavity with large collections in the lesser sac and right subphrenic and subhepatic spaces.

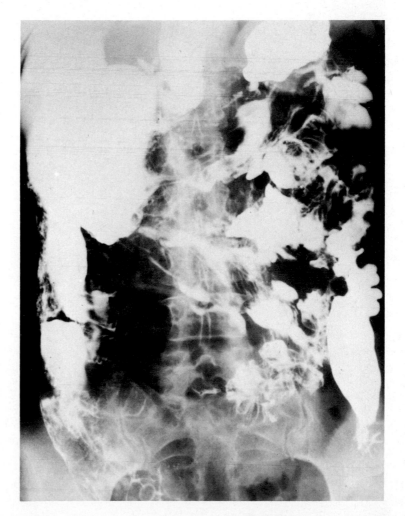

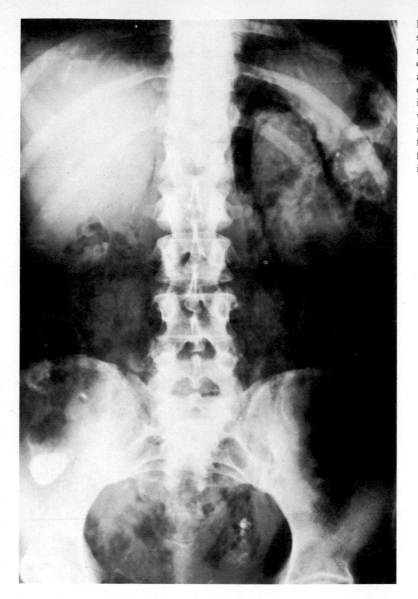

Fig. 4.19 Retroperitoneal emphysema. Air has tracked retroperitoneally, mainly along the left side to outline the psoas and left kidney. Some air is seen in the pelvic soft tissues. The emphysema developed during sigmoidoscopy after a rectal biopsy. The film was taken as a preliminary view for an instant enema, which was not performed. Residual barium in the caecum followed a previous small bowel examination.

this risk, leaving only the very remote danger of contamination of the barium suspension itself. Bacteraemia has been demonstrated during sigmoidoscopy and although the evidence for bacteraemia following barium enema is conflicting, it would seem reasonable to assume that this may occur. Fortunately, it is likely to be a transient phenomenon without clinical significance.

Bowel preparation is not without hazard. Purgation sometimes leads to colonic perforation if a stricture is impacted with faeces and the pressure in the proximal colon then becomes excessive. Water intoxication is a danger, particularly if the patient has become very dehydrated or when very large volumes are used to fill a megacolon in a child. Care should be taken to make sure that only warm water is given because hot water may cause extensive thermal burns to the colon. Detergent or soap enemas should not be used as they cause excess bubbling and poor mucosal coating, and have produced a caustic colitis.

Tannic acid causes marked colonic contraction and precipitates proteins, which may improve the coating of barium. It was banned following reports of death from liver failure in patients who were given tannic acid in the cleansing and barium enemas. Tannic acid is now considered safe to use in a cleansing enema at a concentration of less than 1%, but it should not be used in colitis because of the risk of increased absorption through the inflamed mucosa.

The dangers of balloon catheters

The majority of perforations are due to the use of balloon catheters and may occur in several ways. Laceration of the rectal wall may result from an overdistended balloon, a balloon which is asymmetrical on inflation and thus causes the catheter tip to be impaled on the rectal wall, and the sudden torque reaction secondary to bursting of the balloon.

A narrow rectum may be unable to distend when the balloon is inflated and will split. Balloon catheters should therefore not be used in patients with large rectal tumours or ulcerative colitis, or with non-functional loops which are always very narrow. A balloon catheter may seal the rectum so effectively that undue pressures can be applied to the colon by bulb inflators. The degree of colonic distension is a matter of experience, but there is a high risk that the colon is about to burst if the caecum reaches 8.5 cm in diameter or there is obliteration of the haustra.

Factors predisposing to perforation

Toxic megacolon is an absolute contra-indication to barium enema, because the friability of the colon renders it very susceptible to perforation. There are other situations where there is a slightly increased risk of perforation. A biopsy of the rectal wall weakens the bowel at the point or, if it is too deep, may inadvertently cause a perforation. In general, a ten day interval after a rectal biopsy allows the mucosa to grow over the biopsy site. However, the risk of perforation is very small and it may be more harmful to delay the barium enema. A barium enema may therefore be performed immediately after a rectal biopsy at the discretion of the clinician. Colonoscopic biopsies, which are very small and superficial and biopsies of a tumour do not constitute a hazard. A perforated diverticulum and abscess are usually sealed off by adherent adjacent structures, such as the omentum, and it is rare for the build-up of pressure within the abscess during a barium enema to rupture the abscess and lead to a free perforation. Colostomy enemas, as described above, are associated with an increased risk of perforation.

Effects of the contrast medium

Impaction of barium proximal to a stricture rarely precipitates colonic obstruction, although a recent study has suggested that inspissated barium is no more of a problem than inspissated faeces. Barium remains in the colon in the presence of an ileus. If barium is in an obstructed colon and fluid levels are present, this indicates that the barium is still in a fluid state.

Water-soluble contrast agents are hypertonic and draw a large quantity of fluid into the bowel. This may cause diarrhoea but, if an obstruction is present, gross distension of the caecum may result in perforation. A sudden reduction in circulating blood volume occurs following the administration of a large volume of contrast medium. This is dangerous in neonates and care must be taken in patients with Hirschsprung's disease.

THE RELATIONSHIP OF THE BARIUM ENEMA TO OTHER INVESTIGATIONS

It is a common fallacy to perform a barium enema before a small bowel examination. The small bowel should be examined before the barium enema. The stomach and small bowel will be clear of barium within a few hours and the bowel preparation for the enema will then remove all the barium from the colon. The presence of residual barium indicates inadequate preparation. Both examinations can be performed within a 48 hour period. If the barium enema is performed first, barium will remain in the colon for a number of days and further purgation will be required before a barium meal or small bowel.

It is now standard practice to perform sigmoidoscopy before a barium enema. The diagnostic returns from sigmoidoscopy are high because the rectosigmoid is the commonest site of adenomatous polyps and cancers. If the mucosa is abnormal on sigmoidoscopy, the patient may be spared full bowel preparation before performing an instant enema. The presence of a polyp necessitates a full DCBE to exclude further neoplasia.

Although double contrast enema gives good views of the rectum and distal sigmoid, sigmoidoscopy is not obsolete and remains an essential examination. However, lesions can often be missed because sigmoidoscopy is performed under suboptimal conditions, and the radiologist must carefully examine the distal large bowel despite a negative sigmoidoscopy report.

The rigid sigmoidoscope reaches only as far as the

sigmoid flexure. The flexible sigmoidoscope, on the other hand, passes easily into the descending colon and sometimes reaches the splenic flexure. Use of the flexible sigmoidoscope complements the barium enema by examining the sigmoid segment, the most difficult part of the colon to delineate by barium enema.

The entire colon may be visualized by colonoscopy. Direct inspection of the colon has the advantage of showing colitis at an earlier stage than the barium enema, demonstrating small vascular lesions which are not apparent on barium enema, and enabling distinction to be made between small polyps and adherent faecal residue. However, colonoscopy is time-consuming and it may be very difficult to visualize all the colon in the presence of redundant loops. A good quality double contrast barium enema remains the initial examination of choice and will show the endoscopist the overall configuration of the colon, as well as the site and shape of any lesion. The endoscopist can therefore plan the polypectomy and avoid examining normal colon proximal to the lesion. When the barium enema is negative, and there is a strong clinical suspicion of a lesion, colonoscopy should be performed rather than repeating the barium enema. Used in this way, colonoscopy complements the double contrast barium enema and has the advantages of allowing polypectomy and biopsy to be performed in the investigation of problem cases.

REFERENCES

Ansell G (1973) *Complications in Diagnostic Radiology*, pp. 333–60. Blackwell Scientific Publications, Oxford.

Donowitz M. (1979) Current concepts in laxative action: mechanisms by which laxatives increase stool water. *J. clin. Gastroenterol.*, **1**, 77–80.

Gelfand D. W. (1980) Complications of gastrointestinal radiologic procedures; 1. Complications of routine fluoroscopic studies. *Gastrointest. Radiol.*, **5**, 293–7.

Goldstein H. M. & Miller M. H. (1976) Air contrast colon examination in patients with colostomies. *Amer. J. Roentgenol.*, **127**, 607.

Laufer I. (1979) *Double Contrast Gastrointestinal Radiology*, pp. 495–515, W. B. Saunders Co., Philadelphia.

Miller R. E. (1975) The cleansing enema. *Radiology*, **117**, 483.

Peterson G H. & Miller R. E. (1978) The barium enema; a reassessment towards perfection. *Radiology*, **128**, 315–20.

Thomas B. M. (1979) The instant enema in inflammatory disease of the colon. *Clin. Radiol.*, **30**, 165–73.

Stephens D. H., Mantell B. E. & Kelly K. A. (1979) Radiology of the continent ileostomy. *Amer. J. Roentgenol.*, **132**, 717–21.

Barium Sulphate Suspension as a Contrast Agent   5

NICOLA S. RUSSELL

The first contrast agents to be used in the gastrointestinal tract were bismuth subnitrate and later bismuth subcarbonate. Toxicity resulting from absorption of these compounds, however, soon became apparent. In 1910, Bachem described the advantages of barium sulphate. Although the barium ion is highly toxic, barium sulphate has a low solubility product and the number of free barium ions in a barium meal or enema is therefore negligible. Other heavy metal compounds such as cerium and thorium have been evaluated, but barium sulphate has become the agent of choice for studying the gastrointestinal tract because of its ready availability, high density and low toxicity. The barium sulphate suspensions which are considered to be most suitable for use in gastrointestinal studies are those which provide good demonstration of mucosal surfaces.

The desirable characteristics of a barium sulphate solution

The ideal barium suspension must be dense enough to provide adequate radiographic contrast, yet flow readily over mucosal surfaces to give a uniform coating. It should therefore display the properties of a plastic colloid suspension with a yield point so low that it flows readily under the influence of gravity. The barium should remain suspended after stopping any agitation or stirring, should only form a cake at the bottom of the container very slowly, and it must be easy to resuspend. The suspension should not foam or flocculate. Mucosal coating should be uniform, stable and flexible, without cracking or artefacts. The suspension should be stable over a wide range of pH and in the presence of substances, such as sodium chloride and mucin, which promote flocculation. It must be non-toxic. A compromise in the characteristics of the suspension has to be adopted in general.

THE PHYSICO-CHEMICAL PROPERTIES OF BARIUM SULPHATE SUSPENSION

James (1978) has commented on the lack of available knowledge concerning the physical basis of the properties of barium sulphate suspensions, manufacturers being reluctant to divulge the precise constituents of their preparations. In addition to barium sulphate and water, the suspension contains a variety of additives including agents to inhibit foaming, flocculation and sedimentation, as well as flavouring compounds.

The barium sulphate particles

Particles of barium sulphate are produced either by precipitation or by crushing natural barium sulphate. The solid particles in barium sulphate suspensions have been examined by scanning electron microscopy (Russell & Worthington, unpublished). Commercial barium preparations are divided into two groups on the basis of the morphology of their constituent particles. Some preparations, for example Micropaque and Baritop 100, consist of smooth and nearly spherical particles, suggesting that they are produced by precipitation. The size of most of the particles is between 0.6 μm and 1.4 μm. A second group, which includes EZ-HD and X-Opaque is more likely to be produced by crushing larger crystals, and contains particles which are more irregular in size and shape. In addition to many small particles, a large part of these preparations is in the form of much larger crystals with a diameter of 20–40 μm and occasionally over 100 μm. (Figs. 5.1–5.4).

The nature of the constituent particles in a suspension affects the maximum density of the preparation and the degree of radiographic contrast. The proportion of the volume in a suspension which is occupied by crystals decreases as the crystals become more uniform in size and shape. This is because the number of points of contact between particles is reduced to a minimum while the volume of space between them tends to a maximum. This effect is accentuated with small particles because of the absorption of a layer of water onto the surface of the particles; the finer the particles, the greater is the surface area. When there is a mixture of particles of different sizes and shapes, the suspension is denser because the grains are more closely packed together. Also, increase in particle size results in a reduction of the total surface area and therefore less absorption of water. The result is a less

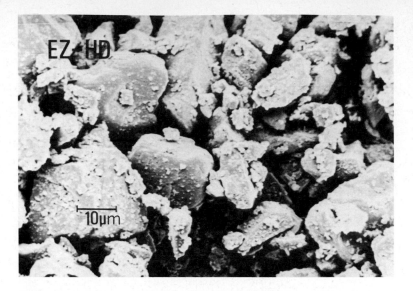

Fig. 5.1 Scanning electron micrograph of the barium preparation EZ-HD. Note the variation in the size and shape of the particles.

viscous and more fluid suspension. A high level of contrast is required to perceive fine radiographic detail, such as the areae gastricae in the stomach (Campbell & Matteil, 1974). Anderson *et al.* (1979) have shown that when a barium sulphate suspension is allowed to flow over and settle on the mucosa for a short period of time, a high proportion of the rapidly sedimenting large particles settle in the grooves, while the tufts are covered less densely with a fraction containing more of the smaller particles (Fig. 5.5). Depressions in the mucosa are therefore radiographically denser than raised areas. Heterogenicity of the barium sulphate particles therefore improves the demonstration of mucosal details in double contrast studies (Russell & Worthington, unpublished).

Water

The type of water added to barium sulphate affects the resultant suspension. Barium sulphate is supplied in two forms for clinical use:

(1) as a ready made up suspension which is used as supplied or watered down;
(2) as dry powder to which tap water is added to produce the suspension.

The degree of hardness of the water added has important effects on the electrochemical properties of the resultant suspension which are relevant to the behaviour of the particles and, therefore, of the suspension as a whole. Dissolved salts in the suspen-

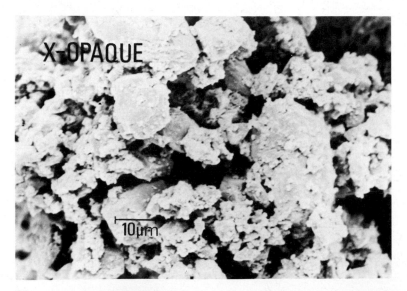

Fig. 5.2 Scanning electron micrograph of the barium preparation X-Opaque showing similar appearances.

Fig. 5.3 Scanning electron micrograph of the barium preparation Micropaque DC to the same scale. In this case the particles appear uniformly small.

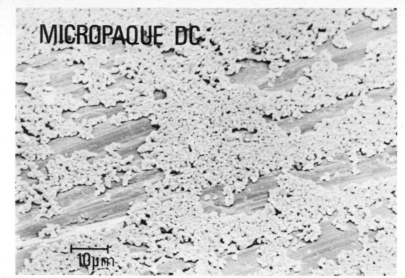

sion have an antifoaming effect. Electrolytes alter the charge on bubbles so that the gas has a positive charge and the liquid a negative charge, resulting in a collapse of bubbles. In a soft water area, where there may be a relatively low concentration of ions, foam formation may be troublesome. In hard water areas, the hot water may be softened and the cold water left untreated.

In addition to the water required to create a suspension, the preparation should contain sufficient water to allow miscibility with gastrointestinal secretions and the dissolving of any gas-producing agents.

Viscosity

The viscosity of a barium sulphate preparation is important, especially in double contrast studies. A low viscosity preparation mixes more easily with liquids already present in the gut lumen and are therefore more readily distributed. The suspension should flow easily over the mucosa as the patient is turned. A suspension which is thick and viscous will form a film which is deeper than the mucosal irregularities, minimizing the degree of radiographic contrast. (Fig. 5.6a). Conversely, a thinly coating suspension of low

Fig. 5.4 Scanning electron micrograph of the barium preparation Baritop 100 at a higher magnification. The particles appear smooth, round, and show little variation in size.

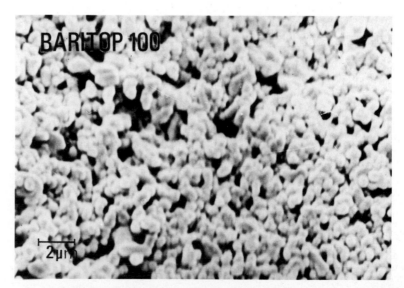

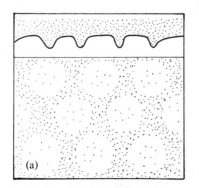

Fig. 5.5 Diagram to show distribution of barium sulphate particles over the mucosal surface.

viscosity is better able to delineate the surface features of the mucosa and particularly pathological irregularities (Gellfand, 1978). (Fig. 5.6b).

Barium preparations may be described as having 'high viscosity' or 'low viscosity', but a study of the rheological properties of different brands shows that a more precise determination of flow characteristics is possible and that the current preparations may be divided into two main groups. The viscosity of the fluid is the ratio of the applied stress to the shear (or the resistance to flow). Newtonian fluids are those that are permanently deformed to a degree directly proportional to the deforming force (Fig. 5.7). Barium sulphate suspensions exhibit non-Newtonian flow. Some preparations have plastic flow, meaning that a minimum shear stress must be applied before the suspension starts to flow. This is thought to be because the individual particles are in close contact, and that some of the interparticle bonds must be broken before the flow can start. X-Opaque and EZ-HD show plastic flow (Anderson *et al.*, 1980). Other preparations show an apparent decrease in viscosity at high shear rates and are described as having pseudoplastic flow. Their shear rate is a complex function and is intermediate between that of the Newtonian fluids and plastic fluids (Fig. 5.3). They appear to have relatively high viscosity at a low rate of shear, which is known as 'false body'. The rate of flow becomes accelerated as the stress is increased, perhaps due to the particles becoming more parallel in orientation with a con-

sequent release of interlocking fluid. Baritop 100 and Micropaque are preparations with pseudoplastic flow. Although X-Opaque, EX-HD, Barosperse and Micropaque all show relatively low viscosity, it is the preparations with plastic flow which produce the best clinical results in upper gastrointestinal contrast studies. This correlation may be related to the ease with which particles can settle out of the suspension.

No similar studies have been reported comparing preparations currently used for barium enema examinations, in relation to their clinical performance and flow properties. Miller & Skucas (1977) measured the density of a selection of barium enema preparations. The density of suspensions was varied by combining two different preparations and changing the barium sulphate:water ratio. Individual preparations which had densities between 6 and 8.5 produced the worst results in practice. The coating of the mucosa tended to be too thin and flocculation, bubbles and flaking of the barium film were problems. These preparations included Micropaque, X-Baryt, Barosperse and Unibaryt C. Intropaque (density 5.5) produced better results, but a mixture of Intropaque and Unibaryt C (with intermediate density) produced the best results with good coating even in patients whose colons contained residual mucus and faeces. It was concluded that variations in local conditions and the techniques of individual radiologists mean that no universally ideal barium sulphate can be made for enemas. Only by experimenting with various combinations of

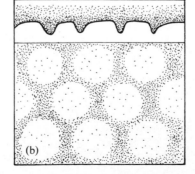

Fig. 5.6 (a) Low density, high viscosity barium; (b) High density, low viscosity barium.

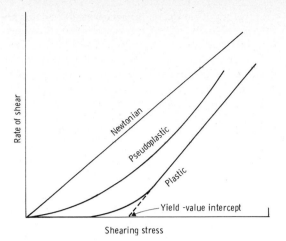

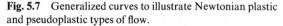

Fig. 5.7 Generalized curves to illustrate Newtonian plastic and pseudoplastic types of flow.

barium preparations and different amounts of water can the radiologist determine which suspension is best suited to use in a given location.

Foam

Foam occurs during a barium enema examination when air is insufflated, and during a barium meal because of the very rapid release of carbon dioxide from effervescent tablets or powders. Bubbles are undesirable as they produce artefacts and may obscure mucosal detail. Foaming is affected by the viscosity of the suspension at the surface and in the bulk of the liquid, and is a function of the interaction between the electrolytes, colloid additives and solid particles in the suspension (Miller & Skucas, 1977). The film forming the bubbles must be sufficiently viscous in itself or it must be stabilized for a persistent foam to form. Many hydrophilic colloids such as soap, proteins and glycoproteins (for example mucin) give quite stable foams with a high surface viscosity. The contents of gastric secretion may therefore affect the foaming of the suspension.

Commercial barium sulphate agents usually contain antifoaming agents, whose nature and efficacy depend on the other additives in the suspension and the nature of the foam-producing substance. Oily substances, such as silicone and oils in very low concentrations, are examples of antifoaming agents. As mentioned earlier, dissolved salts in the suspension also have an antifoaming effect. Bagnall *et al.* (1977) concluded that a dimethyl polysiloxane emulsion preparation is the most suitable for clinical use. Too much antifoam

agent, however, increases the amount of bubble formation and prevents proper wetting of the mucosa by the barium sulphate.

Flocculation

Another problem encountered with barium sulphate suspension is flocculation, the formation of particle aggregates producing a change in the effective particle size. Flocculation may lead to radiographic artefacts (Golden, 1959). The thixotropic behaviour of the suspension is increased by flocculation, which means that the shearing stress to produce a given rate of shear is less when the suspension is slowing down than when the speed is increasing. As there is a slight delay, the suspension does not form its original shape immediately after stirring. If the delay is short, thixotropic flow may approach plastic or pseudoplastic flow. A high level of thixotropic behaviour reduces the speed at which particles settle out of suspension and increases the yield point at which the suspension will flow.

Flocculation is promoted by gentle agitation, lack of a strong negative charge, and a nidus which acts as a nucleus for the formation of a floc. The pH of the conditions in which the barium sulphate is used affects the electrical charge on the surface of the particles. Particles without charge or with dissimilar charges are likely to combine, in certain circumstances, under the influence of attractive electrical forces and so form a floc. Particles bearing similar charges are mutually repulsive and, because the repulsive force usually exceeds the surface forces of attraction, the particles remain separate. Anderson *et al.* (1980) using electrophoretic mobility as an index, studied the effects of pH on the charge of barium sulphate particles. A decrease in pH from pH 7.0 increases the charge on the barium sulphate particles of some preparations (X-Opaque, EZ-HD, Barosperse), which are therefore more stable in an acid medium. Other preparations (Baritop G and Micropaque) show a decreased particle charge when placed in acid medium, and are therefore more prone to flocculation in acid.

The pH is affected by the ionic content of the water used to make up the suspension and by gastrointestinal secretions. The mucous content of secretions may also affect flocculation behaviour when large macromolecules, such as glycoproteins, may form bridges between particles or flocculated particles. Experiments by Roberts *et al.* (1977) have shown that the flocculation effect of mucoprotein may be decreased by increasing the amount of undiluted barium. The flocculating factor is absorbed by some of the barium suspensions so that the excess is unaffected. In follow-through examinations of the small bowel, the causes of flocculation are compounded when an acid suspension enters an alkaline medium containing a different type of mucin. From the studies of Anderson *et al.* (1980), only X-Opaque maintained a relatively high level of electrophoretic mobility at pH 8.0, indicating less likelihood of flocculation when compared to other preparations. Micropaque showed the lowest motility, and therefore charge, while other preparations were intermediate.

Suspension

The particles of barium sulphate eventually settle out when barium sulphate suspension is allowed to stand. The rate of settling of the particles is roughly in accordance with Stoke's Law, which defines the rate of fall of a small sphere in a viscous medium. In a suspension with a wide range of particle size, the largest particles settle out first. Settling out of the barium suspension has advantages and disadvantages. The settling out of the barium sulphate and formation of a cake of solid at the bottom of the container is a problem in preparations which are stored as suspensions. Suspending agents, such as sodium citrate, are therefore added to the suspension (Miller & Skucas, 1977). The effect of sodium citrate is accentuated by sorbitol, although unfortunately citrate ions also stabilize foam. One advantage of preparations which are supplied as powders, and are made up immediately before use, is that there is no necessity to maintain the particles in suspension. The larger particles therefore settle out more readily as the suspension is applied to the mucosa. This is an advantage in examinations of the gastric mucosa, while lower down the gastrointestinal tract suspending agents are useful in maintaining a uniform suspension for single contrast studies and in preventing flocculation.

SUMMARY

In double contrast upper gastrointestinal studies, good demonstration of the mucosal surface requires a radiographically dense medium containing a high concentration of barium sulphate suspension, with a low viscosity for it to flow easily. The suspension should be plastic in behaviour with a low yield point and should contain a proportion of large particles. As the suspension flows smoothly over the mucosa due to its low viscosity, the larger particles settle out of suspension into the grooves. Once settled in the grooves, the suspension is not easily displaced because

the yield point must first be overcome before it will flow. A relatively static film of suspension is therefore obtained which is denser in the grooves than over the areae gastricae, so that a maximum level of contrast is achieved to demonstrate the mucosal pattern. Suspensions composed of small round particles, medium-high density, and adequate suspending agents to prevent flocculation and maintain uniformity of the suspension, are of value in studies of the small bowel. These provide the degree of translucency necessary to examine overlapping loops of bowel and allow the contours of the lumen to be outlined. Preparations such as Baritop 100 or Micropaque are useful for such studies, and may be used as supplied or watered down. In large bowel studies, a medium high density preparation is again useful as it may be used for both single and double contrast studies. The barium sulphate used for double contrast studies must be able to form an even coating over the mucosa which does not crack, dribble, flocculate or foam. The ability of a suspension to resist such behaviour depends on its content, the way it is made up or altered before use, and local variations such as the hardness of the water and the technique of the radiologist. With experience, the radiologist can adapt these factors to suit local conditions. The final and most variable factor is the individual patient. The best suspensions are those which produce good clinical results in the majority of patients, despite the differences between them.

REFERENCES

Anderson W., Harthill J. E., James W. B. & Montgomery D. (1979) Function of size heterogenicity in barium sulphate used as a radiocontrast medium. *J. Pharm. Pharmacol.*, **3**, 54.

Anderson W., Harthill J. E., James W. B. & Montgomery D. (1980) Barium sulphate preparations for use in double contrast examination of the upper gastrointestinal tract. *Brit. J. Radiol.*, **53**, 1150–9.

Bagnall R. D., Galloway R. W. & Annis J. A. D. (1977) Double contrast preparations: an in vitro study of some anti-foaming agents. *Brit. J. Radiol.*, **50**, 546–50.

Campbell F. W. & Matteil L. (1974) Contrast and spatial frequency. *Sci. Amer.*, **231**, 106–14.

Gelfand D. W. (1978) High density, low viscosity barium for fine mucosal detail on double contrast upper gastrointestinal examinations. *Amer. J. Roentgenol.*, **130**, 831–3.

Golden R. (1969) Technical factors in roentgen examination of the small intestine. *Amer. J. Roentgenol.*, **82**, 965–72.

James W. B. (1978) The double contrast meal: new high density barium sulphate powders. *Brit. J. Radiol.*, **1**, 1020–2.

Miller R. E. & Skucas J. (1977) In *Radiographic Contrast Agents*. (Eds. Miller R. E. & Skucas J.) University Park Press, Baltimore.

Roberts G. M., Roberts E. E., Davis R. L. L. & Evans K. T. (1977) Observations on the behaviour of barium sulphate suspensions in gastric secretions. *Brit. J. Radiol.*, **50**, 468–72.

The Biliary Tract

J. P. OWEN

ORAL CHOLECYSTOGRAPHY

Introduction

Abel and Rowntree reported in 1910 that several phenolphthalein compounds were largely excreted by the liver and were found in the gall bladder some hours after ingestion. The work of Rowntree *et al.* (1913) established phenoltetrachlorphthalein as a test of liver function, while Rouse and McMaster (1921) showed that a normal gall bladder was able to concentrate bile. Based on these studies, the first successful cholecystogram was performed in 1923 by Graham and Cole on a fasting dog following the injection of tetrabromphenolphthalein (Graham & Cole, 1924; Graham *et al.*, 1924).

Indications

Oral cholecystography is indicated when the clinical history and examination suggest non-acute gall bladder disease.

In the presence of gall bladder disease, oral cholecystography probably has an accuracy of more than 90% (Wickbom & Rentzhog, 1955; Alderson, 1960; Baker & Hodgson, 1960). The overall accuracy of the examination in detecting gall bladder pathology has, however, never been determined since all patients having oral cholecystograms are not subjected to surgery. It has been shown that a normal cholecystogram does not always exclude gall stones or gall bladder pathology (Gough, 1977).

Contra-indications

Oral cholecystography is contra-indicated in: (1) pregnancy; (2) patients in combined hepatic and renal failure; (3) known hypersensitivity to iodine; (4) a period of less than 14 days after an intravenous cholangiogram; (5) acute cholecystitis.

Since the major pathways for elimination of the oral media are liver and kidney, then the simultaneous failure of both organs is a recipe for potential disaster.

The reasons for avoiding the 14 day period between an oral cholecystogram and an intravenous cholangio-gram will be covered in the section on intravenous cholangiography.

The mechanism of failure of gall bladder opacification in acute cholecystitis has been elegantly investigated by Lasser (1966), who showed that *E. Coli* can deconjugate the conjugated contrast medium in the gall bladder and that the unconjugated contrast medium is rapidly reabsorbed by the gall bladder because of its lipid solubility.

There is a decreased likelihood of the examination being successful when there is elevation of the serum bilirubin, or of the liver alkaline phosphatase even when there is a normal serum bilirubin level. The relationship between elevation of the serum bilirubin or alkaline phosphatase and sub-optimal gall bladder opacification is not surprising since these biochemical parameters may indicate hepatocyte dysfunction, the handling of the contrast medium by the liver depending on intact liver cells (Owen *et al.*, 1980).

The contrast media (Tables 6.1 and 6.2)

Modern oral cholecystographic media are totally unrelated to the iodophthaleins originally used by Graham and his colleagues. They are tri-iodinated benzoic acid derivatives with iodine atoms at positions 2, 4 and 6, and are incompletely substituted with a vacancy at position 5 on the nucleus (Fig. 6.1). In this respect they differ from the completely substituted water-soluble urographic agents (Fig. 6.1). The incomplete substitution with the vacant position causes the media to be bound to protein, which reduces their glomerular filtration and causes them to be preferentially excreted by the liver (Lasser *et al.*, 1962; Lang & Lasser, 1967).

Oral cholecystographic media are absorbed via the small intestinal mucosa but have a variable rate of absorption. In the case of iopanoic acid, which has high lipid solubility but low aqueous solubility, absorption is probably by non-ionic diffusion. Experimental work has shown that the aqueous solubility and hence absorption of iopanoic acid is increased by lowering the hydrogen ion concentration, which increases the degree of ionization (Taketa *et al.*, 1972), and by increasing the bile salt flow (Goldberger *et al.*, 1974), in particular the taurocholate excretion (Berk

Table 6.1 The metabolic pathway of oral cholecystographic media

Site	Activity	Solubility
1. The basic contrast medium		Iopanoic acid—predominantly lipid soluble with weak aqueous solubility The other oral agents are also lipid soluble but have greater aqueous solubility than iopanoic acid
2. Duodenum	To portal vein by non-ionic diffusion Absorption influenced by: a Physical state of the contrast b pH of bowel lumen c Presence of bile salts. (Affects iopanoic acid absorption only)	
3. Portal vein	Binding to serum albumen	No information available about bound moiety
4. Hepatocytes	a Albumen bond broken b Contrast enters hepatocytes—by a rate limiting active transport mechanism c Conjugation with glucuronic acid d To bile via an active transport mechanism	Glucuronide conjugate is water soluble
5. Bile ducts	Transport to gall bladder	Water soluble
6. Gall bladder	Reabsorption of water hence concentration of contrast in bile	Water soluble
7. Fate of contrast medium	a Excretion of unabsorbed contrast in faeces b Deconjugation and entero-hepatic circulation c Excretion of conjugate in faeces d Excretion of conjugate in urine	Lipid soluble Lipid soluble Water soluble Water soluble

Table 6.2 Oral cholecystographic contrast media

Generic name	UK trade name	Molecular weight of salt	Iodine content of salt %	Preparation	Iodine content of preparation
Iopanoic acid	Telepaque (Winthrop laboratories)	571	66.7	Tablets containing 500 mgm Iopanoic acid	2.0 g from 6 tablets
	Cistobil (BDH Pharmaceuticals)	571	66.7	Tablets containing 500 mgm Iopanoic acid	2.0 g from 6 tablets
Sodium Ipodate	Biloptin (Schering)	620	61.4	Capsules containing 500 mgm Sodium ipodate	1.84 g from 6 capsules
Calcium Ipodate	Solubiloptin (Schering)	1234	61.7	Sachet containing 3 g of Calcium ipodate	1.85 g from 1 satchet
Iocetamic acid	Cholebrin (Napp Laboratories)	614	62.0	Tablets containing 500 mgm of Iocetamic acid	1.86 g from 6 tablets
Iopronic acid	Bilimiro (BDH Pharmaceuticals)	673	56.6	Tablets containing 750 mgm of Iopronic acid	2.5 g from 6 tablets

et al., 1980). On the other hand, in the case of the more water-soluble oral media such as sodium tyropanoate and sodium ipodate, there is no such dependence on bile salts (Berk *et al.*, 1977).

The physical state of the oral media in the bowel is also important in determining the rate of absorption.

Goldberger *et al.* (1974) showed that the acid precipitated sodium salt of iopanoic acid, which has small crystals, was more soluble and more readily absorbed than commercially available iopanoic acid which has larger crystals and a smaller surface to weight ratio.

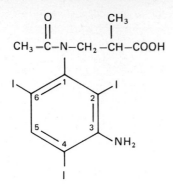

Fig. 6.1 (a) Iocetamic acid (Cholebrin)—a typical oral cholecystographic agent. Note the incomplete substitution at position 5 on the nucleus.

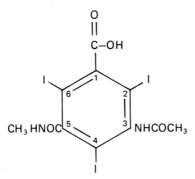

Fig. 6.1 (b) Iothalamic acid (Conray)—a typical urographic agent. Note the complete substitution.

The molecules of contrast media are bound in the portal blood to plasma albumen (Lasser, 1966; Lang & Lasser, 1967), although some unbound contrast medium may be temporarily stored in fat, blood, muscle and other organs including the liver (Dunn & Berk, 1972). Cholecystographic media are removed from the blood by the liver via a rate-limiting active transport process and undergo conjugation with glucuronic acid in the hepatocytes (McChesney & Hoppe, 1954; McChesney, 1964; Lasser, 1966; Naleman, 1967), from where they are actively transported into the bile. The active transport mechanism is overloaded by excessive contrast medium. Above a threshold value, merely increasing the rate of administration of the contrast media to the patient produces no significant change in its biliary excretion rate. Recent studies (Amberg et al., 1980); however, have shown that increasing the total dosage of the contrast media does increase the biliary iodine concentrations of some media, namely iopanoic acid, sodium tyropanoate and sodium ipodate, but not iopronic acid. Amberg et al. (1980) also showed that increased doses

of iopronic acid and sodium ipodate were usually associated with increased biliary excretion rates, the effect being less marked with iopanoic acid and sodium tyropanoate. The glucuronide conjugates are less lipid-soluble than the free acid, which prevents them from being reabsorbed via the bile ducts and gall bladder.

Sperber and Sperber (1971) found the time from oral administration of iopdate to peak concentration in the bile ducts in man to be about 3 hours, within a range of 1–5 hours. In the non-inflamed gall bladder, the glucuronide conjugate is concentrated by reabsorption of water from the bile. The time scale in adults from duodenal absorption to maximum concentration of the conjugate in the gall bladder is 14–19 hours, depending on the particular contrast medium. The optimal time to radiograph patients following oral administration of the contrast media is, therefore, at 3 hours for the bile ducts and 14–19 hours for the gall bladder. In practice, this is usually achieved by giving a divided dose of the contrast medium at 3 and 14 hours before the radiographic examination.

Values for the percentage urinary excretion of a standard dose of the oral contrast media in man show an enormous range of variability; 10–45% for iopanoate and 21–57% for ipodate (McChesney, 1971). False urinary tests for albumen have been recorded after the administration of a number of oral cholecystographic agents (Sanen, 1962).

The non-absorbed contrast medium and the excreted conjugates are both excreted in faeces. Some of the conjugate may be deconjugated by intestinal organisms, being reconverted into the lipid-soluble free contrast medium with some entero-hepatic recirculation.

Patient preparation

There is some controversy regarding dietary preparations for oral cholecystography. Studies have suggested that bile salts are important in promoting the intestinal absorption of iopanoic acid by a postulated allosteric interaction between the bile salts and the carrier for iopanoic acid (Goldberger et al., 1974; Berk et al., 1974). They concluded that stimulating gall bladder emptying by the ingestion of a meal rich in fat, before the iopanoic acid was taken, would increase the amount of bile salt in the intestinal lumen and thus enhance absorption of the contrast medium. No such dependence on bile salts was found with the more water-soluble agents sodium tyropanoate and sodium ipodate (Berk et al., 1977). On this evidence, it would appear that a high fat diet prior to the examination should improve gall bladder visualization with iopanoic acid but not with other, more water-soluble, agents. Clinical studies investigating these claims have, however, given contradictory findings (Mauthe, 1974; Stanley *et al.*, 1974). Most manufacturers recommend a restricted fat intake on the evening before the oral examination, in line with an early clinical study (Whitehouse, 1956), but subsequent series have failed to show any benefits for dietary restriction of fat (Parkin, 1973; Mauthe, 1974).

Patients are often instructed to drink at least 1–2 pints of water after ingestion of the contrast medium, the rationale being to prevent nephrotoxicity from the uricosuric action of the oral cholecystographic agents (Mudge, 1971). Adequate hydration by this means has no deleterious effects on the diagnostic quality of the examination (Bainton *et al.*, 1973).

An instruction to avoid smoking is commonly given to patients before a cholecystogram. The question arises as to whether or not smoking produces any significant effects on the gall bladder which interfere with radiological investigations of the biliary tract. Nicotine could be expected to produce effects on the smooth muscle of the gall bladder and the sphincter of Oddi as well as the secretion of bile (Thompson, J. W., personal communication). Only a limited number of studies have been carried out on the pharmacology of nicotine in relation to the gall bladder.

Since nicotine is capable of activating both the parasympathetic and sympathetic parts of the autonomic nervous system, it is likely that the effects of nicotine on the tone and motility of the gall bladder and sphincteric contraction will be variable and will depend upon the relative contributions of these two opposing systems.

There is convincing evidence that nicotine alters biliary secretion in man. Cigarette smoking has been shown to reduce biliary secretion (Koehler *et al.*, 1947), but to increase biliary flow into the duodenum (Liscia, 1954). It is therefore strongly advisable to stop smoking before radiological investigations of the biliary tract, in order that the responses of the biliary tract to nicotine cannot interfere with contrast opacification.

Normal radiographic technique

There should be a radiographic table with an overcouch tube, undercouch and vertical bucky, and a facility for tomography.

The control film (Fig. 6.2)

An oblique position projects the gall bladder clear of the spine. There are two methods:

1. Left anterior oblique, with the patient prone and the right side raised off the table with 20° of obliquity. The centring point is 7.5 cm to the right of the L3 spinous process and 2.5 cm cephalad to the level of the lower costal margin;
2. Right posterior oblique, with the patients supine and left side raised off the table with 10° of obliquity. Occasionally greater obliquity is required in order to project the bile ducts clear of the spine. The centring point is 7.5 cm to the right of L3 and 4.5 cm cephalad.

A low kilovoltage is preferred for maximum soft tissue differentiation. For a person of average build, using a fast film/screen combination, typical factors are 65–75 kV, 100 mA and 0.2 s.

A short exposure time and the use of compression bands give a sharp radiographic image. The radiographs should include an area bounded laterally by the tissues of the flank, medially by the lumbar spine, superiorly by the dome of the diaphragm, and inferiorly by the right iliac crest.

Giving the contrast medium

The contrast medium is given orally in two divided doses of 3 g each. The first dose is taken about 14 hours before the radiographic examination and should be in a concentrated glucuronated form in the gall bladder at the time of the radiographic study. The second dose is taken 3–4 hours before the examination and this contrast medium should be in a non-concentrated form in the bile ducts at the time of the examination.

The radiographic examination after contrast medium

(1) Prone oblique view as for the preliminary film (Fig. 6.2b). (2) An erect film (Fig. 6.2c) either (a) in the left anterior oblique position with the abdomen towards the cassette and the right side raised away from the cassette, centring to the right of the spine about 5 cm below the centring point for the prone oblique projection, (b) the erect right posterior oblique with the patient's back towards the cassette and the left side raised from the cassette, centring to the left of the spine about 5 cm below the centring point for the prone oblique projection.

The right lateral decubitus view is not a routine part of the examination but is useful if the gall bladder is obscured by bowel gas on the prone or erect radiographs. The patient lies on the right side facing a vertical film, with centring as for the P–A projection to the right of L2 or L3 vertebrae.

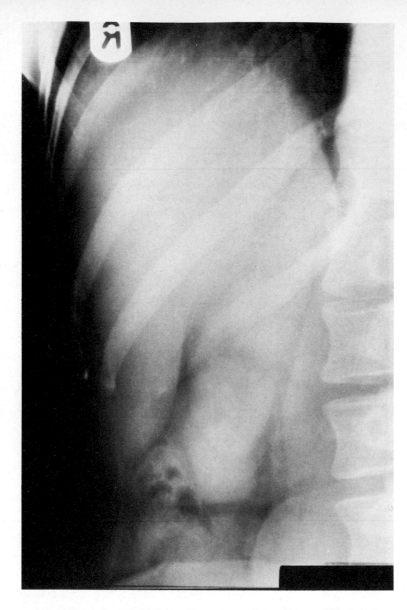

An additional method is to fluoroscope the gall bladder in the erect position and take spot radiographs. In some centres, this is the preferred technique.

The fatty meal or cholecystokinin stimulation

A further, coned, supine oblique radiograph of the gall bladder area is taken 30–60 min after the oral ingestion of a proprietary fatty emulsion such as Prosparol (Fig. 6.2d). The fatty meal invokes the action of endogenous cholecystokinin liberated from the duodenal mucosa. Its main values are: (1) to evaluate gall bladder contractility, (2) to detect small filling defects such as stones or polyps, and (3) to visualize the cystic and common ducts in greater detail.

Cholecystokinin given by the intravenous route has been used to investigate the ill-defined functional disorder referred to as 'biliary dyskinesia', in which it is often claimed that motor dysfunction of the extrahepatic biliary tract produces clinical symptoms such as pain (Ivy, 1947). The theory is that following a slow intravenous injection of cholecystokinin the patient's clinical symptoms are reproduced and the gall bladder contraction must be less than 20–40% of its pre-contracted volume (Goldberg, 1976). The precise values of this technique are currently a matter

re. if poor

Fig. 6.2 (b) Prone oblique radiograph
following contrast medium.

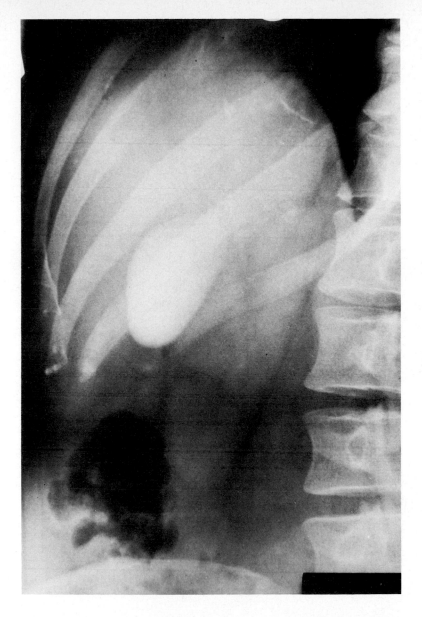

for debate and further investigation, but it does have
some enthusiastic supporters.

The non-opacifying gall bladder

The causes of failure to opacify the gall bladder
include:

1. Failure of the patient to take the contrast medium.
2. Failure to absorb the contrast medium in the
   presence of upper alimentary tract obstruction,
   such as oesophageal stricture and pyloric stenosis;
   in duodenal disease, for instance Crohn's disease
   and lymphoma; post surgery, for example after
   ileal resection; and with acute diarrhoea.
3. Failure to transport the contrast medium. A low
   serum albumin would be a theoretical possibility;
4. Failure to conjugate the contrast medium, for
   example when there is hepatocyte dysfunction.
5. Failure to excrete the contrast medium into the
   bile, namely a failure of active transport.
6. Failure of the contrast medium to reach the gall
   bladder in cases of cystic or hepatic duct obstruction.
7. Failure of the gall bladder to function, as in severe
   chronic cholecystitis.

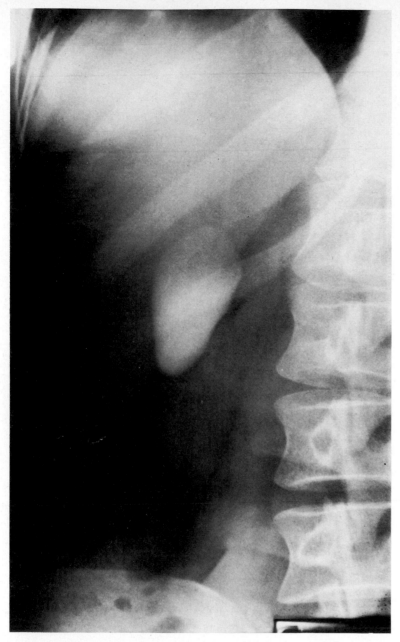

Fig. 6.2 (c) Erect radiograph following contrast medium.

The radiologist should be in possession of adequate clinical details, including operation records, before embarking on the procedure. Ideally, liver function tests and serum albumin levels should be available on all patients, although this is often not feasible. The influence of chronic cholecystitis on absent and suboptimal gall bladder opacification has initiated much interest and research and there is evidence to show that, if liver function is normal, the degree of gall bladder opacification is inversely related to the severity of the chronic cholecystitis (Owen *et al.*,

1980b). The level of serum bilirubin above which the examination is unlikely to succeed is frequently given as 2 mgm% (34 μmol/l). While the evidence for this is anecdotal rather than factual, this level seems to be a reliable guide in practice.

Variation of technique for failure to opacify the gall bladder

A frequent problem of management arises when the gall bladder is not visible after a conventional 6 g dose

Fig. 6.2 (d) Responses of gall bladder
to oral fat.

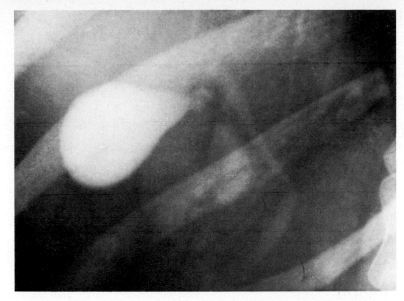

of oral contrast medium. Most centres give a further
6 g of contrast medium in two 3 g doses and ask the
patient to return for further radiographs the next day.
The object is to almost saturate the active transport
mechanism in the hepatocytes without exceeding the
threshold level. Further doses of the contrast medium
would then be merely excreted by the kidneys, which
could prove fatal in patients with a low creatinine
clearance.

If the conventional radiographs still fail to demonstrate the gall bladder, two further procedures may
help:

1. A full size abdominal radiograph in case the gall
   bladder has an ectopic situation.
2. Tomography. A vogue for using multi-section
   cassettes has fallen out of fashion and most centres
   now perform multiple single section cuts. Tomography is performed in the prone oblique position.
   Linear or, where available, circular tomography
   are the movements of choice. Cuts should be taken
   at 0.5 or 1 cm intervals from 7–8 cm, and may
   occasionally have to be as low as 4 cm in the obese.
   The potentials of the technique have been ex-
   hausted if there is failure of all these manoeuvres.
3. Ultrasonography. See 'Investigation of suspected
   Gall Bladder Disease' p. 84.

Complications

Ansell (1978) has recorded the following complications:

1. Minor side effects occur in 50% of cases, and
   include nausea, vomiting, diarrhoea, headaches,
   abdominal pain, dysuria, dizziness and urticaria.
2. Hypotension and collapse has occurred in a few
   cases.
3. Myocardial infarction or cardiac arrest is a very
   rare complication.
4. A minor elevation of serum creatinine is a common
   occurrence.
5. The protein bound iodine is elevated for up to three
   months. A few cases of thyrotoxicosis have been
   attributed to the procedure.

In data collected by the American Medical Association
between 1963 and 1967 (de Nosaquo, 1968), 22
patients developed acute renal failure following the
administration of sodium bunamiodyl (Orabilex) with
death in 9 cases. Orabilex was subsequently withdrawn
from the market. The uricosuric action of the contrast
media may have played a part in inducing the renal
failure (Mudge, 1971).

REFERENCES

Abel J. J. & Rowntree L. G. (1910) On the pharmacological
action of some phthaleins and their derivatives with
especial reference to their behaviour as purgatives. *J.
Pharmacol. exp. Ther.*, **1**, 231–64.
Alderson D. A. (1960) The reliability of Telepaque cholecys-
tography. *Brit. J. Surg.*, **47**, 206, 655–8.
Amberg J. R., Thompson W. M., Goldberger L., Williamson
S., Alexander R. & Bates M. (1980) Factors in the
intestinal absorption of oral cholecystopaques. *Invest.
Radiol.*, **15** (Suppl) S136–S141.

Ansell G. (1978) Complications of X-ray investigations. Adverse Drug Reaction Bulletin No. 71. (Ed. Davies D. M.) Adverse Drug Reaction Research Unit, Shotley Bridge General Hospital.

Baert A. L., Usewils R., Marchal G., Wilms G. & Ponette E. (1981) Contrast enhancement of the liver. In *Contrast Media in Computed Tomography*. (Ed. Felix R., Kazner E. & Wegener O. H.) pp. 259–61. Excerpta Medica, Amsterdam.

Bainton D., Davies G. I., Evans K. T., Gravell I. H. & Abernethy M. (1973) A comparison of two preparation regimens for oral cholecystography. *Clin. Radiol.*, **24**, 381–4.

Baker J. L. & Hodgson J. R. (1960) Further studies on the accuracy of oral cholecystography. *Radiology*, **74**, 239–45.

Berk R. N., Goldberger L. E. & Loeb P. M. (1974) The role of bile salts in the hepatic excretion of iopanoic acid. *Invest. Radiol.*, **9**, 7–15.

Berk R. N., Loeb P. M., Cobo-Frankel A. & Banhart J. L. (1977) The biliary and urinary excretion of sodium tyropanoate and sodium ipodate in dogs: pharmacokinetics, influence of bile salts and choleretic effects with comparison to iopanoic acid. *Invest. Radiol.*, **12**, 85.

Berk R. N., Barnhart J. L. & Goldberger L. E. (1980) The enhancement of iopanoate excretion by taurocholate. *Invest. Radiol.*, **15** (Suppl) S116–S121.

Bryan G. J. (1979) *Diagnostic Radiography*, 3e, pp. 276–8. Churchill Livingstone, Edinburgh.

Cole W. H. (1960) The story of cholecystography. *Amer. J. Surg.*, **99**, 206–22.

Dunn C. R. & Berk R. N. (1972) The pharmaco-kinetics of Telepaque metabolism: the relation of blood concentration and bile flow to the rate of hepatic excretion. *Amer. J. Roentgenol.*, **114**, 758–66.

Goldberg H. I. (1976) Cholecystokinin cholecystography. *Seminars in Roentgenology*, **11**, 175–8.

Goldberger L. E., Berk R. N., Lang J. H. & Loeb P. M. (1974) Biopharmaceutical factors influencing intestinal absorption of iopanoic acid. *Invest. Radiol.*, **9**, 16–23.

Gough M. H. (1977) The cholecystogram is normal—but . . . *Brit. med. J.*, **i**, 960–2.

Graham E. & Cole W. (1924) Roentgenologic examination of the gall bladder. *J. Amer. med. Ass.*, **82**, 613–14.

Graham E. A., Cole W. K. & Copher G. H. (1924) Visualization of gall bladders by the sodium salt tetrabromphenolphthalein. *J. Amer. med. Ass.*, **82**, 1777–8.

Hodgson J. R. (1970) The technical aspects of cholecystography. *Radiol. Clin. N. Amer.*, **8**, 1 pp. 85–97.

Hübener K. N. & Treegut H. (1981) Administration of biliary contrast media in computed tomography. In: *Contrast Media in Computed Tomography*. (Ed. Felix R., Kazner E. & Wegener O. H.) pp. 46–51. A Excerpta Medica, Amsterdam.

Ivy A. C. (1947) Motor dysfunction of the biliary tract. *Amer. J. Roentgenol.*, **57**, 1–11.

Koehler A. E., Hill E. & Marsh N. (1947) The effect of cigarette smoking on malnutrition and digestion. *Gastroenterol.*, **8**, 208, 212.

Lang J. H. & Lasser E. D. (1967) Binding of roentgenographic contrast media to serum albumin. *Invest. Radiol.*, **2**, 396–400.

Lasser E. C., Farr R. S., Fujimagari T. & Tripp W. N. (1962) The significance of protein binding of contrast media in roentgen diagnosis. *Amer. J. Roentgenol.*, **87**, 338–60.

Lasser E. C. (1966) Pharmacodynamics of biliary contrast media. *Radiol. Clin. N. Amer.*, **4**, 511–19.

Liscia G. (1954) Influence de tabac sur les voies biliaires. *Maroc Medical*, **33**, 780.

Loeb P. M. & Berk R. N. (1977) Biliary contrast materials. In *Radiology of the Gall Bladder and Bile Ducts*. (Eds. Berk & Clemett.) pp. 71–100. W. B. Saunders & Co, Philadelphia.

Mauthe H. (1974) The low fat meal in gall bladder examinations. *Radiology*, **112**, 5–7.

McChesney E. W. & Hoppe J. O. (1954) Observations on the metabolism of iodopanoic acid. *Arch. int. Pharmacodyn.*, **99**, 127–40.

McChesney E. W. (1964) On glucuronide formation in the cat. *Biochem. Pharmacol.*, **13**, 1366–8.

McChesney E. W. (1971) Routes and rates of excretion of radio-contrast agents in *International Encyclopedia of Pharmacology and Therapeutics*. (Ed. Knoefel P. K.) Section 76, Vol. I. pp. 335–44. Pergamon Press, Oxford.

Mudge G. H. (1971) Uricosuric action of cholecystographic agents. *New Engl. J. Med.*, **284**, 929–33.

Naleman W. E. P. (1967) Onderzoek Betreffende het Metabolism van Jocetaminazeur in Menselijke Gal en Urine. *Pharmaceutish Weekblad*, **102**, 1039–48.

de Nosaquo N. (1968) Reactions to contrast media. *Radiology*, **91**, 92–5.

Owen J. P., Keir M. J., Lavelle M. I. & Smith P. A. (1980a) Alkaline phosphatase and the oral cholecystogram. *Brit. J. Radiol.*, **53**, 605–6.

Owen J. P., McCarthy J., Makepeace D., Lavelle M. I. & Keir M. J. (1980b) Chronic cholecystitis and the oral cholecystogram. *Clin. Radiol.*, **31**, 671–4.

Parkin G. J. S. (1973) Dietary preparation for oral cholecystography—a critical reappraisal. *Brit. J. Radiol.*, **47**, 452–3.

Rowntree L. G., Hurwitz S. H. & Bloomfield A. L. (1913) Experimental and clinical study of the value of phenoltetrachlorphthalein as a test for hepatic function. *Bull. Johns Hopk. Hosp.*, **24**, 327–42.

Sanen F. J. (1962) Considerations of cholecystographic contrast media. *Amer. J. Roentgenol.*, **88**, 797–802.

Sokoloff J., Berk R. N., Lang J. H. & Lasser E. C. (1973) The role of Y and Z hepatic proteins in the excretion of radiographic contrast materials. *Radiology*, **106**, 519–23.

Sperber I. & Sperber G. (1971) Hepatic excretion of radiocontrast agents. *International Encyclopedia of Pharmacology and Therapeutics* (Ed. Knoefel P. K.)

Section 76, Vol. 1, pp. 165–235. Pergamon Press, Oxford.

Stanley R. J., Melson G. L., Cubillo E. & Hesker A. E. (1974) A comparison of three cholecystographic agents. *Radiology*, **112**, 513–17.

Taketa R. M., Berk R. N., Lang J. H., Lasser E. C. & Dunn C. R. (1972) The effect of pH on the intestinal absorption of Telepaque. *Amer. J. Roentgenol.*, **114**, 767–72.

Whitehouse W. M. (1956) Re-evaluation of the fat free preparatory meal in Telepaque cholecystography. *Amer. J. Roentgenol.*, **76**, 21–3.

Wickbom I. G. & Rentzhog U. (1955) The reliability of cholecystography. *Acta Radiol.*, **44**, 185–200.

INTRAVENOUS CHOLANGIOGRAPHY

Indications

With the advent of safer non-invasive imaging techniques such as ultrasonography, and also the more widespread use of transhepatic cholangiography with the Chiba needle, the traditional indications for intravenous cholangiography will continue to decline. At the present time, the indications are: simultaneous failure of both oral cholecystography and real-time ultrasonography, suspected common bile duct disease in non-icteric patients, and post-cholecystectomy biliary symptoms.

Contra-indications

Absolute contra-indications are pregnancy, known iodine sensitivity, and combined hepatic and renal failure.

In addition, intravenous cholangiography should not be performed within 14 days of an oral cholecystogram. Finby and Blasberg (1964) showed that the administration of the intravenous cholangiographic agent meglumine iodipamide 24 hours after an oral cholecystographic agent dramatically increased the incidence of adverse side effects, with 14% having severe reactions which included severe hypotension. Furthermore, there was a sharp reduction in the number of diagnostic cholangiograms by the competition in the liver for the active transport mechanism, with consequent retention of the intravenous medium in the vascular compartment (Moss et al., 1973).

The contrast media (Tables 6.3 and 6.4)

Intravenous cholangiographic agents are 'coupled compounds' consisting of two substituted benzoic acids linked by a difunctional radical (Fig. 6.3). Each molecule contains six iodine atoms and two available vacant binding sites. They are highly ionized in solution and have a low lipid solubility with a high aqueous solubility which renders them suitable for intravenous injection but not for oral administration (Table 6.3). The two vacant binding sites also cause cholangiographic media to be protein bound and this is a source of their known toxicity (Lasser et al., 1962). Like the oral cholecystographic media, they become bound to serum albumen, with a resultant reduction in glomerular clearance and hence limited renal excretion (Lang & Lasser, 1967). There is, however, evidence that plasma albumen binding itself decreases

Table 6.3 The metabolic pathway of the intravenous cholangiographic media

Pathway	Activity	Solubility
1. The basic contrast media		Predominantly water soluble and highly ionised (Weak lipid solubility)
2. Intravenous administration	Strong binding to serum albumen	No information available about bound moiety
3. Hepatocytes	a Albumen bond broken	
	b Contrast enters hepatocytes	Water soluble
	c To bile in an *unchanged* form by an active-carrier-mediated transport system against a large concentration gradient and limited by a transport maximum	Water soluble
4. Bile ducts	Transport to gall bladder	Water soluble
5. Gall bladder	Reabsorption of water and hence concentration of contrast in bile	Water soluble
6. Fate of contrast medium	a Excretion of the bile transported contrast in faeces	Water soluble
	b Excretion of contrast in urine	Water soluble

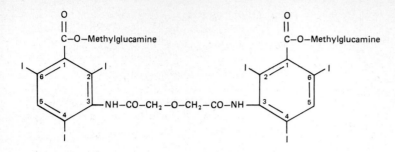

Fig. 6.3 Ioglycamide (Biligram)—a typical i.v. cholangiographic agent. Note the two vacant binding sites at positions 5 on the nuclei.

the hepatic uptake of intravenous cholangiographic agents so that selective liver uptake is a complex process. Some experimental work suggests that the mechanism of liver uptake may be due to binding to hepatic cytoplasmic proteins, but the evidence is not yet conclusive (Sokoloff *et al.*, 1973).

Intravenous cholangiographic agents do not undergo any complex changes, such as glucuronization on passage through the hepatocytes, but their excretion into bile is by an active transport mechanism similar to that of oral cholecystographic agents. The intravenous cholangiographic agents are also choleretic and stimulate water flow across the bile canaliculus without increasing bile salt excretion. The formation of bile occurs in two phases:

1. Canalicular bile flow, in which are excreted most of the water and organic materials;
2. Ductular bile flow which adds water and inorganic ions.

Recent studies (Barnhart, 1980) with the intravenous cholangiographic medium iodoxamate indicate that its choleretic effect is predominantly canalicular in origin and is accompanied by the stimulation of bicarbonate secretion. The active transport mechanism and choleresis impose limits on the degree of

Table 6.4 Intravenous cholangiographic media

Name		Molecular weight	Iodine content of salt (%)	Preparations	Iodine content		Viscosity (cp)		Osmolality at 37°C (osm/kg water)
Generic	Trade				mg/ml	Per ampoule or bottle	20°C	37°C	
Meglumine Iodipamide	Biligrafin* (Schering)	1530	49.8	30% soln. in 20 ml amps.	150	3.0 g	2.7–2.86	1.71–1.81	0.36
	Biligrafin* forte (Schering)			50% soln. in 20 ml amps.	250	5.0 g	8.58–9.12	4.59–4.87	0.58
Meglumine Ioglycamate	Biligram (Schering)	1518.1	50.2	35% soln. in 30 ml amps.	176	5.3 g	2.36	1.86	0.45
	Biligram infusion Schering)			15% soln. in 100 ml vials	85	9.5 g	1.57	1.05	0.25
Meglumine Iotroxinate	Biliscopin (Schering)	1606	47.4	38% soln. in 30 ml amps.	180	5.4 g	3.5	2.1	0.46
	Biliscopin infusion (Schering)			10.5% soln. in 100 ml vials	50	5.0 g	1.3	0.9	0.28
Meglumine Iodoxamate	Endobil infusion (BDH pharmaceuticals)	1678	45	9.91% soln. in 100 ml bottle	45	4.5 g	1.3	0.9	0.148

* No longer available in UK.

opacification of the duct system which is obtained by increasing the administered dose of contrast medium. A list of available media is given in Table 6.4.

Infusion or bolus injection?—the choice

There are two main methods of intravenous cholangiography: bolus injection over about 5–10 min and slow intravenous infusion for 30–60 min. The choice between bolus injection and intravenous infusion has been extensively investigated, often with contradictory results. Earlier studies show a lack of awareness in the fundamental principles which underlie the excretion of cholangiographic media by the liver. These are:

1. that the excretion of the contrast medium by the liver is an active carrier-mediated transport process proceeding against a large concentration gradient;
2. this excretion is limited by a transport maximum;
3. the concentration of the contrast medium in bile depends on the rate of excretion, the choleresis which is stimulated and the basal bile flow.

Loeb (1975) and his colleagues showed in dogs that iodipamide given in bolus injection produced higher plasma concentrations, greater renal excretion but less total biliary excretion than an equal amount infused over a longer period of time. In basic terms, in the case of bolus intravenous injection, if too much contrast medium is injected too quickly into the system, then the liver is overwhelmed and the contrast medium is excreted by the kidneys. However, increasing the dose of contrast medium by intravenous infusion improves the quality of the resulting image but only up to a maximum; the limit being the liver's transport maximum for the contrast medium, after which no further improvement is possible.

Despite some contrary views (Scholz et al., 1975), the available evidence indicates that an infusion technique is preferable to bolus injection. Adequate information regarding the optimal rate of infusion is only available for ioglycamide. The studies of Fuchs and Preisig (1975) and Bell et al. (1978a) indicate a transport maximum for ioglycamide of about 30 mgm/min (range 19.8–40.4 mgm/min). Bell et al. (1978b) suggest that optimal concentrations of iodine in the bile duct are obtainable during intravenous cholangiography if ioglycamide is infused for one hour at a rate of about 4 mgm kg^{-1} min^{-1}. There seems to be universal agreement that there are significantly fewer side effects induced by the infusion technique as compared with bolus injection.

The influence of liver function

Because cholangiographic contrast agents and bilirubin are excreted by the same transport mechanism, elevation of serum bilirubin is associated with a diminution in the biliary concentration of contrast media. It is impossible to give a definite level of serum bilirubin above which the examination will not work, but an indication of the percentage success rate for the examination at varying levels of serum bilirubin has been given by Wise (1962) (Table 6.5).

Table 6.5

Serum bilirubin		% Visualization
mg/100 ml	μmol/l	
1	17.5	92.0
2	34.0	72.0
3	52.0	49.0
4	69.0	28.0
5	85.5	7.0

Table modified from *Intravenous Cholangiography* by Robert E. Wise (1962), Charles C. Thomas.

The use of glucagon in intravenous cholangiography

The smooth muscle relaxant effect of intravenous glucagon has been used to improve the visualization of the ampullary region of the common bile duct during 'T' tube cholangiography. Dyck and Janowitz (1971) reported that intravenous glucagon increased the rate of bile flow in man without a significant change in the electrolyte composition of the bile. It would, therefore, be expected that glucagon, given during intravenous cholangiography, would lead to an increased volume of bile with dilution of the contrast medium. Initial studies by Evans and Whitehouse (1979) showed that, contrary to expectation, i.v. glucagon actually improved the visualization of the biliary tract by ioglycamide. Jarrett and Bell (1980), using the newer contrast agent Iotroxamide (meglumine iotroxinate), showed a temporary increase in the transport maximum for Iotroxamide following i.v. glucagon, although a double blind study failed to show any advantage in clinical practice (Jarrett et al., 1982). Biliary iodine levels following 1 mgm glucagon were only increased for about 5 min while bile flow was increased for about 20 min, so that radiographs taken at 3 min after i.v. glucagon should show enhanced bile duct opacification while radiographs taken 30–60 min post glucagon should show improved gall bladder opacification. Evans and Whitehouse (1980) later

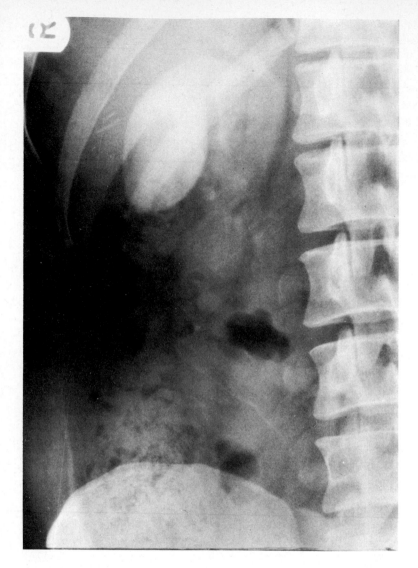

found that a dose of 1 mgm of glucagon was equally effective as 2 mgm in improving visualization of the biliary tree. At present, the exact mechanism of the increased excretion of contrast medium and its efficacy in clinical practice is a controversial issue.

Normal radiographic technique

Patients should be in a fasting state, but well hydrated to reduce the nephrotoxicity of the contrast media. The colon should be cleansed by a suitable aperient to reduce obscuration of the opacified ducts by faeces and colonic gas.

The radiographic technique is essentially the same whichever injection method is employed, differing only in the timing of the individual radiographs. An initial prone oblique (LAO) control radiograph of the gall bladder area using a low kV (50–60 kV) is taken before the administration of contrast medium. If the LAO projection is not possible, an alternative is the supine oblique projection (RPO). The centring point is 7.5 cm to the right of the spinous processes and 2.5 to 3.0 cm cephalad to the level of the lower costal margin (Bryan, 1979).

A further prone oblique radiograph of the gall bladder area is taken 30 min after injection or at the end of infusion (Fig. 6.4a). Linear tomography is performed if the duct system is not clearly shown on the first radiograph. The technique is identical to that outlined in the section on Oral Cholecystography, with the exception that the cuts are usually taken from

(b) 9 cm tomographic cut showing improved resolution of the hepatic ducts and distal common bile duct.

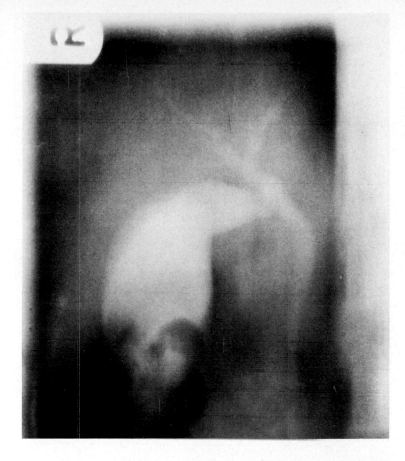

8 cm to 12 cm (Fig. 6.4b). Zonography is preferred by some workers (Bryan, 1979).

Many authors advise continuation of the radiographic examination at 30 min intervals for up to 2 hours after administration of the contrast medium in order to obtain gall bladder opacification (Figs. 6.5a and b). If the gall bladder is visualized, a prone radiograph is taken to show the gall bladder fundus, a supine radiograph for the neck of the gall bladder and Hartmann's pouch, and an erect radiograph to demonstrate the presence of gallstones. It should be noted that the erect radiograph occasionally shows a stratification or layering phenomenon, variously attributed to incomplete mixing of concentrated old bile and contrast laden new bile (Ounjian, 1976; Tada *et al.*, 1974). A 24 hour film in these circumstances allows adequate mixing of the contrast material and bile.

Complications

Deaths attributed to the technique are said to occur once in every 5000 examinations. This is approximately 8 times the risk of death at intravenous urography. It has been suggested that the toxic effects of the intravenous cholangiographic media may be related to their property of pseudocholinesterase inhibition (Lasser, 1966). Hepatotoxicity (Stillman, 1974) and renal failure (Craft & Swales, 1967) have followed high dose of the contrast agents. The nephrotoxicity may be due to the uricosuric action (Mudge, 1971; Sargent *et al.*, 1973) and consequently patients should be adequately hydrated for the examination. Renal failure has occurred in patients with myelomatosis and Ansell (1978) regards Waldenström's macroglobulinaemia as an absolute contraindication to the technique due to the risk of precipitation of the abnormal paraproteins.

REFERENCES

Ansell G. (1978) Complications of X-ray investigations. Adverse Drug Reaction Bulletin No. 71. (Ed. Davies D.M.) Adverse Drug Reaction Research Unit, Shotley Bridge General Hospital.

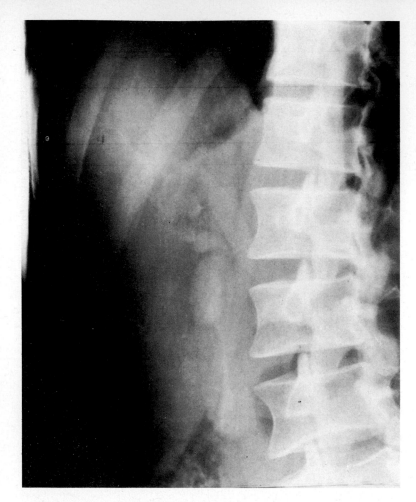

Fig. 6.5 Intravenous cholangiogram—showing value of a delayed radiograph in demonstrating the gall bladder.
(a) Radiograph taken at end of contrast infusion. The common bile duct is faintly demonstrated. The gall bladder is not filled.

Barnhart J. L., Berk R. N. & Combes B. (1980) Changes in bile flow and composition induced by radiographic contrast materials. *Invest. Radiol.*, **15** (Suppl) S124–S131.

Bryan G. J. (1979) *Diagnostic Radiography.* 3e pp. 278–81. Churchill Livingstone, Edinburgh.

Bell G. D., Fayadh M., Frank J., McMullin J. & Fry I. K. (1978a). Ioglycamide (Biligram) Studies in man—relation between plasma concentration and biliary excretion. *Brit. J. Radiol.*, **51**, 111–15.

Bell G. D., Frank J., Fayadh M., Smith P. L. C. & Fry I. K. (1978b) Ioglycamide (Biligram) Studies in man—radiological opacification of the bile duct. A comparison of a number of different methods. *Brit. J. Radiol.*, **51**, 191–5.

Craft I. L. & Swales J. D. (1967) Renal failure after cholangiography. *Brit. med. J.*, **ii**, 736–8.

Dyck W. P. & Janowitz H. D. (1971) Effect of glucagon on hepatic bile secretion in man. *Gastroenterology*, **60**, 400–404.

Evans A. F. & Whitehouse G. H. (1979) The effect of glucagon on infusion cholangiography. *Clin. Radiol.*, **30**, 499–506.

Evans A. F. & Whitehouse G. H. (1980) Further experience with glucagon enhanced cholangiography. *Clin. Radiol.*, **31**, 663–5.

Finby N. & Blasberg G. (1964) A note on the blocking of hepatic excretion during cholangiographic study. *Gastroenterology*, **46**, 276–7.

Fuchs W. A. & Preisig R. (1975) Prolonged drip-infusion cholangiography. *Brit. J. Radiol.*, **48**, 539–44.

Jarrett L. N. & Bell G. D. (1980) Effect of intravenous glucagon on the biliary secretion of a cholangiographic agent in man. *Clin. Radiol.*, **31**, 657–61.

Jarrett L. N., Doran J., Clifford K., Keane D., Knapp D. & Bell G. D. (1982) Glucagon infusion cholangiography. *Brit. J. Radiol.*, **55**, 269–71.

Lang J. H. & Lasser E. C. (1967) Binding of roentgenographic contrast media to serum albumin. *Invest. Radiol.*, **2**, 396–400.

Lasser E. C., Farr R. S., Fujimagari T. & Tripp W. N. (1962) The significance of protein binding of contrast media in roentgen diagnosis. *Amer. J. Roentgenol.*, **87**, 338–60.

(b) Radiograph taken 1½ h later showing delayed filling of a normal gall bladder.

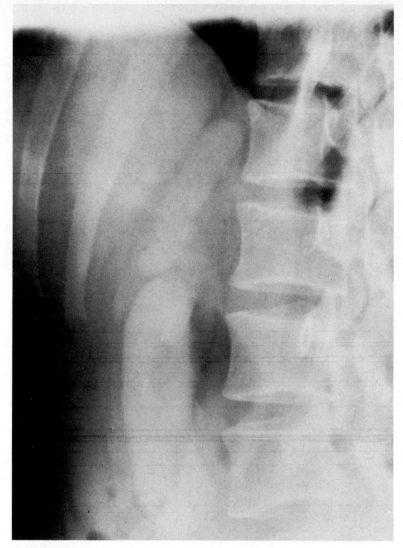

Lasser E. C. (1966) The pharmacodynamics of biliary contrast media. *Radiol. Clin. N. Amer.*, **4**, No. 3, 511–19.

Loeb P. M., Verk R. N., Fled G. D. & Wheeler H. O. (1975) Biliary excretion of iodipamide. *Gastroenterology*, **68**, 554–62.

Moss A. A., Nelson J. & Amberg J. (1973) Intravenous cholangiography. *Amer. J. Roentgenol.*, **117**, 406–11.

Mudge G. H. (1971) Uricosuric action of cholecystographic agents. *New Engl. J. Med.*, **284**, 929–33.

Ounjian Z. J. & Laing F. C. (1976) Stratification in the gall bladder on intravenous cholangiography. *Radiology*, **121**, 591–3.

Sargent E. N., Barbour B. H., Espinosa N. & Meyers H. I. (1973) Evaluation of renal function following double dose infusion intravenous cholangiography. *Amer. J. Roentgenol.*, **117**, 412–18.

Scholz F. J., Johnston D. O. & Wise R. E. (1975) Intravenous cholangiography: optimum dosage and methodology. *Radiology*, **114**, 513–18.

Sokoloff J., Berk R. N., Lang J. H. & Lasser E. C. (1973) The role of Y and Z hepatic proteins in the excretion of radiographic contrast materials. *Radiology*, **106**, 519–23.

Stillman A. E. (1974) Hepatotoxic reaction to iodipamide meglumine injection. *J. Amer. med. Ass.*, **228**, No. 11, 1420–1.

Tada S., Nanjo M., Kino M., Sekiya T., Harada J., Kuroda T. & Anno I. (1979) Various manifestations of stratification phenomenon during intravenous cholangiography. *Clin. Radiol.*, **30**, 457–61.

Wise R. E. (1962) *Intravenous Cholangiography*. p. 21. Charles C. Thomas, Springfield, Illinois.

PER-OPERATIVE CHOLANGIOGRAPHY

In 1918 Reich delineated a biliary fistula with bismuth paste and Cotte in 1929 described opacification of the bile ducts with Lipiodol. Mirizzi in 1932, performed the first cholangiogram on an operating table (Mirizzi, 1932; 1937). The per-operative technique was soon widely employed although it was not universally accepted in the UK for many years (Schulenberg, 1966).

Butsch et al. (1936) undertook the first manometric studies of intrabiliary pressures in humans, using a T tube inserted per-operatively into the common bile duct, and were able to show the effects of various drugs on the sphincter of Oddi. French surgeons, most notably Mallet-Guy (1952), have used manometry in the assessment and management of biliary disease but the technique has never met with universal acclaim.

The operative cholangiogram is one of the most neglected and badly executed radiological investigations. It can lead to diagnostic failures when conducted without scrupulous attention to detail. In the USA ductal stones are overlooked in 3–10% of patients undergoing common duct exploration, mostly due to poor operative cholangiographic technique (Burhenne, 1976). Walker (1975) found clinically unsuspected common duct stones on routine operative cholangiography in 6% of patients. Wheeler (1970) showed that per-operative cholangiography could have prevented several post-operative deaths attributable to needless re-operation and fruitless duct exploration.

Indications

Not only is the technique of value in the per-operative detection of hitherto unsuspected calculi in the intra- and extra-hepatic bile ducts, but it assists the surgeon by demonstrating the biliary duct anatomy (McEvedy, 1970).

Contra-indications

Known hypersensitivity to the contrast medium is a contra-indication. If the surgeon is contemplating a cholecystenterostomy (Burke, 1972) the cystic duct will need to be preserved and per-operative cholangiography is, therefore, not possible.

Technique

Few radiologists enter the operating theatre during the performance of this examination, the control of

which is therefore left to the surgeon and radiographer. There are few operating theatres which have dedicated X-ray units and generators, most examinations having to be performed with mobile generators of 100–300 mA capacity and either portable Bucky units or fine stationary grids. A sterile cover should be fastened over the tube housing to prevent accidental contact with the operating field.

There are a number of cassette tunnels available which allow the radiographic cassettes to be slid easily under the patient. Some operating tables themselves have a space in which to place a cassette. In many situations none of these aids are available. When a grid is required, it should be positioned with the grid lines running at right angles to the long axis of the patient's abdomen.

Ideally, contrast examinations should be performed both before and after duct exploration. The pre-exploratory examination is performed by cannulation of the cystic duct with a thin polythene catheter and the post-exploratory examination usually via a T-tube catheter placed in the common duct.

It is essential to remove all surgical instruments from the operating field, to exclude leaks in the injection system, to irrigate the system with saline, and to make certain that no air bubbles are introduced into the system. The injection tubing must be of sufficient length to exclude the operators hands from the primary X-ray beam.

The patient lies supine on the table and the gall bladder area should be over the film (Fig. 6.6). The choice of water-soluble contrast medium is critical, as too great an iodine content will obscure small stones. Hypaque 25% is the preferred contrast agent and, although not all may be required, at least 20 ml is drawn into the syringe. The contrast medium should be warmed to body temperature. The room should be cleared of all non-essential personnel during contrast injection and those remaining should be protected either by lead aprons or mobile lead screens. Before injecting, the patient should be tilted 20° obliquely to the right in order to project the common duct off the spine. The surgeon should indicate when he is commencing the injection and the anaesthetist suspends the patient's respiration during exposure of the radiograph. Fractionating the contrast injection and taking radiographs with each fraction is recommended, for example at 3, 5–8 and 12 ml (McEvedy, 1970; Le Quesne, 1960; Wall, 1957). A single 10 ml injection should be avoided as this could obscure the terminal portion of the duct and any small filling defects.

The radiographs should be processed immediately and interpreted by a radiologist who may require

Fig. 6.6 Normal per-operative cho-langiogram—There is a vascular clip at the origin of cystic duct following the cholecystectomy. Some contrast has entered the duodenum and refluxed into the duodenal cap.

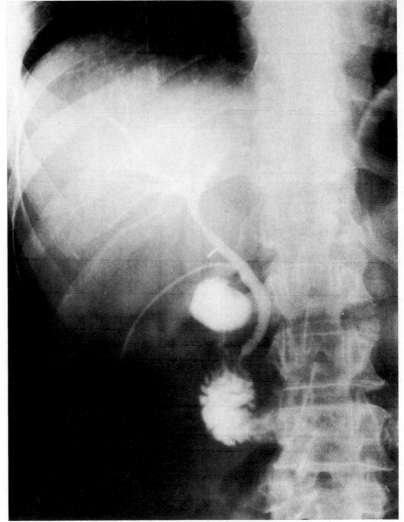

further radiographs. Because of the inherent limitations present in the per-operative situation, it may be impossible to move the patient into differing degrees of obliquity for repeat radiographs. It is, therefore, very important that the operating surgeon prevents air bubbles by careful pre-filling of the syringe and injection tube and examines the duct system before operative manipulation to prevent duct spasm.

An additional method which sometimes removes the need for patient rotation is 'Contact Cholangiography'. A small dental occlusal film, contained in a sterile polythene wrapping, is placed by the operating surgeon behind the duodenum. The X-ray beam is coned to the area of the film and an exposure is made during contrast injection.

Le Quesne (1960) considers that a normal pre-exploratory cholangiogram should show a duct not exceeding an upper limit of 12 mm in diameter, free flow of contrast into the duodenum on all radiographs with the terminal narrow segment of the duct shown on at least one radiograph, an absence of filling defects and no excess retrograde filling of the hepatic ducts.

Occasionally spasm of the sphincter of Oddi mimicks a distal common duct stone (Mujahed, 1972). This effect is abolished by the use of a smooth muscle relaxant such as glucagon (Ferrucci *et al.*, 1976).

Complications

Complications are few and rare but include bile duct rupture and septicaemia. There is a theoretical risk of pancreatitis from reflux of contrast medium into the pancreatic duct.

REFERENCES

Burhenne J. H. (1976) Non-operative extraction of stones from the bile ducts. *Roentgenology of the Gall Bladder and Biliary Tract.* (Ed. Felson B.) pp. 74, Grune and Stratton.

Burke M. (1972) Routine per-operative cholangiography. *Brit. J. Hosp. Med.,* **7,** 237–9.

Butsch W. L., McGowan J. M. & Walters W. (1936) Clinical studies on the influence of certain drugs in relation to biliary pain and to the variation in intrabiliary pressure. *Surg. Gynec. Obstet.,* **63,** 451–6.

Cotte M. G. (1929) Sur l'exploration radiologique de voies biliaires avec injection de Lipiodol après cholecystostomie ou choledocotomie. *Bull. Mem. Soc. Nat. Chir. (Paris),* **55,** 863–71.

Ferrucci J. T., Wittenberg J., Stone L. B. & Dreyfuss J. R. (1976) Hypotonic cholangiography with glucagon. *Radiology,* **118,** 466–7.

Le Quesne L. P. (1960) Discussion on cholangiography. *Proc. roy. Soc. Med.,* **53,** 851–60.

Mallet-Guy P. (1952) Value of per-operative manometric and roentgenographic examination in the diagnosis of pathologic changes and functional disturbances of the biliary tract. *Surg. Gynec. Obstet.,* **94,** 385–93.

McEvedy B. V. (1970) Routine operative cholangiography. *Brit. J. Surg.,* **57,** 277–9.

Mirizzi P. L. (1932). La colangiografia duvante las operaciones de las vias biliares. *Bol. Soc. argent. Ciruj. Buenos Aires,* **16,** 1133–61.

Mirizzi P. L. (1937) Operative cholangiography. *Surg. Gynec. Obstet.,* **65,** 702–10.

Mujahed Z. & Evans A. (1972) Pseudocalculus defect in cholangiography. *Amer. J. Roentgenol.,* **116,** 337–41.

Reich A. (1918) Accidental injection of bile ducts with petrolatum and bismuth paste. *J. Amer. med. Ass.,* **71,** 1555.

Schulenberg C. A. R. (1966) *Operative Cholangiography.* Butterworth, London.

Walker J. H. (1960) Operative cholangiography: The obligation of the radiologist to the surgeon and his patient. *Amer. J. Roentgenol.,* **125,** 490–1.

Wall C. A. & Peartree S. O. (1957) Practical value of operative cholangiography. *J. Amer. med. Ass.,* **164,** 236–8.

Wheeler M. H., Raksasook S. & Williams J. A. (1970) Operative cholangiography. Its effect on the practice of cholecystectomy. *Brit. med. J.,* **iv,** 161–4.

POST-OPERATIVE CHOLANGIOGRAPHY ('T' TUBE CHOLANGIOGRAPHY)

Following explorations to the common bile duct, a drainage tube is usually left *in situ* in the common duct to promote bile drainage. A contrast examination via this drainage tube is performed 7–10 days after the operation.

Indications

Post-operative T-tube cholangiography allows an assessment of the intra- and extra-hepatic bile ducts prior to removal of the 'T' tube.

Contra-indications

Known hypersensitivity to the contrast medium is a contra-indication to the technique.

Technique

Post-operative cholangiography is a simple and quick procedure which is performed by a radiologist in the X-ray department on a fluoroscopic unit with an undercouch tube.

A control radiograph of the gall bladder area is a prerequisite. A clamp is temporarily applied to the 'T' tube. Patients should be warned that they may experience some discomfort in the right hypochondrium during the injection of contrast medium, especially when there is obstruction of the duct system. A small needle is inserted into the tube proximal to the clamp, followed by the aspiration of air bubbles and bile. Contrast medium, for instance Hypaque 25%, is warmed to body temperature and is injected, spot radiographs being taken in varying degrees of obliquity (Fig. 6.7).

These radiographs are processed immediately and assessed by the radiologist. If the duct system contains any translucencies which may be due to air bubbles, there are some helpful manoeuvres:

1. Air bubbles will rise upwards when the patient is brought into a semi-erect position.
2. The patient may be turned on to his right side in the head-down position, and 50 ml of saline are forcefully injected into the tube, the cholangiogram being repeated when the patient is turned onto his back.

The 'pseuodo-calculus' phenomenon due to sphincteric spasm is occasionally seen in postoperative cholangiography, the appropriate technique for dealing with this situation being the same as that outlined in the section on per-operative cholangiography.

Complications

Duct rupture and septicaemia are rare complications of post-operative cholangiography.

Fig. 6.7 Normal postoperative 'T' tube cholangiogram—Some contrast has refluxed into the pancreatic duct.

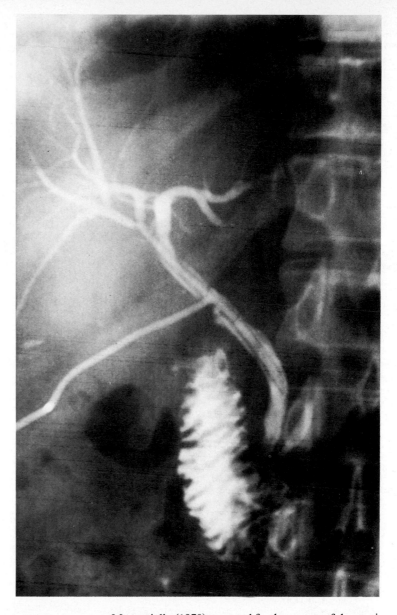

Modifications of the basic technique

It is still possible to overlook residual calculi in the biliary tract despite a meticulous surgical and per-operative cholangiographic technique. Second surgical operations to remove retained stones are complicated by a higher morbidity and mortality than the primary surgical procedure. Non-operative techniques for the removal of these stones offer an attractive alternative to surgery.

Mondet (1962) described a method of extracting stones using specially designed forceps introduced along the track left by the post-operative 'T' tube.

Mazzariello (1970) reported further successful experience with Mondet's technique. Other methods for removing retained calculi have employed irrigation with saline (Lamis *et al.*, 1969) aspiration by catheters, and the use of anti-spasmodics. Magarey (1971) improved the technique by using a Dormia ureteric basket to grasp the retained stones. This method was refined by Burhenne (1973).

The optimum time for the technique is not less than four weeks, and preferably about five weeks, after initial biliary surgery (Burhenne, 1974). A prerequisite is the use of an indwelling 'T' tube catheter of not less than No.16 French gauge, the sinus tracks from smaller catheters being too narrow to permit instrumentation. Localization of the stones by 'T' tube cholangiography precedes removal of the 'T' tube. Catheterization of the sinus track is usually possible for at least 48 hours after 'T' tube removal. A steerable catheter (Medi-Tech Inc., Watertown, Mass., USA) is then guided through the sinus track and its tip is advanced beyond the retained stone. The Dormia basket is then fed through the lumen of the steerable catheter and the catheter is withdrawn. The basket is first opened and slowly withdrawn, never being advanced, until it engages the stone which is then extracted through the sinus track. Stones of more than 10 mm in diameter usually require fragmentation either by forceful traction of the open basket into the proximal part of the sinus track or by closure of the basket within the duct system (Burhenne, 1974).

Complications of the technique include the creation of false sinus passages, septicaemia, vagal stimulation with shock, and pancreatitis.

In the hands of experienced operators the success rate of the technique is as high as 96% (Burhenne, 1974) but as low as 58% in centres treating only a few patients (Mason, 1980).

REFERENCES

Burhenne H. J. (1973) Non-operative retained biliary tract stone extraction. *Amer. J. Roentgenol.*, **117**, 388–99.
Burhenne H. J. (1974) The techniques of biliary duct stone extraction. *Radiology*, **113**, 567–72.
Lamis P. A., Letton A. H. & Wilson J. P. (1969) Retained common duct stones: a new non-operative technique for treatment. *Surgery*, **66**, 291–6.
Magarey C. J. (1971) Non-surgical removal of retained biliary calculi. *Lancet*, **i**, 1044–6.
Mason R. (1980) Percutaneous extraction of retained gallstones via the T tube track—British experience of 131 cases. *Clin. Radiol.*, **31**, 497–9.
Mazzariello R. (1970) Removal of residual biliary tract calculi without re-operation. *Surgery*, **67**, 566–73.
Mondet A. (1962) Tecnica de la extraccion incruenta de los calculos en la litiasis residual del coledoco. *Bol. Soc. Ciruj.*, *Buenos Aires*, **46**, 278–90.

PERCUTANEOUS TRANSHEPATIC CHOLANGIOGRAPHY

The first percutaneous transhepatic cholangiogram (PTC) is credited to Huard and Do-Xuan-Hop (1937) who introduced Lipiodol into the biliary tree. In 1952, Carter and Saypol described an anterior percutaneous approach into the left lobe of the liver using a No.17 spinal needle in a case of obstructive jaundice. In the same year Leger et al. (1952) described a further 14 cases. Prioton et al. (1960) used a posterior approach in order to direct the needle into the extraperitoneal segment of the liver in an attempt to contain any resultant leakage of bile.

These methods did not meet with universal acclaim and most operators preferred an anterior subcostal approach using a 20 gauge steel needle over which was drawn a flexible polyethylene tube (George et al., 1965; Mujahed & Evans, 1966). In the 1960s and early 1970s percutaneous transhepatic cholangiography was restricted to the immediate preoperative period because of the risks of bile leakage, haemorrhage and septicaemia (Zinberg et al., 1965; Machado, 1971).

In 1974, Kunio Okuda, working in Chiba University Hospital, Japan, reported his experience with a fine 23F gauge flexible needle, subsequently known as the 'Chiba needle' (Okuda et al., 1974). The following description is restricted to the use of this needle since the Chiba needle technique has now replaced the other methods as a primary diagnostic procedure. The principal advantages of the Chiba needle over the older sheathed needle are due to its flexibility and narrow calibre.

Indications

PTC is used to distinguish intrahepatic cholestasis from extrahepatic obstruction and to determine the site and, if possible, the nature of an extrahepatic biliary duct obstruction.

Contra-indications

Strong contra-indications to the use of PTC are coagulation problems, for example a platelet count of less than $100 \times 10^9/l$ ($100\,000/mm^3$) and a prothrombin time of less than 60% of the control value, biliary infection, hypersensitivity to contrast medium, severe heart disease and a respiratory problem which renders the patient unable to hold his breath.

Okuda (1974) also included as contra-indications a poor general condition of the patient, extreme jaundice, ascites, and moderate to severe anaemia. He also considered that PTC should not be performed immediately after a severe attack of abdominal pain.

Technique

The Chiba needle is made of flexible stainless steel and is 15 cm in length, with outer and inner diameters of respectively 0.7 mm and 0.5 mm, and a bevel angle of 30°. The procedure is usually performed under local anaesthesia, except in very young children and uncooperative adults. Patients may require sedation but it is unwise to administer any drugs in the presence of liver failure. The choice of sedative should be discussed with the referring clinician before the procedure. It is preferable to starve the patient.

If the patient is suspected of having a biliary obstruction, it is important to give a suitable antibiotic, such as i.v. gentamicin 120 mgm, in order to prevent an ascending cholangitis. Some authors give antibiotic cover to all their patients in this way (Okuda et al., 1974; Jain et al., 1977). It is essential to check the prothrombin time and platelet count and to screen the patient for hepatitis B surface (Australia) antigen before commencing the procedure. Parenteral vitamin K is given in some centres to all jaundiced patients (Fraser et al., 1978).

The examination is performed on a fluoroscopy unit with image intensification and facilities for spot radiographs with both supine and horizontal X-ray beams. The subject lies supine on the fluoroscopy table. It is worthwhile to screen the upper abdomen in order to locate the inferior hepatic border during suspended respiration. A supine control radiograph of the right hypochondrium is sometimes recommended, centring in the mid-clavicular line 2.5–5 cm above the lower costal margin (Bryan, 1979).

The skin surface of the lower right chest and right hypochondrium is cleaned with a suitable antiseptic solution and sterile drapes are placed over the surrounding areas. The skin and subcutaneous tissues down to the liver capsule are infiltrated with 1% lignocaine. A small incision is made in the skin at the optimum puncture site as determined by preliminary screening, usually in the mid-axillary line of the right seventh of eight intercostal space. The needle is inserted parallel to the plane of the table and advanced during suspended respiration through the right lobe of the liver on a line above the gall bladder and the junction of the right and left hepatic ducts. The point to which the needle tip is inserted may be determined by placing a metal marker on the skin over the xiphisternum and using this as a guide (Fraser et al., 1978), or by introducing a duodenal tube and aiming at the midpoint on the vertical line drawn from the vertex of the tube to the diaphragm (Okuda et al., 1974). In practice, it has been found satisfactory to introduce the needle until it is judged to have reached the level of the right border of the spine (Jain et al., 1977). The patient does not need to maintain suspended respiration, because of the flexible needle. A 20 ml syringe is filled with Hypaque 45% and is

connected via a long plastic anaesthetic extension set to the needle, thus avoiding irradiation to the hands of the operator. A small quantity, approximately 0.5 ml, of contrast medium is injected via the needle under the screen control. Injection into the hepatic blood vessels leads to rapid instantaneous clearing of the contrast medium, while entry into a lymphatic vessel shows a slower but complete clearing of contrast medium. A persisting curvilinear collection of contrast medium is seen if the needle tip lies in the subcapsular space of the liver. The injection of contrast medium into the biliary tree leads to slow centrifugal flow and the persistent delineation of a short section of the duct system (Fig. 6.8).

If a biliary radicle has not been cannulated, the needle is withdrawn in increments of 0.5–1.0 cm with further small injections of contrast medium. An alternative method is to withdraw the needle whilst continually injecting the contrast medium (Jain et al., 1977; Fraser et al., 1978). An arbitrary decision is made to abandon the procedure in the event of failure to repuncture the liver at differing angulations on a further three occasions (Lavelle et al., 1977), although some authors are prepared to make up to 10 insertions in cases without bile duct dilatation (Fraser et al., 1978). While the biliary tract may be delineated via the Chiba needle, in patients who do not have dilated intrahepatic ducts, the failure of the technique in itself casts doubt on the diagnosis of bile duct obstruction and a subsequent surgically treatable lesion. In a successful puncture, at least 20 ml of contrast medium should be injected before removal of the needle.

Some authors recommend suction and removal of bile with replacement of an equal volume of contrast medium in those cases with a dilated and obstructed biliary system (Fig. 6.9), but this may not be possible with the small gauge needle. The injection site is sealed with collodion and covered with a light sterile dressing.

Radiographs are immediately taken in the A–P, lateral and oblique projections. The patient is then encouraged to lie on the left side to promote drainage of the bile ducts, further radiographs being taken up to two hours after the procedure. These delayed radiographs are very useful in demonstrating the gall bladder and the site of common bile duct obstruction. Erect radiographs are particularly helpful in demonstrating the point of obstruction because the dilated common bile duct is frequently bowed anteriorly, which impairs its complete delineation in the supine position.

If extravasation of contrast medium has occurred into the liver parenchyma or in the subcapsular space of the liver, a delayed radiograph often shows

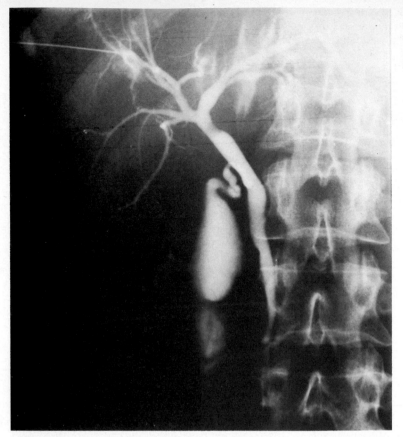

Fig. 6.8 Normal percutaneous transhepatic cholangiogram. There is filling of gall bladder and cystic duct. Some subcapsular contrast overlies the left hepatic duct.

reabsorption to have occurred and permits an unobscured view of the biliary ducts and gall bladder.

The patient should remain in bed and be carefully monitored for pulse, blood pressure and temperature and the wound inspected regularly for at least 24 hours.

Modifications of the basic technique

The diagnostic technique has been modified to provide biliary drainage in cases of obstructive jaundice. This may be a temporary measure to aid surgical management and diminish the incidence of post-operative complications, in particular renal failure. Permanent biliary drainage is used when surgery is contraindicated or to give palliation. The drainage procedure is preceded by PTC.

External biliary drainage

A biplane screening facility is especially helpful. Nakayama *et al.* (1978) recommended horizontal insertion of the needle 1 cm posterior or 1 cm anterior to the PTC puncture to enter respectively the right or left hepatic ducts. The sheathed needle, which was used for PTC in the past (Dooley *et al.*, 1979), and a 17 gauge steel needle with mandrin (Nakayama *et al.*, 1978) have been used to enter the biliary tract prior to drainage. A guide wire is then advanced along the teflon sheath or steel needle into the bile duct. A catheter is then inserted over the guide wire, which is then removed, and is secured to the skin surface. Long-term external drainage is complicated by cholangitis and by water, electrolyte and bile salt loss.

Combined internal/external biliary drainage

(Ring *et al.*, 1978; Ferrucci *et al.*, 1980.) An attempt is made to pass a special rotary torque control guide wire, with a curved right-angle memory tip, through the biliary obstruction and into the duodenum. A catheter is then inserted over the guide wire until its tip lies in the duodenal lumen, followed by removal of the guide wire. Occlusion of the catheter is prevented by numerous side holes, situated proximal and distal to the obstruction, over the distal 10–12 cm of the catheter. A pigtail configuration to the catheter provides anchorage in the duodenum. The catheter is

Fig. 6.9 Percutaneous transhepatic cholangiogram. 74 year old man with weight loss and jaundice. The intrahepatic ducts and common bile duct are dilated and the common bile duct is totally occluded distally. Note the incidental finding of gall stones in the gall bladder. Pathology—carcinoma head of pancreas.

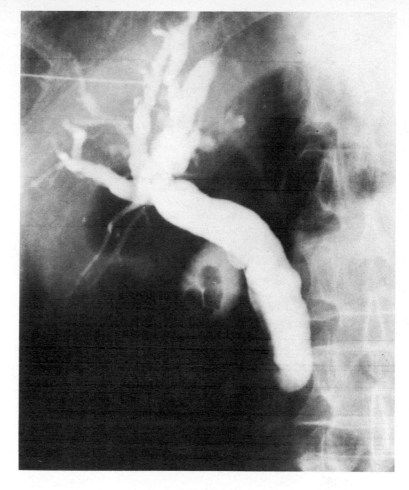

initially allowed to drain externally for 3–4 days, following which the catheter is clamped and bile drains into the duodenum.

Internal biliary drainage

(Burcharth *et al.*, 1979.) This is provided by the insertion of a permanent endoprosthesis into the lumen of a stricture, following a percutaneous transhepatic puncture. The endoprostheses are made of polyethylene or teflon, and are 10–25 cm in length with an internal diameter of 1.5–3 mm, and have multiple side holes. Following the percutaneous transhepatic insertion of a guide wire, the endoprosthesis is pushed through the obstruction by an introducer catheter so that its ends lie proximal to the obstruction and in the duodenum. (Burcharth *et al.*, 1979.) Two coaxial catheters have been used by Hoevels and Ihse (1979) in the insertion of the endoprosthesis. Bile is drained externally via a catheter for a few days after the procedure. The presence of ductal calculi is a contra-indication to endoprosthesis insertion. Recorded complications include cholangitis, local wound abscess, biliary peritonitis, external bile fistulae, and bleeding.

Complications

The commonest complications of PTC are a leakage of bile into the peritoneal cavity, intraperitoneal haemorrhage and septicaemia.

Other reported complications include hypotension and the formation of a blood-bile fistula. The overall incidence of serious complications for the Chiba technique is 3.4% (Harbin *et al.*, 1980). Harbin *et al.* (1980) have estimated that the incidence of serious complications using the fine needle, excluding sepsis which had a 1.4% incidence in their series, has been reduced by a factor of 2.6 compared to the old sheathed needle technique. While the attendant risks of the procedure are small, and routine laparotomy is not indicated, the procedure should *never* be performed if surgical help is not immediately available.

REFERENCES

Bryan G. J. (1979) *Diagnostic Radiography*, 3e, pp. 285–7. Churchill Livingstone, Edinburgh.

Burcharth F., Jensen L. I. & Olsen K. (1979) Endoprosthesis for internal drainage of the biliary tract. *Gastroenterology*, **77**, 133–7.

Carter F. R. & Saypol G. M. (1952) Transabdominal cholangiography. *J. Amer. med. Ass.*, **148**, 253–5.

Dooley J. S., Dick R., Irving D., Olney J. & Sherlock S. (1981) Relief of bileduct obstruction by the percutaneous transhepatic insertion of an endoprosthesis. *Clin. Radiol.*, **32**, 163–72.

Elias E. (1976) Progress report: cholangiography in the jaundiced patient. *Gut*, **17**, 801–11.

Ferrucci J. T., Mueller P. R. & Harbin W. P. (1980) Percutaneous transhepatic biliary drainage. *Radiology*, **135**, 1–13.

Fraser G. M., Cruikshank J. G., Sumerling M. D. & Buist T. A. S. (1978) Percutaneous transhepatic cholangiography with the Chiba needle. *Clin. Radiol.*, **29**, 101–12.

George P., Young W. B., Walker J. G. & Sherlock S. (1965) The value of percutaneous cholangiography. *Brit. J. Surg.*, **52**, 779–83.

Harbin W. P., Mueller P. R. & Ferrucci J. T. (1980) Transhepatic cholangiography: complications and use patterns of the fine needle technique. *Radiology*, **135**, 15–22.

Hoevels J. & Ihse I. (1979) Percutaneous transhepatic insertion of a permanent endoprosthesis in obstructive lesions of the extrahepatic bile ducts. *Gastrointest. Radiol.*, **4**, 367–77.

Huard P. & Do-Xuan-Hop (1937) La ponction transhépatique des canaux biliaires. *Bull. Soc. méd. Chir. Indochine*, **15**, 1090–1100.

Jain S., Lond R. G., Scott J., Dick R. & Sherlock S. (1977) Percutaneous transhepatic cholangiography using the 'Chiba' needle—80 cases. *Brit. J. Radiol.*, **50**, 175–80.

Lavelle M. I., Owen J. P., McNulty S. & Hamlyn A. N. (1977) Initial experience of percutaneous transhepatic cholangiography using a fine gauge needle. *Clin. Radiol.*, **28**, 453–6.

Léger L., Zara M. & Arvay N. (1952) Cholangiographie et drainage biliaire par ponction transhépatique. *Presse Med.*, **60**, 936–7.

Machado A. L. (1971) Percutaneous transhepatic cholangiography. *Brit. J. Surg.*, **58**, 616–24.

Mujahed Z. & Evans J. A. (1966) Percutaneous transhepatic cholangiography. *Radiol. Clin. N. Amer.*, **4**, No. 3, 535–45.

Nakayama T., Ideda A. & Okuda K. (1978) Percutaneous transhepatic drainage of the biliary tract. *Gastroenterology*, **74**, 554–9.

Okuda K., Tanikawa K., Emura T., Kuratomi S., Jinnouchi S., Urabe K., Sumikoshi T., Kanda Y., Fukuyama Y., Musha H., Mori H., Shimokawa Y., Yakushiji F. & Mastsuura Y. (1974) Nonsurgical, percutaneous transhepatic cholangiography—Diagnostic significance in medical problems of the liver. *Amer. J. dig. Dis.*, **19**, 21–35.

Prioton J. B., Vialla M. & Pous J. G. (1960) Nouvelle technique de cholangiographie trans-parieto-hépatique. *J. Radiol. Électrol.*, **41**, 205.

Ring E. J., Oleaga J. A., Frieman D. B., Husted J. W. & Lunderquist A. (1978) Therapeutic applications of catheter cholangiography. *Radiology*, **128**, 333–8.

Zinberg S. S., Berk J. E. & Plasencia H. (1965) Percutaneous transhepatic cholangiography: its use and limitations *Amer. J. dig. Dis.*, **10**, 154–69.

RELATIONSHIP OF RADIOLOGICAL INVESTIGATIONS OF THE BILIARY TRACT TO EACH OTHER AND TO OTHER TECHNIQUES

Investigations of the biliary tract fall into the following categories: Investigation of suspected gall-bladder disease; Investigation of cholestatic jaundice; Investigations of per-operative and post-operative patients.

Investigation of suspected gall-bladder disease

The choice of imaging technique after the plain abdominal radiograph initially rests between oral cholecystography, ultrasonography and cholescintigraphy.

Although an overall accuracy of over 90% has been claimed for oral cholecystography in the diagnosis of gall-bladder disease (see p. 60), its accuracy in detecting gall stones is only about 75% (Alderson, 1960; Baker & Hodgson, 1960). On the other hand, B mode grey-scale ultrasonography offers a 90–98% accuracy in detecting gall stones (Thal *et al.*, 1978; Wolson & Goldberg, 1978; Lee *et al.*, 1980). Real-time ultrasonography has similar accuracy with the added benefit of an increased speed of performance (Cooperberg & Burhenne, 1980). A study by Walker (1981) showed that a high level of operator experience was not necessary to achieve a high success rate in the ultrasonic diagnosis of gall stones.

The oral cholecystogram gives diagnostic information that ultrasonography cannot rival in the evaluation of gall-bladder wall diseases such as adenomyomatosis, diverticula and septa (Brit. med. J., 1981). However, ultrasonography has been useful in the diagnosis of emphysematous cholecystitis

(Blaquière et al., 1981), cholesterol polyps (Ruhe et al., 1979) and papillary adenoma (Carter et al., 1978).

Non-opacification of the gall-bladder by single dose oral cholecystography has been reported in 4.7% to 25% of examinations (Achkar et al., 1969; Mujahed et al., 1974). In a study comparing oral cholecystography with ultrasonography (Bartrum et al., 1976), 60% of the non-opacifying gall-bladders contained gall stones and ultrasonography detected 93% of them. An earlier study (Goldberg et al., 1974) correctly predicted 81% of gall stones in non-opacifying gall bladders. A contrasting study (Harbin et al., 1979) found that failure to demonstrate the non-opacified gall-bladder by ultrasonography indicated a high level of gall-bladder pathology, excluding the rare entity of congenital absence of the gall-bladder.

Ultrasonography has shown excellent diagnostic potential in the diagnosis of acute cholecystitis, where oral cholecystography is contra-indicated (Croce et al., 1981; Dillon & Parkin, 1980), and in assessing the size and complications of gall-bladder carcinoma (Dalla-Palma et al., 1980).

Newer hepatocyte mediated radio-pharmaceuticals such as Tc 99m labelled HIDA (N- [2, 6-dimethyl-phenylcarbamoylmethyl] imino-diacetic acid) have been claimed to be of value in the diagnosis of acute cholecystitis (Weissmann et al., 1979) although the evidence is not yet conclusive. Studies using Tc 99m PIPIDA (paraisopropylimidodiacetic acid), a substance closely allied to HIDA, have shown that gall-bladders imaged by this agent, and which subsequently failed to contract in response to cholecysto-kinin, had low-grade chronic cholecystitis (Topper et al., 1980). Radionuclide scintigraphy seems to have some value in the diagnosis of gall-bladder wall disease but has no application in the direct demonstration of gall stones in the gall-bladder lumen.

Investigation of cholestatic jaundice

The differentiation must be made between intra-hepatic cholestasis, when surgery is not usually feasible, and extra-hepatic obstruction, which is generally amenable to surgery. Oral cholecystography and i.v. cholangiography have little to offer in the management of jaundice for the basic reason that success is less likely with increasing parenchymal cell failure.

Hepato-biliary imaging using Tc 99m diethyl IDA (NoC- [2, 6, diethylacetanilide] iminodiacetic acid) has been claimed by Pauwels et al. (1980) to discriminate between hepato-cellular and obstructive jaundice in 90% of cases, although the reliability of

the test declines with increasing severity of the jaundice. The main advantages in using Tc 99m labelled iminodiacetic acid derivatives over i.v. cholangiography are that they are considerably less toxic, dynamic data is obtainable (Nielsen et al., 1978), they can be used with serum bilirubin levels of up to 250 mol/l (Oster-Jorgensen et al., 1979), and information is also obtained about the liver, kidneys and bowel (Cheng et al., 1979).

Grey scale ultrasonography differentiates dilated from non-dilated intrahepatic ducts with almost 100% accuracy (Taylor & Rosenfield, 1977) and may also detect duct stones. Sometimes, however, intrahepatic biliary duct dilatation may be absent in the presence of obstruction (Thomas, 1980), and the diameter of the common hepatic duct may be a more reliable indication of obstruction. (Cooperberg et al., 1980). While computed tomography (CT) is reliable and accurate in differentiating obstructive from non-obstructive jaundice and in determining the cause of the obstruction (Levitt et al., 1977), it is not yet widely available and its precise place in the scheme of management is uncertain. In some centres CT competes with ultrasonography as the first line investigation, but elsewhere CT is only used if ultrasonography is either equivocal or impracticable due to surgical sutures or wounds (Whalen, 1979).

In patients with dilated intrahepatic bile ducts, percutaneous transhepatic cholangiography (PTC) is probably the next investigation of choice and will identify the site but not always the cause of the obstruction (Owen, 1980). Patients with non-dilated intrahepatic ducts should then be investigated by endoscopic retrograde cholangiopancreatography (ERCP) (Elias, 1976), although this technique may also show the distal extent of obstructions which have been demonstrated by PTC.

Investigations of per-operative and post-operative patients

In the per-operative situation the operative cholangiogram is unrivalled in its application and the immediate post-operative patient is best examined by the indwelling 'T' tube.

The patient who has had biliary surgery some years before presents a difficult challenge. Clinicians often request i.v. cholangiography to assess the ducts but its value in such an assessment has recently been questioned by Goodman et al. (1980). These authors regard the accuracy of i.v. cholangiography to be so low that they recommend its replacement by ERCP or transhepatic cholangiography. Ultrasonography,

CT and radionuclide scintigraphy seem logical aids to the investigation of these patients and, in cases of suspected obstructive jaundice, may be used along the lines suggested in the preceding section.

REFERENCES

Achkar E., Norton R. A. & Siber F. J. (1969) The fate of the non-visualised gallbladder. *Amer. J. dig. Dis.*, **14**, 80–3.

Alderson D. A. (1960) The reliability of Telepaque cholecystography. *Brit. J. Surg.*, **47**, 206, 655–8.

Baker H. L. & Hodgson J. R. (1960) Further studies on the accuracy of oral cholecystography. *Radiology*, **74**, 239–45.

Bartrum R. J., Crow H. C. & Foote S. R. (1976) Ultrasound examination of the gallbladder. An alternative to 'double-dose' oral cholecystography. *J. Amer. med. Ass.*, **236**, 1147–8.

Blaquiere R. M. & Dewbury K. C. (1982) The ultrasound diagnosis of emphysematous cholecystitis. *Brit. J. Radiol.*, **55**, 114–16.

British Medical Journal (1981) Editorial: Echoes from the gallbladder, **283**, 3.

Carter S. J., Rutledge J., Hirch J. H., Vracko R. & Chikos P. M. (1978) Papillary adenoma of the gallbladder: ultrasonic demonstration. *J. clin. Ultrasound*, **6**, 433–5.

Cheng T. H., Davis M. A., Seltzer S. E., Jones B., Abbruzzese A. A., Finberg H. J. & Drum D. E. (1979) Evaluation of hepatobiliary imaging by radionuclide scintigraphy, Ultrasonography and contrast cholangiography. *Radiology*, **133**, 761–7.

Cooperberg P. L. & Burhenne J. H. (1980) Real-time ultrasonography: diagnostic technique of choice in calculous gallbladder disease. *New Engl. J. Med.*, **302**, 1277–9.

Cooperberg P. L., Li D., Wong P., Cohen M. M. & Burhenne H. J. (1980) Accuracy of common hepatic duct size in the evaluation of extrahepatic biliary obstruction. *Radiology*, **135**, 141–4.

Croce R., Montali G., Solbiati L. & Marinoni G. (1981) Ultrasonography in acute cholecystitis. *Brit. J. Radiol.*, **54**, 927–31.

Dalla Palma L., Rizzatto G., Pozzi-Mucelli R. S. & Bazzocchi M. (1980) Grey-scale ultrasonography in the evaluation of carcinoma of the gallbladder. *Brit. J. Radiol.*, **53**, 662–7.

Dillon E. & Parkin G. J. S. (1980) The role of upper abdominal ultrasonography in suspected acute cholecystitis. *Clin. Radiol.*, **31**, 175–9.

Elias E. (1976) Cholangiography in the jaundiced patient. *Gut*, **17**, 801–11.

Goldberg B. B., Harris K. & Broocker W. (1974) Ultrasonic and radiographic cholecystography. *Radiology*, **111**, 405–9.

Goodman M. W., Ansel H. J., Vennes J. A., Lasser R. B. & Silvis S. E. (1980) Is intravenous cholangiography still useful? *Gastroenterology*, **79**, 642–5.

Harbin W. P., Ferruci J. T., Wittenber J. & Kirkpatrick R. H. (1979) Non-visualised gallbladder by cholecystosonography. *Amer. J. Roentgenol.*, **132**, 727–8.

Lee J. K. T., Melson G. L., Koehler R. E. & Stanley R. J. (1980) Cholecystosonography: accuracy, pitfalls and unusual findings. *Amer. J. Surg.*, **139**, 223–8.

Levitt R. G., Sagel S. S., Stanley R. J. & Jost R. G. (1977) Accuracy of computed tomography of the liver and biliary tract. *Radiology*, **124**, 123–8.

McNeil B. J. & Adelstein S. J. (1976) Determining the value of diagnostic and screening tests. *J. nucl. Med.*, **17**, 439–48.

Mujahed Z., Evans J. A. & Whalen J. P. (1974) The non-opacified gallbladder on oral cholecystography. *Radiology*, **112**, 1–3.

Nielson S. P., Trap-Jensen J., Linberg J. & Nielsen M. L. (1978) Hepato-biliary scintigraphy and hepatography with Tc 99m diethyl-acentanilido-iminodiacetate in obstructive jaundice. *J. nucl. Med.*, **19**, 452–7.

Oster-Jorgensen E., Petersen S. A. & Schoubye J. (1979) Hepato biliary scintigraphy with Tc 99m HIDA in patients with jaundice. *Acta Radiol. Diagn.*, **20**, 299–310.

Owen J. P. (1980) Analysis of the signs of common bile duct obstruction at percutaneous transhepatic cholangiography. *Clin. Radiol.*, **31**, 271–6.

Ruhe A. H., Zachman J. P., Mulder B. D. & Rime A. E. (1979) Cholesterol polyps of the gallbladder: ultrasound demonstration. *J. clin. Ultrasound*, **7**, 386–8.

Taylor K. J. W. & Rosenfield A. T. (1977) Grey-scale ultrasonography in the differential diagnosis of jaundice. *Arch. Surg.*, **112**, 820–5.

Thal E. R., Weigelt J., Landay M. & Conrad M. (1978) Evaluation of ultrasound in the diagnosis of acute and chronic biliary tract disease. *Arch. Surg.*, **113**, 500–3.

Thomas J. L. & Zornoza J. (1980) Obstructive jaundice in the absence of sonographic biliary dilatation. *Gastrointest. Radiol.*, **5**, 357–60.

Topper T. E., Ryerson T. W. & Nora P. F. (1980) Quantitative gallbladder imaging following cholecystokinin. *J. nucl. Med.*, **21**, 694–6.

Vecchio T. J. (1966) Predictive value of a single diagnostic test in unselected populations. *New Engl. J. Med.*, **274**, 1171–3.

Walker T. M. (1981) Ultrasound of the gallbladder; experience in a district hospital. *Brit. med. J.*, **282**, 1452–3.

Weissmann H. S., Frank M. S., Bernstein L. H. & Freeman L. M. (1979) Rapid and accurate diagnosis of acute cholecystitis with 99m Tc—HIDA cholescintigraphy. *Amer. J. Roentgenol.*, **132**, 523–8.

Whalen J. P. (1979) Radiology of the abdomen: impact of new imaging methods. *Amer. J. Roentgenol.*, **133**, 585–618.

Wolson A. H. & Goldberg B. B. (1978) Grey-scale ultrasonic cholecystography. *J. Amer. Med. Ass.*, **240**, 2073–5.

Endoscopic Retrograde Cholangiopancreatography (ERCP) 7

A. F. EVANS

Endoscopic retrograde cholangiopancreatography (ERCP) was first performed in Japan (Oi, Takemoto & Kondo, 1969). The technique has become increasingly used throughout the world during the last decade. Although ERCP was introduced as a purely diagnostic procedure, recent technical advances in instrumentation have added a therapeutic dimension.

Indications

The principal application for ERCP is in the evaluation of suspected pathology in the pancreas or biliary duct system. The technique allows biopsy, brushing, and aspiration of the biliary or pancreatic ducts, while papillotomy and/or common bile duct stone removal are other extensions of the procedure.

The indications may be considered under three headings:

1. *Obstructive jaundice of unknown aetiology* To demonstrate extrahepatic causes such as stones, tumours, strictures, as well as sclerosing cholangitis.
2. *Suspected pancreatic disease*, particularly pancreatitis and neoplasms.
3. *Unexplained severe abdominal pain* of suspected biliary or pancreatic origin.

Contra-indications

Contra-indications to ERCP include oesophageal stenosis, gastric outlet obstruction, thoracic aortic aneurysm and severe pulmonary disease. ERCP should be avoided in patients with either hypersensitivity to contrast media or with known Australia antigen hepatitis. Acute cholangitis is a contra-indication unless a stone in the common bile duct is thought to be the cause, in which case the stone may be removed during the procedure. ERCP should not be performed during and within four weeks of an episode of acute pancreatitis, or in the known presence of a pseudocyst.

Technique

A close rapport between the endoscopist and radiologist is required to obtain the best possible radiographic record of the examination.

Radiographic equipment

The examination must be performed in the X-ray Department (Bauene *et al.*, 1972), in a room containing high quality radiographic equipment and which is large enough to accommodate readily all the necessary apparatus and personnel.

A conventional screening unit with an under-couch tube is preferable to an over-couch remote control unit, which may cause excessive radiation exposure to the endoscopist. The table top should be capable of being tilted from the upright to at least a 15° head-down position. The X-ray tube should have a small focal spot (0.3–0.6 mm) and a high MaS and KV facility. A combination of rare earth screens and high-speed film is used to reduce exposure time and minimize the effect of patient movement. An over-couch tube is required for delayed radiographs.

Endoscopic equipment

The basic endoscopic kit consists of a side viewing endoscope, such as the Olympus BJIT; together with its cold light source, suction apparatus and cannulation catheters (Fig. 7.1).

Dormier baskets, sphincterotomy knives and a diathermy unit should be available to allow therapeutic techniques to be performed after the diagnostic procedure (Fig. 7.2).

A lignocaine spray is required for pharyngeal anaesthesia and syringes of various sizes should be included on the trolley. Drugs available should include pethidine, Omnopon, atropine, diazepam and Buscopan. A suitable contrast medium should be to hand. Resuscitation equipment should always be available in case of cardio-respiratory collapse.

Contrast media

Numerous workers (Oi *et al.*, 1969; Classen, 1972; Cotton *et al.*, 1972) have described preferences for various contrast agents, none of which is ideal. Conray 280 (meglamine iothalamate 60%) is generally satisfactory for delineating the pancreatic duct and the normal biliary tree, with the option of dilution with saline to a 30% solution for opacification of the dilated common bile duct. The newer non-ionic contrast agents require further evaluation but Osnes *et al.*

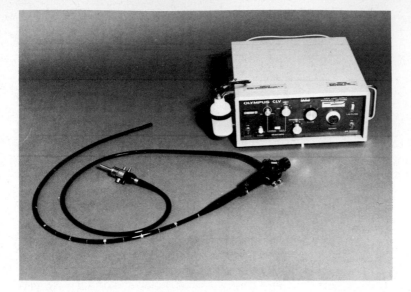

Fig. 7.1 Olympus cold light source and side viewing endoscope.

(1977) have found metrizamide to cause less pain and a lower rise in serum amylase on pancreatography than a conventional contrast medium with the same iodine concentration. The pressure of injection should be sufficient to fill but not over-distend the pancreatic or biliary ducts. The normal pancreatic duct volume is of the order of 2–5 ml whereas 8–12 ml are required to fill the normal biliary tract. Much larger volumes may be required to adequately demonstrate the biliary system if there is free filling of the gall bladder.

Procedure

The patient should be reassured by prior explanation of the procedure. A chest radiograph and barium examinations of the oesophagus and stomach are essential to exclude an aortic aneurysm and oesophageal or gastric outlet obstruction. An abdominal radiograph will show the presence of pancreatic calcification. The patient is starved for six hours prior to the examination.

The patient lies on the fluoroscopy table. A Butterfly needle is used to provide an intravenous line into the arm. Sedation is provided by opiates or intravenous diazepam. If the patient becomes uncooperative during the administration of diazepam, as sometimes happens with alcoholics, it is necessary to change immediately to another sedative. The onset of ptosis or dysarthria usually indicates adequate sedation, but the requisite dosage varies from one patient to another. Intravenous atropine is given immediately before the examination to control salivation.

Plain radiographs of the hepato-biliary area are obtained to assess radiographic factors prior to subsequent radiography. Endoscopy is then performed in the left lateral position. The stomach is insufflated, the pylorus is identified and negotiated, and the duodenal bulb is inspected (Salmon *et al.*, 1972) before a paralytic ileus is obtained by intravenous hyoscine-n-butyl bromide (Buscopan) or glucagon. The latter, being a choloretic agent, may cause easier identification of the ampulla.

The ampulla of Vater is usually located half way down the postero-medial wall of the second part of the duodenum, but may be situated anywhere between the post-bulbar region and the third portion of the duodenum. It is necessary to obtain an en face view of the papilla in order to successfully cannulate the ampulla. Once cannulation has been obtained, 1–2 ml of contrast medium is slowly injected under fluoroscopic control. The field size should be kept to a minimum to obtain maximum detail. Reflux of contrast medium into the duodenum indicates a failure of cannulation and requires repositioning of the cannula. If the pancreatic duct is opacified, a slow injection of contrast medium proceeds under constant fluoroscopic control. Radiographs are obtained when the pancreatic duct is delineated to its tail (Fig. 7.3). The injection is stopped when lateral branches of the pancreatic duct are seen or when the patient complains of pain. The patient is gently turned as necessary so that the endoscope does not obscure ductal detail on further radiographs. Having obtained radiographs of the duct system, the instrument is retracted into the stomach and over-couch films of the pancreatic area are obtained in the prone oblique and antero–posterior positions. These radiographs must be quickly obtained as contrast medium is very rapidly evacuated from

Fig. 7.2 Examples of instruments which may be passed through the endoscope.
(a) Upper—sphincterotomy knife closed
Lower—dormier type basket closed

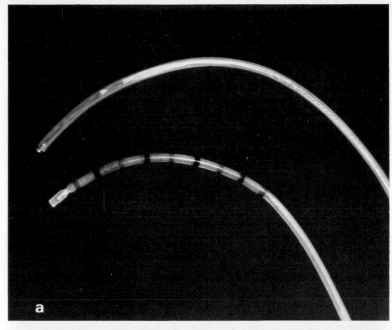

(b) Upper—sphincterotomy knife open
Lower—basket open

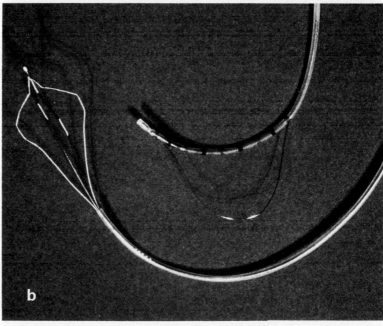

the normal duct system (Cotton *et al.*, 1972). Extravasation of contrast medium into the parenchyma of the pancreas, with the consequent risk of pancreatitis, is avoided by stopping the injection as soon as fine pancreatic radicles are seen.

Additional smooth muscle relaxation, by further injection of intravenous Buscopan or glucagon, may be required during the procedure in order to maintain an ileus.

Cholangiography is often more difficult to attain than pancreatography, but skilled endoscopy usually allows successful cannulation of the common bile duct. Once the common bile duct has been cannulated, the contrast medium is injected under fluoroscopic

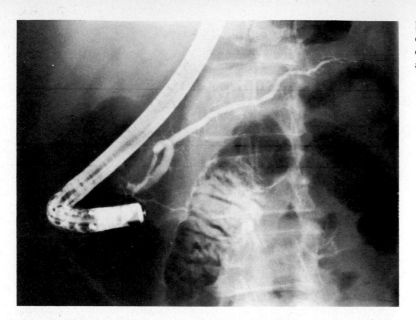

Fig. 7.3 Complete filling of the pancreatic duct out to the tail with side duct filling. There is also delineation of a small accessory pancreatic duct.

control until there is adequate filling of the biliary tree. Great care must be taken not to introduce air bubbles as these may cause diagnostic difficulties. It is good practice to obtain sequential radiographs during filling of the common bile duct because small calculi may become obscured in the distended duct (Whitaker, 1968). With the cannula *in situ*, under-couch radiographs are obtained in the left lateral and left anterior oblique projections (Fig. 7.4). The endoscope is removed as soon as there is adequate opacification of the biliary system and over-couch radiographs are then taken of the biliary tract. Delayed radiographs, including erect views, may be required to assess fully the biliary ductal system (Fig. 7.5).

Burwood *et al.,* (1973) found video recording to be useful in documenting both pancreatic duct and common bile duct filling.

Bauerle (1972) has used a suspended 'C' arm unit, which allows a large range of projections without moving the patient.

If there is simultaneous filling of both pancreatic and bile ducts, it is important to obtain adequate under-couch radiographs during the procedure. Selective cannulation of one or other duct may require repeated injections of contrast medium. It is advisable to aspirate this contrast medium as it may promote peristalsis which makes cannulation more difficult and may obscure diagnostic detail on subsequent radiography.

The patient should be nursed in the lateral position in the immediate post-procedure phase, until there is a full return of pharyngeal sensation.

Special problems

Those patients requiring ERCP and who have had previous gastric or duodenal surgery present difficulties for endoscopy because of alterations in the entrance to the duodenum or in the position of the ampulla. Fluoroscopic monitoring of the endoscope may be useful in these circumstances but, since fibre-optic endoscopes are damaged by X-radiation, the exposure time should be kept as short as possible.

After sphincterotomy or choleduodenostomy, it may only be possible to fill the intrahepatic ducts in the head-down position. Both these operations may make it extremely difficult, if not impossible, to cannulate the pancreatic duct. The presence of a duodenal diverticulum occasionally causes endoscopic difficulties.

Variations on basic technique

Endoscopic transduodenal papillotomy (Classen & Demling, 1974) has become increasingly used in the last four or five years. Selective duct cannulation allows pure pancreatic juice or bile to be collected for biochemical and cytological analysis (Endo *et al.,* 1974; Osnes *et al.,* 1975; Hatfield *et al.,* 1976). Seifert *et al.* (1977) have described intraductal biopsy of the pancreatic duct, while Tsuchiya *et al.* (1978) have reported transendoscopic needle biopsy during ERCP Calculi in the common bile duct may be removed by a dormier basket. A prosthesis may be inserted through a biliary obstruction.

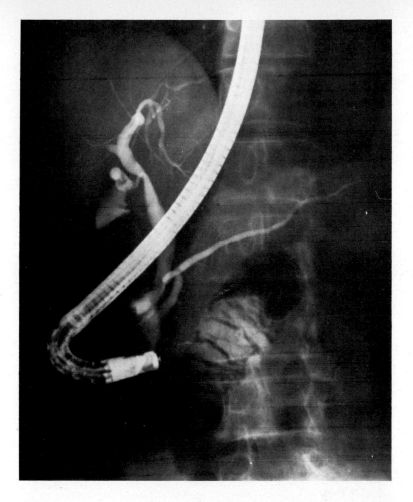

Fig. 7.4 Simultaneous filling of the pancreatic duct and the biliary system demonstrating the common bile duct, intrahepatic ducts and cystic duct. The contracted gallbladder is completely filled.

Complications

The hazards and complications of ERCP include those of upper gastrointestinal fibre-endoscopy in addition to complications which specifically result from cannulation of the ductal system. ERCP has the highest complication rate of all upper gastrointestinal diagnostic endoscopic procedures (Silvis *et al.*, 1976).

Hazards of endoscopy

1. Inhalation of vomit may occur and cause aspiration pneumonia (Blumgart *et al.*, 1972; Cotton *et al.*, 1972; Taylor *et al.*, 1972). This risk is minimized by keeping the patient in the prone or prone oblique position throughout the examination.
2. Perforation of the oesophagus or stomach is possible, although the risk of this occurring is lessened by awareness of abnormalities demonstrated on previous barium examination.
3. Impaction of the fibrescope has occurred during endoscopy due to inversion of the endoscope in the oesophagus or duodenum (Kavin, 1970).
4. An acute abdomen may be simulated after endoscopy (Moldow, 1971) due to the forcible introduction of a large volume of air into the stomach, leading to considerable acute distension of the small bowel. The resultant severe abdominal pain, distension and tenderness may mimick a visceral perforation.
5. Bleeding from oesophageal varices has been reported in one case (Bilbao *et al.*, 1976).
6. Cross-infection is always a possibility with an inadequately sterilized endoscope.

Hazards unique to ERCP

Bilbao *et al.* (1976), in a survey of 10 000 cases, found a 3% incidence of complications and a 0.15% mortality rate. A much lower complication rate was noted in experienced hands. Complications include:

(a) Asymptomatic elevation of the serum amylase has

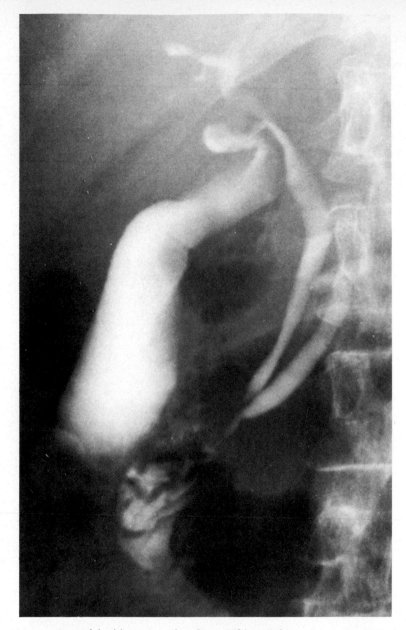

Fig. 7.5 Over-couch radiograph depicting the common bile duct and cystic duct with the gall bladder. The proximal portion of the pancreatic duct is emptying into the duodenum.

a reported incidence varying from 25% to 73% (Cotton *et al.*, 1972; Katon, 1974) and is usually related to over-filling of the pancreatic duct.

(b) Pancreatitis is the most significant complication of ERCP, occurring in approximately 1% of examinations (Silvis *et al.*, 1974; Bilbao *et al.*, 1976). The illness is not generally severe, although one case of fatal pancreatitis has been reported (Anman, 1973) and a pseudocyst has resulted in another patient (Galvan & Klotz, 1973). The risk of pancreatitis following ERCP is reduced if injection into the pancreatic duct is made very

slowly under constant fluoroscopic control and is terminated as soon as there is visualization of branch ducts.

(c) A 0.3% incidence of pancreatic sepsis and abscess formation with a 20% mortality rate has been reported following pancreatography by Bilbao *et al.* (1976). It is now generally agreed that pseudocysts should not be completely opacified by contrast medium. When found, antibiotics should be given and surgical drainage considered within 24 hours of opacification.

(d) Cholangitis has been reported in 0.8% of patients

undergoing ERCP by both Cotton *et al.* (1972) and Bilbao *et al.* (1976). Although the cause is not fully understood, obstruction of the biliary tree is usually present. It is recommended that a surgical consultation should be obtained prior to ERCP in patients with jaundice. If obstruction is demonstrated, decompression by sphincterotomy during the procedure or surgical drainage soon afterwards is the recommended course of action.

(e) While no serious reactions to contrast media have been reported following ERCP, contrast medium does enter the systemic circulation and is excreted by the kidneys (Nelson *et al.*, 1972). There is, therefore, a potential risk of hypersensitivity reaction to the contrast medium.

Relationship to other diagnostic techniques

Within the selection criteria, ERCP allows a precise definition of the cause and nature of biliary and pancreatic disease by means of a single diagnostic study. Barium studies offer very little in terms of a definitive diagnosis in the acutely ill patient with a progressive disease which is thought to originate within the biliary or pancreatic systems. Ultrasonography is of great value in some cases, being non-invasive, but does not always give the definitive diagnosis. The widespread use of percutaneous transhepatic cholangiography (PTC) using the Chiba needle (Hinde *et al.*, 1977) has led to a reduction in the use of ERCP in some centres. PTC will confirm the presence of biliary obstruction and will often show the site and cause of the obstruction. When PTC is contra-indicated, for instance in the presence of sepsis or severe abdominal pain, fibre-optic endoscopy combined with ERCP is an appropriate alternative.

There is a close link between diagnostic and therapeutic procedures in patients suffering from biliary tract or pancreatic disease. A large group of patients with obstructive jaundice, who are at risk from abdominal surgery, benefits from ERCP and external or internal biliary drainage. PTC and percutaneous drainage is easier to perform than ERCP and a radiologist familiar with catheter techniques should be able to accomplish this procedure. The pancreas is still a difficult organ to visualize consistently, but the availability of high resolution ultrasonography and/or computed tomography precludes the need for ERCP in many cases. In general, however, the therapeutic procedures which are available via the endoscope will mean that ERCP will have a considerable place in both diagnosis and therapy for some time to come. The range of diagnostic and therapeutic techniques which are available in the biliary tract and pancreas must be seen in the light of conventional surgery. The hazards of emergency surgery are considerable in these circumstances, so that alternative measures which will temporize and allow a later elective procedure are important in patient management.

REFERENCES

Anman R. W., Deyhle P. & Butikofer E. (1973) Fatal necrotizing pancreatitis after per oral cholangio-pancreatography. *Gastroenterology*, **64**, 320.

Bauerle H., Grassman P. H., Classen M. & Deraling L. (1972) The use of radiographic techniques in gastro-enterological endoscopy. *Electromedicia*, **4**, 109–14.

Bilbao M. K., Dotter C. T., Lee T. G. & Katon R. M. (1976) Complications of endoscopic retrograde cholangio-pancreatography—a study of 10 000 cases. *Gastroenterology*, **70**, 314.

Blumgart L. H., Salmon P., Cotton P. B., Davies G. T., Burwood R., Beales J. S. H., Laurie B., Skirving A. & Read A. E. (1972) Endoscopy and retrograde choledochopancreatography in the diagnosis of the jaundiced patient. *Lancet*, **ii**, 1269–73.

Burwood R. J. (1972) Communication to British Society of Digestive Endoscopy. Scientific Meeting on Cannulation of the Papilla of Vater, London.

Classen M. (1972) Endoscopy '72—Communication to Symposium on Digestive Endoscopy, University of Bristol, 1972.

Classen M. & Demling L. (1974) Endoskopische Sphinkterotomie der papilla Vaten und Stemextraktion an dem Ductus Choledochus. *Dtsch. Med. Wsch.*, **99**, 496–7.

Cotton P. B., Salmon P. R., Blumgart L. H., Burwood R. J., Davies G. T., Lawrie B. W. & Read A. E. (1972) Cannulation of papilla of Vater via fiberduodeno-scope. *Lancet*, **i**, 53–8.

Cotton P. B. (1972) Progress report: cannulation of the papilla of Vater by endoscopy and retrograde cholangiopancreatography ERCP. *Gut*, **13**, 1104.

Endo Y., Morri T., Tarnura M. & Okuda S. (1974) Cytodiagnosis of pancreatic malignant tumours by aspiration, under direct vision, using a duodenal fibrescope. *Gastroenterology*, **67**, 944–5.

Galvan A. & Klotz A. P. (1973) Is transduodenal pancreatography ever contraindicated? A case report of provoked pancreatitis and pseudocyst. *Gastrointestinal Endoscopy*, **20**, 28.

Hatfield A. R. W., Smitties A., Wilkens R. & Levi A. J. (1976) Assessment of endoscopic retrograde cholangio-pancreatography (ERCP) and pure pancreatic juice cytology in patients with pancreatic disease. *Gut*, **17**, 14–21.

Hinde G. de B., Smith P. M. & Craven J. I. (1977) Percutaneous cholangiography with the Okuda needle. *Gut*, **18**, 610–14.

Katon R. M., Lee T. G., Parent J. A., Bilbao M. K. & Smith F. W. (1974) Endoscopic retrograde cholangiopancreatography (ERCP), experience with 100 cases. *Amer. J. dig. Dis.*, **19**, 295.

Kavin H. & Schneider J. (1970) Impaction of a fibreoptic gastroscope in the oesophagus, an unusual complication of gastroscopy. *S. Afr. Med. J.*, **44**, 478–9.

Moldow R., Wayne J. D., Cohen N. (1971) Pseudo acute abdomen following gastroscopy. *Gastrointestinal Endoscopy*, **17**, 117–18.

Nelson J. A. (1972) Absorption of iodipamide from the biliary system of the rabbit. *J. Pharm. Pharmacol.*, **24**, 993.

Oi I., Takenoto T. & Kondo T. (1969) Fibreduodenoscopy, Direct observation of the ampulla of Vater. *Endoscopy*, **1**, 101–3.

Osnes M., Serck-Hanssen A. & Myren J. (1975) Endoscopic retrograde brush cytology of the biliary and pancreatic ducts. *Scand. J. Gastroenterol.*, **10**, 829–31.

Osnes M., Skjennald A. & Larsen S. (1977) Comparison of a new non-ionic (metrizamide) and a dissociable (me-trizoate) contrast medium in endoscopic retrograde pancreatography (ERP). *Scand. J. Gastroenterol.*, **12**, 821–5.

Salmon P. R., Brown P., Htut T. & Read A. E. (1972) Endoscopic examination of the duodenal bulb. Clinical evaluation of the forward and sideviewing fibreoptic systems in 200 cases. *Gut*, **13**, 170–5.

Seifert E., Urokame Y. & Elster K. (1977) Duodenoscopic guided biopsy of the biliary and pancreatic ducts. *Endoscopy*, **9**, 154–61.

Silvis S. E., Nebel O., Rogers G., Sugawa C. & Mandelstam P. (1974). Endoscopic complication—results of 1974 meeting of the American Society for Gastrointestinal Endoscopy Survey. *J. Amer. med. Ass.*, **235**, 928.

Taylor P. A., Cotton P. B., Towey R. M. & Gent A. E. (1972) Pulmonary complications after oesophagogastroscopy using diazepam. *Brit. med. J.*, **i**, 666.

Tsuchiya R., Henmi T., Kondo N., Akashi M. & Horada N. (1977) Endoscopic aspiration biopsy of the pancreas. *Gastroenterology*, **73**, 1050–2.

Whitaker P. H., Parkinson & Howell Hughes J. (1968) Television fluoroscopy for operative cholangiography. An analysis of 150 cases. *Clin. Radiol.*, **19**, 368–78.

SECTION 2
THE CARDIOVASCULAR SYSTEM

Arteriography

T. A. S. BUIST

THE INDICATION FOR ARTERIOGRAPHY

Arteriography is an invasive procedure which carries an element of discomfort for the patient and some risk of complications. It is therefore important to assess carefully the indications for the investigation in the individual patient and its influence on case management. Where there is doubt concerning the need for arteriography, the case should be fully discussed with the referring clinician. The patient's overall condition should be reviewed with particular attention to adverse factors such as advanced age, low cardiac reserve or cardiac failure, recent myocardial infarction, hypertension, severe arteriosclerosis, impaired renal function, dehydration, and a history of previous reaction to contrast medium. It is important to weigh the potential benefit of the examination against the possibility of complications, especially in patients who have additional risk factors.

CONTRA-INDICATIONS TO ARTERIOGRAPHY

A previous severe reaction to contrast medium may contra-indicate angiography. Cardiac failure, coagulation defects, severe anaemia and dehydration should be corrected before arteriography. Recent myocardial infarction and severe hypertension are relative contra-indications. Local arterial disease or soft tissue infection may preclude the use of a particular vessel for catheterization.

THE ANGIOGRAPHY/SPECIAL PROCEDURES ROOM

Arteriographic examination should be carried out in a specialized room with equipment appropriate for the different types of angiography and for other special procedures which are required in that hospital. Fluoroscopy with high quality image intensification and television monitors is essential. A film changer with a versatile control system and facilities for exposing at least three films per second are desirable. Single plane filming is adequate in most circumstan-

ces, but departments carrying out a large number of neuro-radiological investigations may justify the more complex and expensive simultaneous biplane installation. Large field serial film changers, up to 130 cm in length, are available for use primarily in pelvic and lower limb arteriography. The standard 35×35 cm AOT or Puck cut film changer with an automatic, synchronized table movement control system is, however, a generally satisfactory alternative. Photofluorography with 100 or 105 mm roll or cut film imaging is a useful additional facility with the advantages of lower patient radiation dose, low film cost, and a convenient and quick method of filming what is shown on the fluoroscopic screen. The anatomical detail of small vessels seen by this method, particularly in selective arteriographic studies, is less than one would expect from a good quality large serial film system. Cine-angiographic facilities are of particular value in coronary and cardiac angiography. Video tape recording systems allow immediate replay of fluoroscopic images, such as test injections, and are often used in conjunction with cine filming, particularly in coronary arteriography. The resolution of present video-tape recorders is less than that provided by film systems.

An important part of the angiographic equipment is the catherization table. This requires a floating top with multi-directional movement and is integrated with the fluoroscopic and filming system. If magnification studies are required, up and down movement of the table or film changer is necessary. Modern angiographic tables with rotating fluoroscopic and filming systems on a C or U suspension have the advantage of providing multi-directional imaging facilities without moving the patient and easy magnification (Levin & Dunham, 1982).

The quality and reliability of angiography has increased greatly with the use of modern electronically controlled contrast injectors. The exact amount and rate of contrast material injection is pre-determined and automatically coordinated with the filming system. These injectors are capable of delivering contrast medium at high speed through small catheters, although it is essential that they are operated with great care. Maximum pressure settings are chosen in relation to the strength of the particular catheter. Modern injectors incorporate a facility for varying the

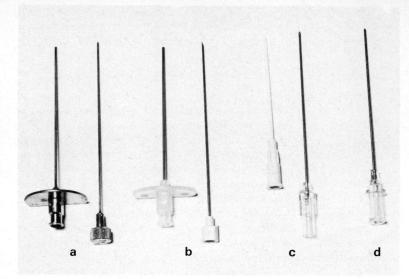

Fig. 8.1 Needles commonly used for percutaneous arterial catheterization.
(a) 7 cm 18 gauge thin wall arterial cannula and stylet
(b) Similar cannula with plastic hub (disposable)
(c) 5 cm bevelled needle with close fitting 18 gauge plastic cannula (disposable)
(d) 7 cm 18 gauge simple short bevelled needle (disposable)

a   b   c   d

time during which the injection builds up to its full delivery rate, which avoids recoil of the catheter tip in selective angiography.

Emergency resuscitation apparatus should be available in or close to the angiography room. This should include facilities for giving oxygen, suction equipment, a laryngoscope, endotracheal tubes and airways. A defibrillator and ECG machine should also be available. It may be appropriate to incorporate the resuscitation equipment with general anaesthetic apparatus and for these to be supervised by a specialist anaesthetist.

A range of appropriate angiographic needles, cannulae, catheters, guide wires, dilators, sheaths, connecting tubes and taps should be organized and kept within the angiographic room. The various contrast agents, infusion fluids and drugs which may be required should also be immediately available.

ANGIOGRAPHY STAFF

The practice of vascular radiology cannot be entirely free from hazard, careful attention to every detail of technique being necessary to keep the incidence of complications to an absolute minimum. The experience of the operator is another important factor in the avoidance of complications. It is essential that radiologists carrying out angiographic procedures should be well trained in these techniques and have obtained sufficient supervised experience before undertaking vascular examinations on their own. Repeated film series are not only expensive but may subject fragile patients to additional dangers from an

excess of contrast medium. It is therefore important that radiographers should also have an adequate period of supervised training and experience in the vascular room before assuming responsibility for this work. Nurses in the angiography and special procedures room play a very important part in the care of the patient, assist the radiologist, and organize and maintain the wide range of materials, instruments and apparatus which are required in angiography. Radiologists, radiographers and nurses working as a well-organized team achieve the best possible results.

EQUIPMENT FOR PERCUTANEOUS CATHETERIZATION

Selection of correct catheterization equipment is an essential part of successful and safe arteriography. Percutaneous catheterization is carried out using a technique based on that described by Seldinger (1953). The essential requirements are a needle, a guide wire and a catheter. These must be matched so that there is a good fit between the needle and guide wire and between the guide wire and the tapered catheter tip.

Needles

A variety of needle assemblies are available for arterial puncture (Fig. 8.1). The needle commonly used is approximately 7 cm long, has an outer 18 gauge thin-walled cannula, and an inner pointed or bevelled stylet. The original thick-walled arterial cannula is more traumatic and should no longer be used. A simple sharp needle, with a bore just large enough for the guide wire, is preferred by many radiologists and may make it easier to puncture only the anterior arterial wall.

Guide wires

The guide wire has two basic functions. First it leads the catheter through the puncture site, soft tissues and arterial wall, and into the lumen. Secondly, having been passed onward from the point of arterial entry, it leads the catheter over atheromatous plaques, irregularities and tortuosities with minimal trauma during catheter advancement. Guide wires are made with two inner cores of straight wire, around which a tightly coiled outer wire is wound. One of the inner wires tapers and terminates a few centimetres from the end, leaving a more flexible tip. The other inner wire is firmly secured at each end to protect the wire from breakage, a safety feature which should exist in all modern guide wires. The wires are made with straight or J shaped tips and both types should be available. The J shaped tip is particularly used in older patients, when atheroma or arterial tortuosity is likely. The flexible curved tip passes over surface irregularities with minimal risk of damage. Teflon-coated guide wires facilitate passage, particularly when polyurethane catheters are used. The guide wire must closely fit the catheter tip and pass closely, but freely, through the puncture needle. Commonly used guide wire diameters in adults are 0.89 and 0.97 mm. The guide wire should be at least 20 cm longer than the catheter being used. Guide wires can be coated with benzylkonium heparin precipitate to deter thrombus formation (Amplatz, 1971).

Manipulation of the catheter tip into position for selective angiography is often facilitated by the use of guide wires. Sometimes wires with variable tip stiffness (moveable core guide wires) are particularly helpful when catheter placement is difficult.

Catheters

Most catheters are now manufactured and supplied to order in a variety of sizes complete with preformed curves, a tapered tip to fit closely a standard guide wire, and a Luer Lok connection. They are made of polyethylene, teflon, polyurethrane or dacron and contain barium, bismuth or lead salts to render them radio-opaque. Different catheter materials have particular qualities and the choice of catheter depends on the requirements of the particular situation. Teflon catheters are suitable for mainstream injections. They have a low coefficient of friction and are very strong.

They are able to withstand high pressure, so that small thin-walled teflon catheters can deliver contrast medium very rapidly for aortography. However, such catheters have very little torque control, are difficult to reshape, and are unsuitable for selective catherization. Teflon can be autoclaved.

Polyethylene catheters are easily shaped in steam, a hot air jet or sterile hot water, have good torque control and are suitable for selective angiography. Polyethylene and the softer polyurethane catheters are available with wire mesh incorporated in their walls to provide additional torque for manipulation in selective angiography. Polyurethane catheters are more difficult to reshape, have a rubbery surface texture, and need to be used with teflon-coated guide wires. Polyethylene and polyurethane catheters require gas or cold sterilization.

The outer diameter of the catheter chosen should generally be the smallest that can deliver contrast medium at the required speed, the catheter also having suitable characteristics for manipulation and positioning. Catheter sizes from 5 to 7 French gauge are commonly used in adults. The largest diameters are required for mainstream aortic injections of viscous contrast media through longer catheters. Mainstream catheters must withstand high pressures but should have thin walls to facilitate rapid delivery of contrast medium. The smaller sizes are used for selective injections. Catheter sizes between 3 and 5 French gauge should be used for infants and small children. Tapered catheter tips may tear and damage the artery on entry. This is avoided by using a close-fitting guide wire and by the passage of a short rigid tapered tube (a dilator) of appropriate size before the catheter. Side holes increase the delivery rate when the end hole is significantly smaller than the inner diameter of the catheter and are therefore necessary in mainstream aortic catheters. In smaller selective catheters, it is resistance along the full length of the catheter that limits the delivery of contrast medium. The main value of side holes close to the tip of selective catheters is to increase stability during injection, thus reducing the tendency to catheter recoil and sub-intimal injection. With modern contrast medium injectors, acceleration of injection may be controlled to avoid recoil and side holes are usually unnecessary for stabilization in selective angiography. Side holes predispose to thrombus formation in the catheter tip.

Taps and connectors between the contrast medium injector and the catheter should have relatively large diameters to minimize flow resistance. All connecting tubes and connectors require Luer Lok fittings and must withstand maximum injection pressures.

CONTRAST MEDIA

Contrast media for angiography should have relatively high density, low viscosity and very low toxicity. The sodium and methylglucamine salts of diacetrizoate, metrizoate and iothalamate are commonly used. Methylglucamine salts cause less discomfort and less neurotoxicity but their high viscosity may limit the delivery rate through small catheters. Contrast media should be heated to body temperature before injection to reduce viscosity.

The choice of contrast medium depends on the arteriographic requirements of the particular situation. Mainstream aortography, celiac and superior mesenteric angiography are carried out with media containing 350–400 mg I/ml. Contrast media containing 280–300 mg I/ml and consisting mainly of methylglucamine salts are preferable for selective angiography in other areas. Ioxaglate (Hexabrix) and the non-ionic materials iopamidol (Niopam) and iohexol (Omnipaque) have recently become available and produce significantly less discomfort and less toxicity for the patient. Although significantly more expensive than conventional contrast media at present, there is much to be said for using non-ionic contrast agents, such as iopamidol or iohexol in concentrations of 300–370 mg I/ml, routinely in angiography.

Although most of the adverse effects which can result from intravascular contrast media are not clearly related to dose, and modern media are generally well-tolerated, attention must still be paid to the total volume of contrast medium injected during the full examination. This should not exceed approximately 4 ml/kg of standard contrast medium, or 5 ml/kg of non-ionic contrast medium.

PREPARATION OF THE PATIENT

The patient is, if possible, admitted to hospital on the day before arteriography. A full physical examination is performed and recorded, with particular attention to the peripheral pulses and the blood pressure. If the patient is on anticoagulant therapy, this is stopped and the prothrombin time is checked. A coagulation screen is carried out when there is any reason to suspect a bleeding disorder.

Before carrying out arteriography, it is important for the radiologist to inform the patient in general terms as to what the procedure involves and why it is necessary. After providing an opportunity for discussion, the patient is asked to sign a statement of informed consent for the procedure. In emergency cases, the first contact between patient and radiologist may be in the angiography room, and it is important to take time to inform and reassure him.

No food is allowed for at least 8 hours before arteriography, but dehydration must be avoided and the patient is encouraged to take simple fluids unless general anaesthesia is required. Both groins are shaved. The axillae are prepared if axillary artery catheterization is anticipated. An anxiolytic drug, such as diazepam may be prescribed on the ward if the patient appears unusually apprehensive, but it is otherwise usually best to delay premedication until immediately before the procedure. For most patients, premedication with intravenous diazepam, 5–10 mg, is useful and adequate. Pethidine 50–100 mg intravenously, and cyclizine, 50 mg intramuscularly, are often more effective as an immediate premedication. An intravenous fluid infusion is initiated in advance if there is any question of dehydration, a history of previous reaction to contrast medium or other situations which may require immediate drug therapy.

It is important that ward medical and nursing staff should know which angiographic procedure is planned for a particular patient.

CATHETERIZATION SITES

The common femoral artery is the most suitable and most widely used artery for catheter introduction, giving access to the aorta and all its branches, including those in the neck and upper and lower limbs, and to the left ventricle. The femoral artery is technically the easiest route, is most comfortable for the patient, and has the lowest incidence of local complications. Femoral or iliac artery stenosis, occlusion or previous surgery may contra-indicate femoral catheterization, the axillary artery then being the alternative of choice. Brachial artery catheterization has advantages for certain types of cardiac and neuro-angiography and may also be cannulated percutaneously for examination of the arm and hand, although the axillary approach is safer and preferable for other purposes. Direct percutaneous translumbar cannulation or catheterization of the abdominal aorta is usually a simple alternative for abdominal aortography or lower limb arteriography when the femoral approach is precluded by vascular disease.

THE TECHNIQUE OF FEMORAL ARTERY CATHETERIZATION

All lower limb pulses should be checked when the patient is on the angiographic table. If one femoral pulse is distinctly stronger than the other, this is usually chosen for catheterization. If the femoral pulses are equal, the right side is used by a right-handed operator. A test film should be taken to confirm exposure and positioning in the main area of filming, and to identify radio-opaque features and artefacts such as vascular calcification or residual contrast medium from previous radiological examinations.

Both groins, which should have previously been shaved, are prepared with a skin disinfectant such as chlorhexidine and are draped with sterile covers. The radiologist, having scrubbed and donned a sterile gown and gloves, then proceeds using an aseptic technique. Equipment on the sterile tray is checked, ensuring that the needle, guide wire and catheter fit correctly and are of correct length.

The femoral artery is palpated with the index finger and middle fingers. A point for arterial puncture is chosen approximately 2–4 cm below the inguinal ligament. Local anaesthetic is infiltrated 2 cm distal to this point, first raising a small weal in the skin and then infiltrating deep to the skin anteriorly and on each side of the femoral artery at the level of puncture. Five millimetres of 2% lignocaine is usually adequate but more may be required in obese patients. Infiltration of local anaesthetic should follow the expected oblique line of catheterization from skin surface to artery. A 2 mm incision is made at the skin entry point with the tip of a scalpel blade. The arterial pulse is palpated above this point, with two or three finger tips pressing firmly, and the thin wall 18 gauge arterial needle assembly is introduced at an angle of 30–45° through the skin and soft tissues to the artery. Particularly in slim patients, it is usually possible to feel the needle tip in contact with the anterior arterial wall and to then thrust the needle through this into the lumen. If the anterior wall cannot be distinctly felt, it may be necessary to pass the needle through the anterior and posterior walls and thus transfix the artery. The base of the needle pulsates directly up and down when the needle is in the artery. Rotatory pulsation indicates that it is medial or lateral to the artery and requires to be repositioned. The stylet is removed and the cannula is then slowly withdrawn until a good position within the artery is indicated by a strong pulsatile flow of blood from the needle. A poor flow indicates that the cannula is poorly positioned and should be adjusted until a good flow is obtained. The base of the cannula is then depressed slightly and the flexible end of the guide wire is gently introduced into the artery and advanced approximately 20 cm. If a simple 18 gauge thin-walled needle without stylet is used, entry into the arterial lumen is followed by immediate pulsatile

flow back. The base of the needle should then be depressed toward the skin surface and the guide wire inserted in the same way. The cannula or needle is then removed while finger pressure is applied over the arterial puncture site and the catheter is slid over the guide wire into the artery (Fig. 8.2). Introduction of a

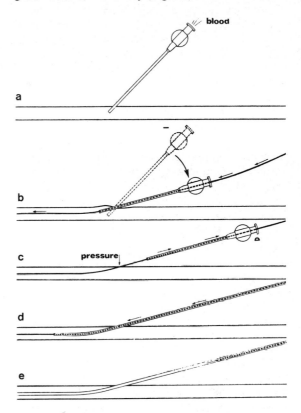

Fig. 8.2 Percutaneous insertion of arterial catheter
(a) Cannula (or needle) tip well positioned in lumen of artery and free backflow of blood
(b) Base of cannula depressed and flexible end of guide wire advanced through it.
(c) Cannula removed leaving guidewire in the artery. Digital pressure over puncture site prevents bleeding
(d) Catheter inserted over guide wire
(e) After positioning catheter tip at injection site, the guide wire is removed.

firm plastic vessel dilator over the guide wire before the catheter is introduced facilitates catheter entry and reduces the incidence of damage to the catheter tip and artery. The dilator should be of similar size or slightly smaller than the catheter, and is inserted with forward thrust and rotation.

The guide wire must not be advanced against resistance. If it does not pass freely through the cannula or needle, the latter is not properly positioned in the artery. If resistance is met during advance of the wire within the artery, the wire should be monitored fluoroscopically and not forced onward. Catheters should always be advanced within arteries over a guide wire with the flexible wire tip leading. The final position of the catheter tip is chosen under fluoroscopic control. The guide wire is then withdrawn, the catheter is flushed with heparinized saline and a small amount of contrast medium is injected by hand to confirm that the catheter tip is free and in a correct position before pressure injection.

Special attention must be given to catheterization of infants and small children. The examination usually requires to be carried out under general anaesthesia. Arteries in children are particularly prone to develop spasm and secondary thrombosis. Arterial puncture should be performed with an 18 or 20 gauge thin wall needle which facilitates puncture of the anterior wall alone. The needle is carefully advanced until pulsatile arterial blood flows through it, indicating that it is in the lumen. The base of the needle is then depressed and a small diameter guide wire is introduced carefully through the needle. The needle is removed and a narrow gauge dilator is introduced over the guide wire with rotatory movement. This is then withdrawn and the catheter is inserted over the wire into the lumen. Catheters greater than 6 French outer diameter should not be used in children.

Irrigation of the catheter during the procedure is important to prevent clot formation. Continuous flushing is effective with single end hole catheters, but fails to irrigate the tip when side holes are present. A closed continuous flushing system with manifold and stopcocks allows alternate pressure monitoring, catheter flushing and contrast medium injection. This is particularly helpful in cardiac angiography and can also be used for pressure controlled vessel puncture, but the pressure measurement system is cumbersome and unnecessary for most types of general and selective arteriography. The catheter should be flushed with heparinized saline or dextrose solution. A suitable fluid for catheter flushing is 250–500 units of heparin added to 500 ml of either 0.9% saline or 5% dextrose solution. The catheter should be flushed frequently with approximately 5 ml of heparinized fluid at a time. A little blood should be aspirated back into the syringe on each occasion before flushing. The quantity of fluid used should be monitored and kept to a minimum, particularly in patients with low cardiac reserve. Systemic heparinization has been advocated to reduce the incidence of thrombosis on the catheter and guide wire and in the access artery (Wallace et al., 1972). As soon as the catheter has been positioned 3000–5000 units of heparin are injected through it.

Although not in general use, this method has particular value for prolonged selective angiography, when there is predisposition to thrombosis (narrowed arteries, arterial spasm and slow flow), and during selective cervico-cephalic angiography where the development and separation of even tiny fragments of thrombus may be a serious complication. Post-catheterization bleeding at the puncture site is not usually a problem but, if necessary, is controlled by injecting 10 mg of protamine sulphate for every 1000 units of heparin given.

At the conclusion of the examination, the catheter is withdrawn while firm digital pressure is applied at the arterial puncture site. Pressure is continued after catheter withdrawal and should be firm enough to prevent bleeding without completely occluding the femoral pulse. Compression should be maintained for a minimum of 10 minutes and until haemostasis is secure. The time required for compression depends on many factors which include catheter size, duration of the procedure, the amount of catheter manipulation which has taken place, arterial disease, systemic blood pressure, and the use of anticoagulants.

After-care of the patients

At the conclusion of the procedure, it is important to check distal pulses and the condition of the limb below the puncture site. The patient is kept recumbant and is returned to the ward for complete bed rest for 24 hours. Observation of the puncture site for evidence of bleeding or haematoma formation and recording of pulse and blood pressure should take place every 15 minutes for 4 hours and then 4 hourly for 24 hours. Pressure dressings over the puncture site are not generally necessary and make observation difficult. A small adhesive dry dressing is usually sufficient. This may be supplemented with compression from a sandbag applied over the puncture site during the patient's transfer to the ward.

AXILLARY ARTERY CATHETERIZATION

The axillary artery is more superficial than the femoral artery and is usually easy to puncture and catheterize. It is, however, a smaller vessel than the femoral artery and is situated close to brachial plexus. Prolonged procedures and catheters larger than 7 French gauge should be avoided and catheter changes should be kept to a minimum, because the axillary artery is more prone to spasm than the femoral artery. Haematoma formation in this area may result in nerve damage.

Indications

Because of the significantly higher incidence of complications from axillary catheterization, this route should only be used when femoral catherization is contra-indicated or impossible and the translumbar approach is not an appropriate alternative. If both axillary arteries are patent and accessible, the side for catheterization depends on the region to be examined. Catheterization of the left axillary artery is performed for the investigation of the descending thoracic aorta, abdominal aorta, pelvis and lower extremities. Selective splanchnic and renal angiography is also better from the left side and is usually straight-forward from this approach. Catheterization of the right axillary artery is used for arteriography of the ascending aorta for selective studies of the head and neck. This vessel may also be used for selective coronary angiography and left ventriculography.

Contra-indications

Axillary catheterization is contra-indicated in the presence of significant subclavian or axillary artery disease. If femoral catheterization is contra-indicated due to arterial disease, it is likely that the axillary and subclavian arteries are also diseased and the translumbar approach is then preferable to axillary catherization for arteriography of the aorta and lower extremities.

Technique

Preparation of the patient is similar to that for the femoral approach, except that the axillae are shaved. The patient lies supine on the angiography table with the arm raised to a right angle, the elbow flexed, and the hand externally rotated. It may be necessary to tie the hand to help maintain this position or for the patient to rest his head on the hand. The axillary artery can be palpated against the neck of the humerus in this position. The point of the arterial puncture should, if possible, be just below the axillary fold. As with femoral artery catheterization, the area is prepared with skin antiseptic and is draped with sterile towels. Local anaesthetic is infiltrated into the skin 1–2 cm below the point of arterial entry. A 2 mm skin incision is made and the thin wall arterial needle is introduced, in the line of the artery, at an angle of approximately 30° to the skin surface. The artery is stabilized between two finger tips while the needle is inserted. Although the axillary artery is more superfi-

cial than the femoral, it is also smaller and more mobile. Puncture of only the anterior wall is difficult and the artery is often transfixed. The needle is then gently drawn back and, when free blood flow occurs, a guide wire is inserted and advanced 8–10 cm along the arterial lumen. The needle is then withdrawn and a small plastic dilator is introduced over the guide wire. The dilator is then replaced by the catheter which is advanced with a J tipped guide wire leading. Fluoroscopic control is important in this region as it is easy inadvertently to enter branch arteries. The position must be carefully checked if any resistance is encountered while advancing the guide wire, because even minor intimal damage can be dangerous when close to the origin of cerebral arteries.

Catherization of the thoracic and abdominal aorta from the left axillary artery is readily accomplished in young patients. With advancing age, the angle that the subclavian artery makes with the aortic arch becomes increasingly sharp and the guide wire and catheter tend to pass into the ascending aorta. It may be difficult to induce the catheter to turn into the descending aorta, but this manoeuvre can usually be achieved by inserting a catheter with a curved tip which is directed towards the descending aorta. The guide wire can then be fed downward and the catheter will follow when the stiff portion of the wire is well into the descending aorta.

Careful digital pressure over the arterial puncture site is important to avoid haematoma after axillary artery catheterization.

SELECTIVE CATHETERIZATION

Selective arterial studies provide optimal arteriographic detail of a localized region or organ, avoiding the overlap by other opacified vessels which may obscure important detail on main stream aortography. The contrast injection rate in selective arteriography should approximately equal the normal blood flow rate in the particular artery, in order to achieve maximum opacification in that vessel and its branches. Most selective catheterization is performed with pre-curved catheters directed from the aorta into the branch artery under fluoroscopic control. An alternative system employs a flexible straight catheter, the tip of which is curved for direction into the branch artery by the introduction of a pre-shaped guide wire or a guide wire whose tip can be curved (deflected) by external control. (Hawkins & Melichar, 1977; Rosch & Grollman, 1969.)

A combination of pre-curved catheter and shaped guide wire or tip deflecting guide wire is often useful

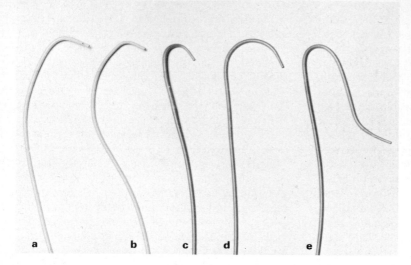

Fig. 8.3 Examples of some commonly used pre-shaped selective arterial catheters.

(a) Renal shape. End hole and two opposing side holes close to catheter tip.

(b) Cobra shape. Combination of two curves helps to stabilize catheter in aortic branch during contrast injection, and also facilitates advance for super selective catheterization.

(c) 1.5 cm J curve. Commonly used for inferior mesenteric and ipsilateral internal iliac arteriography.

(d) 3 cm J curve. Commonly used for renal, coeliac, superior mesenteric and adrenal arteriography.

(e) Sidewinder shape. Suitable for catheterization of renal and most splanchnic aortic branches.

for highly selective (super-selective) catheterization of more distal branch arteries. Co-axial catheter systems may also be used for highly selective angiography. The outer firm catheter is pre-shaped to enter the origin of the aortic branch and, through this first catheter, a flexible small inner catheter is passed further into the branch artery.

When pre-shaped selective catheters are used, the primary curve at the distal end of the catheter is chosen to match the angle that the branch artery makes with the aorta. A more proximal curve may help to advance and maintain the catheter within the branch artery (Fig. 8.3). When the aorta is ectatic, wider curves are required for stability during contrast medium injection. Although arterial catheters should always be as small as possible, good torque control is required for manipulation and there should be sufficient radio-opacity for clear visibility on fluoroscopy. Sizes from 5 to 7 French gauge are commonly used. The injection rate and volume of contrast medium depend upon the blood flow and size of the vascular bed. High injection rates tend to produce catheter recoil. This can be offset by placing the catheter well into the selected branch, using appropriate shape and width of curve on the catheter so that it rests against the opposite side of the aorta, and by prolonging the acceleration phase of the contrast medium injection. Side holes near the tip of the catheter also help to produce stability but they predispose to thrombus formation.

Selective arteriography, particularly in the abdomen, should be preceded by main stream aortography. This reveals the position and condition of branch artery origins and developmental variations of arterial anatomy which might otherwise complicate the

performance and confuse interpretation of selective arteriography.

After studying the aortogram, an appropriate catheter is chosen for the selective arteriogram. Although polyethylene catheters are usually supplied pre-shaped, they can be re-shaped or modified after heating in steam, hot air or sterile boiling water.

A guide wire is then re-introduced through the aortogram catheter which is withdrawn and replaced by the selective catheter.

TRANSLUMBAR AORTOGRAPHY

Indications

The principal indication for translumbar aortography is the investigation of the lower abdominal aorta, pelvic and lower limb arteries in patients where the femoral catheter approach is precluded by arterial disease. For this purpose, the aorta is entered at the level of the third lumbar vertebra. High puncture at T12–L1 level can be carried out to visualize the upper abdominal aorta in patients with severe aortic disease below that level. It is also possible to introduce, by the translumbar route, a catheter which can be advanced upwards for thoracic aortography when the femoral and axillary routes are contra-indicated (Stocks *et al.*, 1969).

Contra-indications

Bleeding from the aortic puncture site is inevitable after this procedure as local compression is not possible. Bleeding disorders, anticoagulant therapy and severe hypertension are therefore contra-indications to translumbar aortography. Abdominal aortic aneurysms and aortic grafts should not be punctured by the translumbar approach but, if necessary, high translumbar puncture may still be possible in these cases.

Technique

Although some radiologists prefer the routine use of general anaesthesia, translumbar aortography can be carried out satisfactorily with local anaesthesia in most patients. A plain film of the abdominal area is useful to identify relevant abnormalities such as lumbar scoliosis or aortic calcification, the latter sometimes demonstrating tortuosity or displacement of the aorta. A lateral plain film should also be obtained when there is a suspicion of abdominal aortic aneurysm. When the procedure is being carried out under local anaesthesia, the patient may be premedicated with oral diazepam in the ward 1–2 hours beforehand and is given pethidine 50–100 ml intravenously and cyclizine 50 ml intramuscularly immediately before the procedure. Peripheral pulses are examined and the patient is placed in the prone position on the angiographic table. Translumbar aortography may be carried out with a 17.5 cm 16 gauge short-bevelled translumbar needle with fitting stylus, although a 22 cm needle and stylus with close fitting outer plastic sheath is preferable (Fig. 8.4). For standard low translumbar aortography, the aorta is entered at the level of the third lumbar vertebra (L3) from a left postero–lateral approach at right angles to the aorta or with slight cranial angulation. The skin entry point is chosen 2–4 cm above the iliac crest and 9–11 cm (approximately one hand's breadth) lateral to the mid-line. Local anaesthetic is infiltrated into and below the skin in a line directed towards the abdominal aorta at L3 level. A 20 cm 20 gauge needle is suitable and is directed at approximately 45° from vertical towards the left side of aorta immediately anterior to the spine. It is often helpful to direct the needle first on to the anterior margin of the vertebral body, then to withdraw it a few centimetres and then advance it slightly anterior to the vertebra. The needle position may then be checked with fluoroscopy and a total of approximately 10 ml of 2% lignocaine is infiltrated at that site and along the needle track before it is withdrawn. The translumbar needle assembly is then inserted along the same track. Pulsation can be felt when the needle is closely apposed to the lateral wall of the aorta and it is then pushed sharply into the lumen. The stylet is then

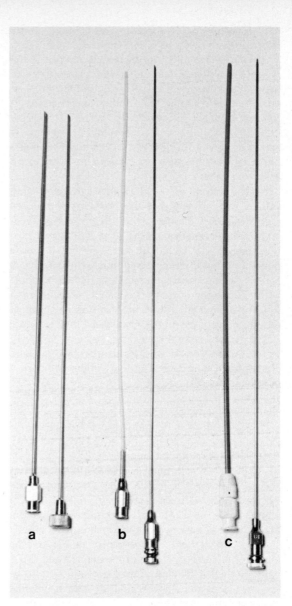

Fig. 8.4 Translumbar needle and plastic sheath-needle assemblies.
(a) 17.5 cm 16 gauge short bevelled translumbar needle with fitting stylus.
(b) 22 cm 18 gauge teflon sheath with matching needle and stylus.
(c) 22 cm 18 gauge polyethylene sheath with matching needle and stylus.

removed. The needle is withdrawn slightly and, if necessary, repositioned if free backflow of blood is not obtained. A small hand injection of contrast medium is made under fluoroscopic control when good back flow occurs to confirm that the needle tip is well positioned in the lumen and clear of branch artery origins before pressure injection is carried out. If a plastic sheath cannula is being used, the inner needle is removed and a J-tipped guide wire is inserted. The plastic cannula is passed over the guide wire and further up into the aorta. Another test injection of contrast is made to make sure that the tip of the cannula is suitably placed for the aortogram. If required, downward direction of the plastic cannula can be achieved using a pre-curved guide wire or tip deflector system.

High translumbar cannulation is carried out in a similar way, except that the needle is introduced approximately 2 cm below the 12th rib with a slight cranial angulation to enter the aorta at T12 level.

Although the technique of translumbar aortic puncture is usually simple and quick, difficulties can arise in patients with spinal scoliosis, tortuosity of the aorta, narrowing of the aortic lumen, or occlusion at the level of puncture. These problems may necessitate repositioning of the needle, usually at a higher level.

The patient is kept in bed for 24 hours following translumbar arteriography. Pulse and blood pressure are recorded quarter hourly for 4 hours and then 4 hourly for 24 hours.

BRACHIAL ARTERY PUNCTURE

Brachial artery cannulation or catheterization is used to study the vertebral and right carotid circulations and in some cardiac investigations (see Chapters 8–12 and 18–20). Direct cannulation of the brachial artery can also be used for arteriography of the forearm and hand. For this purpose the technique is usually simple. The patient is positioned supine on the angiography table with the arm extended and externally rotated. After skin preparation and draping of the lower arm and elbow region, the site of brachial artery puncture is chosen at a point where the pulse is distinctly palpable in the lower third of the arm above the cubital fossa. Five millilitres of 2% lignocaine is infiltrated and a small skin incision is made approximately 1.5 cm distal to the chosen site of arterial puncture. The puncture is then made with the needle directed in the line of the artery, making an angle of approximately 20° with the skin surface. A 5 cm needle assembly with a close fitting 18 gauge outer plastic sheath is useful for this procedure. The operator stabilizes the artery with the finger tips of his other hand during insertion of the needle. It may be necessary to transfix the vessel but, if it can be distinctly felt, it is often possible to puncture only the anterior wall. The needle is withdrawn and the plastic

sheath is very slowly pulled back until there is a free back-flow of blood. A short straight guide wire is then inserted beyond the tip of the plastic sheath, which is then slid over the wire up into the artery. The base of the cannula is then fixed to the skin surface with sterile tape. The guide wire is withdrawn and a plastic connecting tube, which has previously been filled with heparinized saline, is attached to the cannula for perfusion before the injection of contrast medium.

ARTERIOGRAPHY OF THE EXTREMITIES (Table 8.1)

The commonest indication for peripheral arteriography is the assessment of atherosclerosis causing stenosis or occlusion and sometimes aneurysm or dissection. Peripheral arteriography is also used for the evaluation of congenital vascular malformation, arteritis, embolism, and in the investigation of bone and soft tissue tumours.

LOWER EXTREMITY ARTERIOGRAPHY

Femoral artery catheterization with the injection of contrast medium into the lower abdominal aorta is the preferred technique for lower extremity arteriography. Radiographs must show the lower abdominal aorta and the arteries of the pelvis and both lower limbs. The translumbar approach is usually preferable to axillary catheterization when the femoral approach is contra-indicated or impossible due to disease of the lower abdominal aorta or ilio-femoral arteries. The injection of contrast medium through a short plastic cannula inserted into the femoral artery is a simple alternative technique when the problem is confined to one extremity.

Bilateral lower limb arteriography, using the femoral approach, can be carried out with a 50 cm, 6 French gauge, thin wall straight teflon catheter with an end hole and ten side holes (Fig. 8.5). It is introduced over a 100 cm flexible J tipped guide wire, 0.89 or 0.97 mm in diameter, and is positioned in the lower abdominal aorta with all the side holes above the bifurcation.

The position of the catheter tip, if this method has been used, is confirmed fluoroscopically with a small test injection of contrast medium. Blood flow rates in the lower limbs are unpredictable and frequently unequal in the presence of arterial disease. To overcome this difficulty, and to keep repeated injections of contrast medium and film series to a minimum,

Table 8.1 Arteriography of the extremities

Examination	Contrast medium	Contrast volume	Injection rate	Filming delay	Film programme
Bilateral lower limb arteriography (aortic injection above bifurcation)	Iopamidol 300, Iohexol 300 or Ioxaglate 320 or equivalent	100 ml	14 ml/s	3 s	Films at 1/s with 2 films in each of 4 or 5 positions (35 × 35 cm film changer and moving table top)
Single lower limb arteriography (femoral artery injection)	Iopamidol 300, Iohexol 300 or Ioxaglate 320 or equivalent	35 ml	8–10 ml/s	1 s	Films at 1/s 2 films in each of 3 or 4 positions (35 × 35 cm film changer and moving table top)
Upper limb arteriography (subclavian artery injection)	Iopamidol 300, Iohexol 300 or Ioxaglate 320 or equivalent	25 ml	8 ml/s	0.5 s	2 films/s for 2 s in 1st position, 1 film/s for 2 s in 2nd position, 1 film every 2 s for 8 s in 3rd position (35 × 35 cm film changer and moving table top)
Forearm and hand arteriography (brachial artery injection)	Iopamidol 300, Iohexol 300 or Ioxaglate 320 or equivalent	15 ml	5 ml/s	2 s	1 film/s for 10 s (single position)

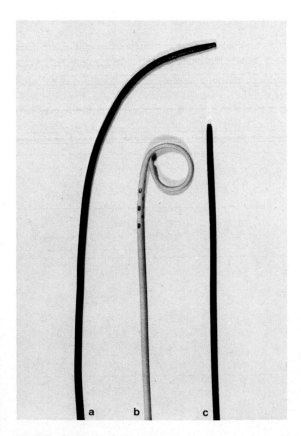

Fig. 8.5 Mainstream aortic catheters.
(a) 100 cm 7F teflon catheter with distal curve, end hole and ten side holes. Suitable for arch aortography from femoral artery approach.
(b) 100 cm 7F polyurethane catheter with pig-tail tip and multiple side holes. Suitable for left ventricular and aortic mainstream arteriography.
(c) 50 cm 6F teflon straight catheter with end hole and ten side holes. Suitable for abdominal aortography.

a relatively large volume of contrast medium is injected at a slow rate with initial delay in the onset of filming. This method is more important when using a serial 35 × 35 cm film changer with automatic table movement. The discomfort produced by the injection of contrast medium into limb arteries is greatly reduced by the use of non-ionic contrast media instead of conventional ionic agents. Approximately 100 ml of contrast medium is injected at a rate of 14 ml/s, with 2.5 s delay between the onset of injection and the commencement of filming. Two radiographs may be exposed at each of 4 or 5 consecutive positions at a rate of 1/s (Fig. 8.6). Although this sequence is satisfactory in the majority of cases, it requires modification for individual patients when the blood flow is unusually slow or fast. The inclusion of the pelvis and both lower limbs on each exposure when a 130 cm large field serial film changer is used largely overcomes the problem of unequal lower limb flow rates, the injection of a smaller volume of contrast medium (approximately 50 ml) then being satisfactory. It is important, in the assessment of vascular disease, to visualize inflow and outflow of the affected areas. A separate abdominal aortogram may be required if the lower abdominal aorta is diseased, particularly when there is an aortic aneurysm. When the lower abdominal aorta is occluded, important collaterals originate from the high lumbar and intercostal arteries and the peripheral run-off can best be seen when these vessels are opacified with a contrast injection in the upper abdominal or lower thoracic aorta.

A steep oblique or lateral view is indicated when there is doubt about the presence or severity of an arterial stenosis in the A–P projection. Oblique views are particularly helpful for assessing stenosis of the iliac arteries and at the origin of the deep femoral artery.

A 5 cm needle assembly with close fitting 18 gauge outer plastic sheath is suitable for single lower limb arteriography. This is introduced percutaneously in a retrograde direction into the common femoral artery and approximately 35 ml of contrast medium is injected at 8–10 ml/s (see Table 8.1).

UPPER LIMB ARTERIOGRAPHY

Preliminary arch aortography may be indicated if disease is suspected at the origin of the subclavian or innominate arteries or if the origins of these vessels are found to be anomalous. In most cases only selective arteriography is required. Percutaneous catheterization of the femoral artery is the preferred approach for upper limb arteriography. A 100 cm 6 or 7 French gauge polyethylene catheter with precurved tip and a single end hole, the Headhunter No. 1 shape being suitable (Fig. 8.7), is manipulated into the subclavian artery. Approximately 25 ml of contrast medium is injected at 8 ml/s and serial A–P radiographs of the axilla, arm, forearm and hand are taken. Additional series in lateral or oblique projections are obtained if required (see Table 8.1).

Contrast filling of arteries in the distal forearm and hand is often delayed by reactive vaso-constriction, even with non-ionic contrast media. This can be overcome by warming the hand and forearm with an electric heating pad which is withdrawn immediately before the injection. If arteriography of only the forearm and hand is required, the catheter is advanced and contrast medium is injected into the brachial artery at approximately 8 cm above the elbow. Alternatively, direct percutaneous cannulation of the brachial artery may be carried out and contrast medium is injected at the same level (see Table 8.1).

ARTERIOGRAPHY OF THE THORACIC AORTA (Table 8.2)

Thoracic aortography is indicated before conducting selective catheter arteriography of the carotid and vertebral arteries for vascular disease. It is also used in the investigation of suspected abnormalities of the thoracic aorta itself; such as a congenital anomaly,

Table 8.2 Arteriography of the thoracic aorta and arch branches

Examination	Contrast medium	Contrast volume	Injection rate	Filming delay	Film programme
Thoracic aortography (ascending aortic injection)	Iopamidol 370, Iohexol 350 or equivalent	60 ml	30 ml/s	0.5 s	3 films/s for 3 s 1 film every 2 s for 6s
Common carotid arteriography	Iopamidol 300, Iohexol 300 or equivalent	10 ml	7 ml/s	0.2 s	2 films/s for 3 s 1 film/s for 3 s 1 film every 2 s for 4 s
Internal carotid arteriography	Iopamidol 300, Iohexol 300 or equivalent	8 ml	6 ml/s	0.2 s	2 films/s for 3 s 1 film/s for 3 s 1 film every 2 s for 4 s
External carotid arteriography	Iopamidol 300, Iohexol 300 or equivalent	6 ml	4 ml/s	0.2 s	2 films/s for 3 s 1 film/s for 3 s 1 film every 2 s for 4 s
Vertebral arteriography	Iopamidol 300, Iohexol 300 or equivalent	5–6 ml	4 ml/s	0.2 s	2 films/s for 3 s 1 film/s for 3 s 1 film every 2 s for 4 s
Innominate arteriography	Iopamidol 300, Iohexol 300 or equivalent	20 ml	10 ml/s	0.2 s	3 films/s for 2 s 1 film/s for 3 s

atherosclerotic or post-arteritic stenosis, aneurysm, dissection or rupture.

Catheterization by the percutaneous femoral approach is preferred, but axillary catheterization is an alternative. The right axillary artery is generally preferred as it provides better access than the left axillary artery for subsequent selective studies of brachio-cephalic vessels. High translumbar puncture of the abdominal aorta, with the introduction of a small teflon catheter which can be advanced over a guide wire into the ascending aorta, is another method which may be considered when there is a contra-indication to femoral and axillary catheterization.

A 100 cm 7 French gauge thin wall teflon catheter with end hole and multiple side holes, or a similar catheter with a pigtail tip, are used from the femoral approach (Fig. 8.5). From the axillary approach, a 50 cm 6 French gauge teflon catheter with an end hole and multiple side holes is satisfactory. The reduced resistance associated with the shorter catheter length enables the smallest catheter to deliver contrast medium sufficiently fast for even thoracic aortography. Good opacification of the thoracic aorta in most adults is provided by 60 ml of iopamidol 370 or iohexol 350 delivered at 30 ml/s (Table 8.2). Films are obtained in the 60° right posterior oblique projection. Additional series in the 45° left posterior oblique and A–P projections may be required if there is still doubt about the presence, nature or extent of an aortic arch lesion, particularly when dissection or traumatic rupture of the aorta is suspected. Two oblique views should also be obtained in the investigation of cervical cerebrovascular disease if subsequent selective catheterization is contra-indicated or impossible.

SELECTIVE CERVICO-CEPHALIC ARTERIOGRAPHY

Indications for selective carotid and vertebral arteriography include intracranial investigations (see Central Nervous System, p. 285) and the investigation of vascular disease and tumours in the neck and face. Arch aortography should usually precede selective studies when arterial disease is suspected, in order to identify anomalies or disease at the origins of the aortic arch branches (Fig. 8.7). Marked atheromatous irregularity at the origin of the carotid, innominate or vertebral arteries is a contra-indication to selective catheterization because of the danger of dislodging thrombus into the cerebral circulation. Selective arteriography by direct percutaneous puncture is safer in this situation. Following thoracic arch aortography, the catheter is exchanged for a 100 cm 7 French gauge

preshaped polyethylene or polyurethane catheter with a single end hole. Various catheter shapes are available for use in this region (Fig. 8.8). The Headhunter No. 1 shape is suitable for transfemoral catheterization of the subclavian, carotid and vertebral arteries in most patients with normal or only mildly diseased arteries. The Headhunter No. 3 and various sizes of Sidewinder are useful for entry into tortuous or unusually angled aortic branch origins. The catheter tip should if possible be advanced well into the selected branch artery, led over a guide wire. If this is impossible due to pronounced tortuosity or a dilated aortic arch, contrast medium may have to be injected just distal to the vessel origin (Hinck et al., 1967; Simmons et al., 1973).

A 50 cm 6 French gauge catheter with a shepherd's crook or small Sidewinder shape is suitable from the axillary approach.

Selective carotid arteriograms are obtained in A–P and lateral projections and vertebral arteriograms in Towne's and lateral projections (see Table 8.2). Evaluation of vascular disease in the neck is incomplete without views of the intracranial vessels, the coexistance of intracranial arterial disease having an important influence on treatment.

In the assessment of arterio-venous malformations and tumours of the face and neck, it is usually advisable to carry out highly selective arteriography of the external carotid artery or its branches. This gives improved detail and avoids unnecessary injections of contrast medium into the intracranial circulation (Fig. 8.9). Superselective catheterization is also essential for embolization therapy.

ARTERIOGRAPHY OF THE ABDOMINAL AORTA (Table 8.3)

Abdominal aortography may be indicated in the investigation of abnormalities of the aorta itself and of its branch arteries. It is also the first part of a selective arteriographic examination of abdominal organs and the retroperitoneum.

Percutaneous transfemoral catheterization is the preferred approach. If this is contra-indicated or impossible, axillary artery catheterization may be a satisfactory alternative provided there is not significant disease of the axillary and subclavian arteries. Percutaneous translumbar aortography is often a simpler and safer alternative when the femoral approach is contra-indicated and subsequent selective arteriography is not required (see p. 104).

A straight 50 cm 6 French gauge thin wall teflon catheter with an end hole and multiple side holes is

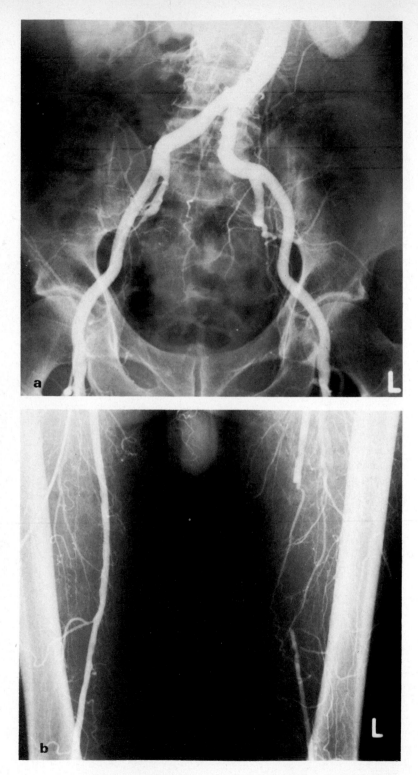

Fig. 8.6 (a) (b) (c) and (d) Lower extremity arteriography. Serial 35 × 35 cm films at four levels after slow large volume injection of contrast into lower abdominal aorta via transfemoral catheter. There is occlusion of left superficial femoral artery and diffuse disease within distal leg arteries.

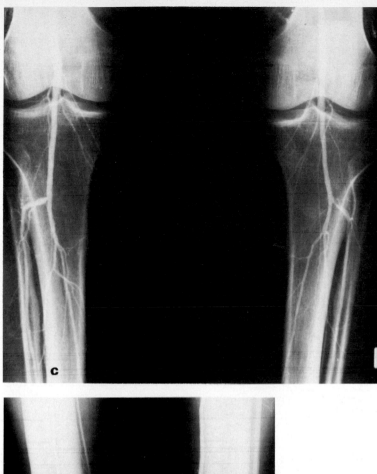

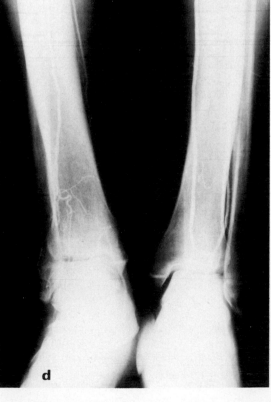

Table 8.3 Arteriography of the abdominal aorta and branches

Examination	Contrast medium	Contrast volume	Injection rate	Filming delay	Average film programme
Abdominal aortography (upper abdominal or lower thoracic aortic injection)	Iopamidol 370, Iohexol 350 or equivalent	50 ml	25–30 ml/s	0.5 s	3 films/s for 2 s 1 film/s for 3 s 1 film every 2 s for 6 s
Selective renal arteriography	Iopamidol 300, Iohexol 300 or equivalent	12 ml	6 ml/s	0.5 s	3 films/s for 2 s 1 film/s for 3 s 1 film every 2 s for 6 s
Selective coeliac arteriography	Iopamidol 370, Iohexol 350 or equivalent	50–70 ml	8–10 ml/s	0.5 s	2 films/s for 3 s 1 film/s for 3 s 1 film every 2 s for 18 s (to include portal venous phase)
Selective superior mesenteric arteriography	Iopamidol 370, Iohexol 350 or equivalent	50–70 ml	8 ml/s	0.5 s	1 film/s for 6 s 1 film every 2 s for 24 s (to include portal venous phase)
Selective inferior mesenteric arteriography	Iopamidol 370, Iohexol 350 or equivalent	25 ml	4 ml/s	0.5 s	2 films/s for 3 s 1 film/s for 3 s 1 film every 2 s for 12 s
Selective splenic arteriography	Iopamidol 370, Iohexol 350 or equivalent	50–60 ml	6 ml/s	0.5 s	1 film/s for 10 s 1 film every 2 s for 16 s (to include venous phase)
Selective hepatic arteriography	Iopamidol 370, Iohexol 350 or equivalent	40–50 ml	6 ml/s	0.5 s	2 films/s for 3 s 1 film/s for 4 s 1 film every 2 s for 6 s
Selective gastro-duodenal arteriography	Iopamidol 300, Iohexol 300 or equivalent	10–15 ml	5 ml/s	0.5 s	2 films/s for 3 s 1 film/s for 4 s 1 film every 2 s for 4 s
Selective dorsal pancreatic arteriography	Iopamidol 300, Iohexol 300 or equivalent	10 ml	2–5 ml/s	0.5 s	2 films/s for 3 s 1 film/s for 4 s 1 film every 2 s for 4 s
Selective left gastric arteriography	Iopamidol 300, Iohexol 300 or equivalent	10–15 ml	5 ml/s	0.5 s	2 films/s for 3 s 1 film/s for 4 s 1 film every 2 s for 4 s
Selective adrenal or inferior phrenic arteriography	Iopamidol 300, Iohexol 300 or equivalent	4–8 ml	Hand injection judged from fluoroscopy		2 films/s for 3 s 1 film/s for 4 s 1 film every 2 s for 4 s

suitable for the transfemoral approach. The low resistance associated with this relatively short catheter enables contrast medium to be delivered at a rate of 30 ml/s. For abdominal aortography, this catheter is positioned with its tip in the lower thoracic aorta. A 7 French gauge catheter with a pigtail tip and multiple side holes is an alternative (Fig. 8.5). While a pigtail catheter reduces the retrograde injection of contrast medium into the thoracic aorta it is inclined to develop thrombus within its distal curve and is less convenient

for subsequent catheter exchange. A 65 mm catheter is often necessary to reach the lower thoracic aorta, from the axillary approach, but an adequate injection rate of 25 ml/s can still be achieved with a 6 French thin wall catheter (Table 8.3).

Radiography of the abdominal aortogram is carried out in the A–P projection alone in most cases (Fig. 8.10). An additional lateral projection is indicated when it is necessary to visualize distinctly the origins of the splanchnic arteries (Fig. 8.11) or to assess the

Fig. 8.7 Catheter shapes commonly used for selective arteriography of aortic arch branches.
(a) Headhunter Number 3.
(b) Headhunter Number 1.
(c) Sidewinder.

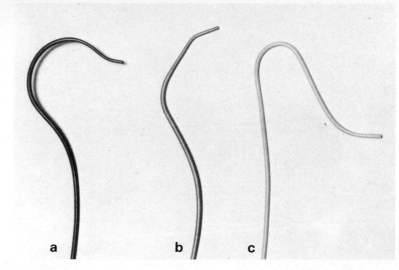

full extent of aortic disease, particularly dissection or aneurysm, when this is uncertain from the A–P series. Renal artery origins are usually shown adequately in the A–P projection, but overlap by splanchnic branches and uncertainty about stenosis at the renal artery orifice may necessitate additional views. A 20° right posterior oblique projection is then likely to be most helpful.

RENAL ARTERIOGRAPHY

Renal arteriography is indicated for the diagnosis and assessment of many forms of renal vascular disease, particularly in the context of reno-vascular hypertension and renal failure, when percutaneous angioplasty or revascularization surgery are being considered. It may also be indicated in the assessment and management of renal trauma, space-occupying masses in the kidney, and for the assessment of kidneys before and after transplantation.

The percutaneous transfemoral approach is preferred, but axillary catheterization may be a satisfactory alternative when necessary. Preliminary abdominal aortography demonstrates the overall abdominal vascular anatomy and any variations, anomalies or disease in the arteries. Supplementary renal arteries are common, arising at any level between the lower thoracic aorta and the iliac arteries, and must be recognized before performing and interpreting selective arteriograms (Fig. 8.12). The diameter, shape and condition of the aorta and renal arteries, as shown on the aortogram, influences the choice of catheter for selective arteriography. The aortic mainstream catheter, preferably 6 French gauge, is then

exchanged for a pre-shaped polyethylene or polyurethane selective catheter of similar size. A simple distal J curve is usually satisfactory, but many configurations, such as the Cobra or Sidewinder, can be used and may be helpful when the renal artery origin is unusually angled or deformed (Fig. 8.3). The selective catheter is then positioned with its tip in the renal artery, proximal to the first renal artery branch. The catheter should have a sufficiently wide distal curve to enable the shaft of the catheter to rest against the opposite aortic wall and deter recoil during contrast medium injection (Fig. 8.13). Contrast medium, e.g. 12 ml of iopamidol 300, or similar, is injected at 6 ml/s. Filming is carried out in the A–P projection, but additional oblique views can be very useful in elucidating or localizing abnormalities which are suspected or shown on the A–P series. The 45° posterior oblique projection shows the kidney in profile while the opposite oblique shows it en face. Renal artery origins may be shown by reflux of contrast medium during selective injections, but are often best seen on aortography.

Artefactual arterial stenosis may appear on selective renal arteriograms at the site of the catheter tip. This occurs most frequently in young patients, is due to arterial spasm, and is absent on the aortogram. Film sequences are shown in Table 8.3.

ARTERIOGRAPHY OF THE GASTROINTESTINAL TRACT, LIVER, SPLEEN AND PANCREAS

Arteriography of the gastrointestinal tract, liver, spleen and pancreas is indicated for the diagnosis and

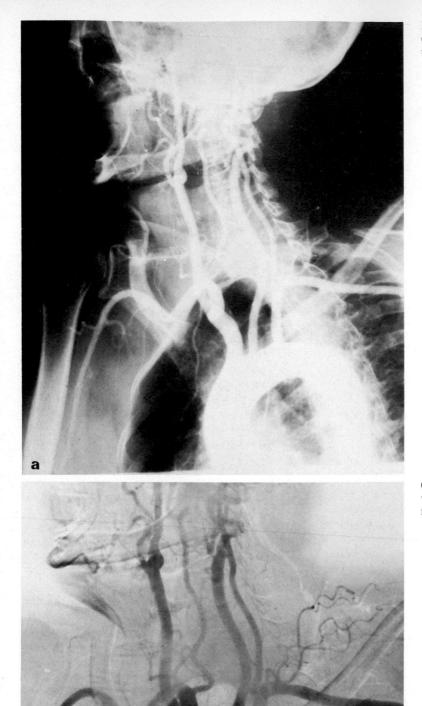

Fig. 8.8 Thoracic arch aortography. (a) Right posterior oblique projection to show brachio cephalic arteries.

(b) Photographic subtraction film of (a) which gives improved detail of contrast filled arteries.

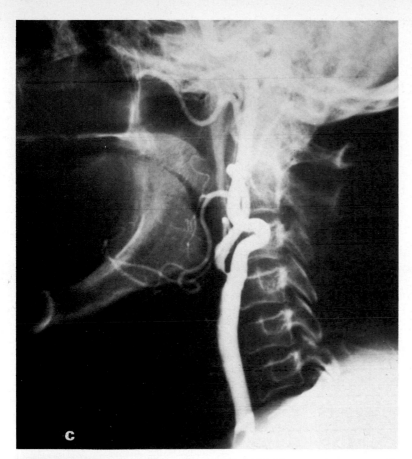

(c) Selective left common carotid arteriograms. Lateral view shows tight external carotid stenosis and tortuosity of internal carotid artery in the neck. (Same case as a and b.)

c

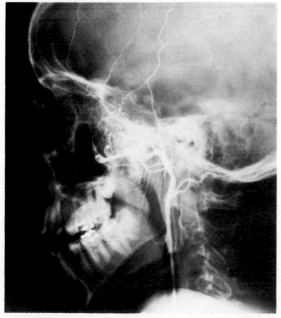

assessment of vascular disease, particularly when there is haemorrhage or evidence of ischaemia. It can also be the most sensitive method for identifying uncommon, highly vascular intestinal tumours such as leiomyomata and hamartomata, which may cause intestinal haemorrhage while being too small to be recognized by other investigations. While tumours and other space-occupying masses of liver and pancreas are usually assessed by radionuclide scanning, ultrasound and computed tomography, important information on the extent and resectability of hepatic and pancreatic tumours may be obtained from arteriography and portal venography. Certain tumours with characteristically high angiographic vascularity, such as hepatoma and islet cell tumour of the pancreas, may be recognized by arteriography when still very small. Arteriography also has an important

Fig. 8.9 Selective upper left external carotid angiography. A 100 cm 7F polyethylene catheter with Headhunter number 1 shape, introduced via the femoral artery, has been advanced into the upper part of the left external carotid artery. A hand injection of 8 ml of iopamidol 300 demonstrates profuse tumour circulation in a nasopharyngeal angiofibroma supplied mainly by the maxillary artery. (Arteriography before pre-operative embolization.)

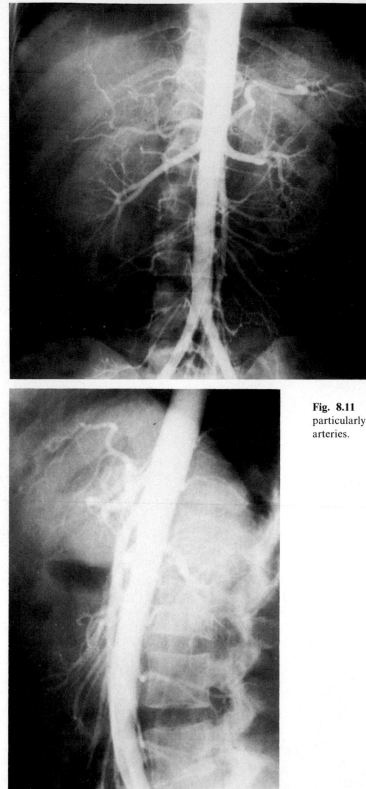

Fig. 8.10 Abdominal aortogram. A–P view. 50 ml of iopamidol 370 was injected at a rate of 30 ml/s through a 50 cm 6F straight teflon catheter with end and multiple side holes, introduced via the right femoral artery.

Fig. 8.11 Abdominal aortogram. Lateral view showing particularly the origins of coeliac and superior mesenteric arteries.

Fig. 8.12 Renal arteriography. Abdominal aortography before selective renal arteriography.

(a) Arterial phase. Single right renal artery. On the left side there is a main renal artery arising at normal level and a small supplementary lower pole renal artery which arises from the aorta immediately above the bifurcation.

(b) Parenchymal phase showing distinct nephrograms. The left kidney is developmentally larger than the right.

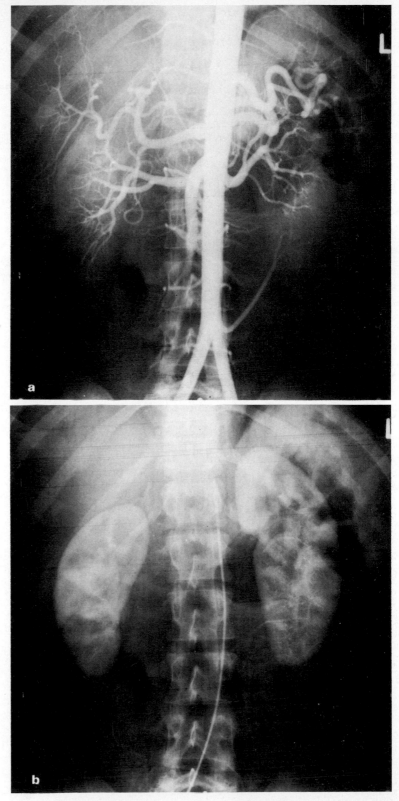

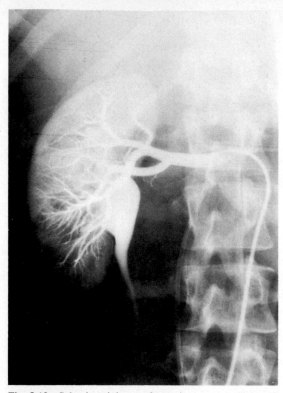

Fig. 8.13 Selective right renal arteriograms. A 65 cm 6F polyethylene catheter with 3 cm diameter J curve, introduced from the femoral approach is positioned in the right renal artery. The catheter shaft rests against the opposing aortic wall to resist recoil during injection of 12 ml of iopamidol 300 at a rate of 6 ml/s.

place in the investigation of patients with portal hypertension. Detailed selective arteriography is an essential part of interventional vascular procedures such as intra-arterial vasoconstrictor perfusion or embolization in the management of gastrointestinal haemorrhage, the embolization of tumours and percutaneous angioplasty of splanchnic artery stenosis.

Catheterization from the femoral artery is the preferred approach. When there is acute angulation of coeliac and superior mesenteric artery origins from the aorta, catheterization from the axillary artery provides the easiest access to these vessels and may be indicated when highly selective arteriography of coeliac or superior mesenteric branches is required but has been unsuccessful from the femoral artery.

Preliminary abdominal aortography is particularly helpful in the presence of anomalous arteries, stenosis of coeliac or mesenteric origins, or aortic disease. If selective studies or coeliac, superior and inferior mesenteric arteries are intended, however, the total dose of contrast medium and the duration of the examination may be justifiably reduced by omitting aortography in the knowledge that no important abnormality of the splanchnic arterial system will be missed if all three vessels are examined selectively.

A 65 cm 6 or 7 French gauge precurved polyethylene or polyurethane catheter with a single end hole is suitable. The ideal distal curve depends on aortic width, the angle and direction of the splanchnic branch, and whether superselective distal branch catheterization is also a requirement.

A simple 3 cm diameter single distal J curve is usually satisfactory for coeliac and superior mesenteric arteriography (Figs. 8.14 & 8.15). The Cobra shape may be more satisfactory when the artery arises from the aorta at a wider angle. The Sidewinder configuration is suitable for most coeliac and superior mesenteric arteriograms and has the additional capability of advancement into distal branches for highly selective (superselective) angiography.

A simple 1.5 cm diameter single distal J curve is usually suitable for inferior mesenteric arteriography (Fig. 8.3).

The inferior mesenteric artery is not always identified on abdominal aortography, but can usually be located with the selective catheter at the left anterolateral aspect of the aorta at the level of L3 (Fig. 8.16).

Radiography of selective coeliac, superior mesenteric and inferior mesenteric arteriograms is carried out in the A–P projection, additional oblique views being obtained for further elucidation or localization of abnormalities.

For coeliac or superior mesenteric arteriography, approximately 50 ml of iopamidol 370 or similar contrast medium is injected at 8 ml/s on average. Variation in volume and speed of injection depends on individual vessel size and flow rate. When visualization of the spleno-portal venous system is required, the volume of contrast medium for coeliac or superior mesenteric arteriography is increased to 65 or 70 ml. The venous phase can be enhanced by infusing a vasodilator such as 60 µg of prostaglandin $F_2\alpha$ into the superior mesenteric artery immediately before the selective injection of contrast medium (Legge, 1977).

Twenty-five millilitres of iopamidol 370 is usually adequate for selective inferior mesenteric arteriography (see Table 8.3).

Superselective arteriography of hepatic, splenic, left gastric, gastro-duodenal and dorsal pancreatic arteries may be required for detailed examination of these areas and before embolization therapy. Various catheter guide wire systems are suitable, but 65 cm 6 French gauge polyethylene catheters with pre-shaped primary and secondary distal curves as described by

Fig. 8.14 Selective coeliac angiography. A 65 cm 6F polyethylene catheter with 3 cm diameter J curve introduced via the right femoral artery, is positioned in the coeliac artery. 60 ml of iopamidol 370 has been injected at 10 ml/s.
(a) Arterial phase.

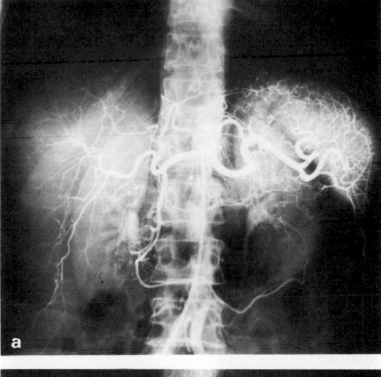

(b) Venous phase showing splenic and portal veins.

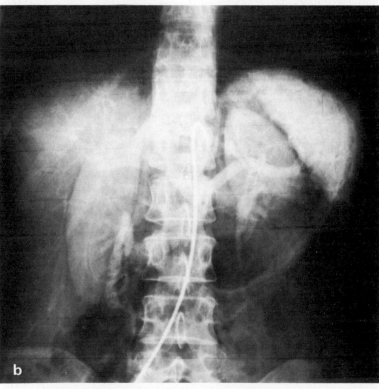

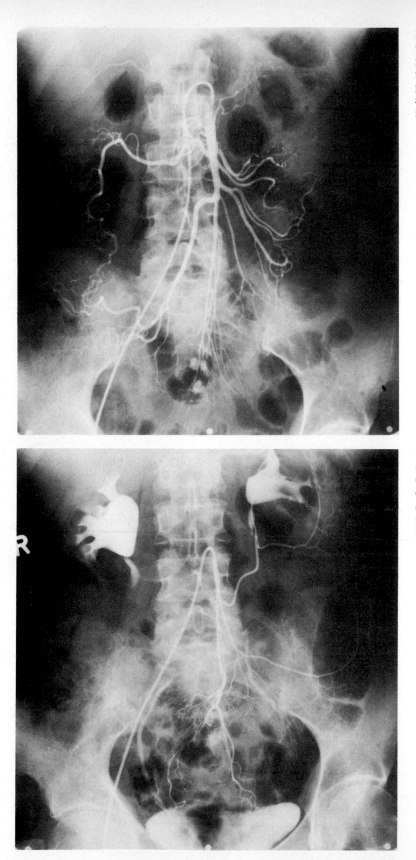

Fig. 8.15 Selective superior mesenteric arteriography—early arterial phase. Catheter and technique similar to coeliac angiography, with catheter positioned in the superior mesenteric artery. 50 ml of iopamidol 370 is being injected at 8 ml/s.

Fig. 8.16 Selective inferior mesenteric arteriography. A 65 cm 6F polyethylene catheter with 1.5 cm diameter J curve introduced via the right femoral artery is positioned in the inferior mesenteric artery. 25 ml of iopamidol 370 is injected at 4 ml/s.

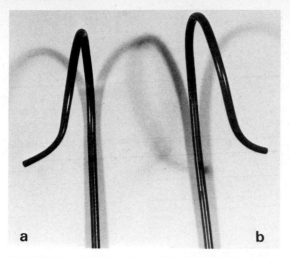

Fig. 8.17 Pre-shaped catheters with primary and secondary end curves.
(a) For hepatic artery catheterization
(b) For splenic artery catheterization.

Rosch and Grollman (1969), (Fig. 8.17) or the Sidewinder shape, are often successful and are relatively easy to use (Fig. 8.18). After the introduction of these catheters into the aorta, the distal curves have to be reconstituted by either rotation in the aortic arch or by using a catheter tip deflecting system. Super-selective catheterization of superior mesenteric artery branches is accomplished with similar multiple curved catheters introduced over an exchange guide wire which has been placed deep within the superior mesenteric artery. Average values for contrast medium volume, flow rates and film sequences are shown in Table 8.3.

ADRENAL ARTERIOGRAPHY

Vascular studies of the adrenal glands include arteriography, venography and adrenal vein sampling. These procedures are usually used for the localization or diagnosis of adrenal tumours when indicated after examination by ultrasound or computed tomography. Adrenal venography and venous sampling are more sensitive examinations than arteriography in the recognition of small tumours or hyperplasia of the adrenal gland. When a retroperitoneal mass has been discovered, arteriography is particularly valuable for confirming that it is of adrenal origin. Adrenal carcinoma, neuroblastoma, ganglioblastoma, and phaeochromocytoma are usually highly vascular and well shown by arteriography. Phaeochromocytomata, when multiple or ectopic, can also be localized with

aortography followed by appropriate selective arteriography. Patients with phaeochromocytomata should previously be stabilized on alpha and beta adrenergic blocking drugs to prevent reactive hypertensive episodes during the examination. When a functioning adrenal adenoma is suspected on the basis of clinical and biochemical findings, localization of even small tumours can often be achieved with computed tomography. If confirmation is necessary, it is most accurately obtained from selective adrenal venography and venous sampling.

The typical adrenal blood supply arises from three arteries. The inferior adrenal usually arises as a branch of the renal artery, the middle adrenal arises from the aorta, and the superior adrenal artery from the inferior phrenic artery which in turn may be a branch of the coeliac artery or arise directly from the aorta. The adrenal arteries are small, show frequent variations of the typical anatomical pattern, and anastomose freely with renal capsular and other retroperitoneal arteries. Catheterization is carried out from the femoral approach and abdominal aortography should precede selective arteriography. In the presence of a hypervascular adrenal gland or adrenal mass, one or more of the adrenal arteries is seen on the aortogram to be enlarged and this facilitates subsequent selective arteriography (Rossi, 1968).

Visualization of the inferior adrenal artery may be adequately achieved on selective renal arteriography, but is improved by infusing 5–10 μg of adrenalin in aqueous solution into the renal artery before contrast injection. Constriction of the renal, but not the adrenal, circulation occurs and provides preferential filling of the adrenal artery (Kahn, 1965). Middle adrenal and inferior phrenic arteries may usually be catheterized with a 6 or 7 French gauge selective catheter, with a 2.5–3 cm diameter distal J curve or with the Cobra head configuration (Fig. 8.19). The volume and rate of contrast injection depends on the size and flow rate within the artery. This should be assessed fluoroscopically and the contrast medium is injected by hand (see Table 8.3).

PELVIC ARTERIOGRAPHY (Table 8.4)

Arteriography of the pelvis is indicated in the assessment of primary vascular disease in this area and usually forms part of bilateral lower limb arteriography when contrast medium has been injected into the lower abdominal aorta. Localized arteriography of the pelvic area, supplemented when necessary by selective arteriography of the iliac arteries and their branches, is sometimes indicated in

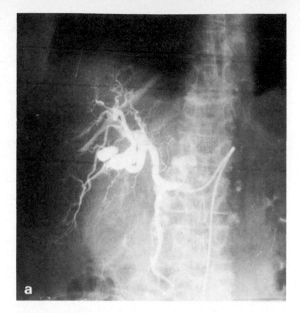

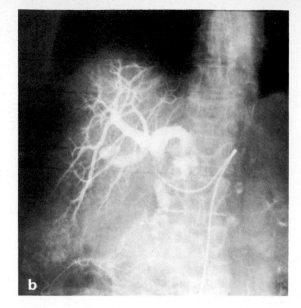

Fig. 8.18 Superselective right hepatic arteriography with sidewinder end shape, introduced via the femoral artery and advanced from the coeliac artery.
(a) Arterial phase showing a post traumatic arterio-portal venous fistula in the right lobe of liver.

(b) Venous phase showing contrast filling of portal venous branches via the fistula which was successfully closed by highly selective arterial embolization.

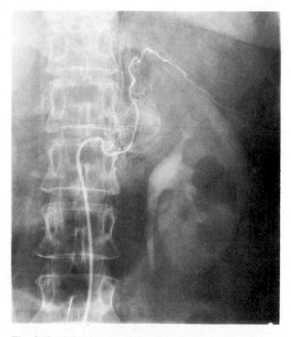

Fig. 8.19 Selective arteriography of enlarged left middle adrenal artery. A 6F polyethylene catheter with 2.5 cm diameter J curve has been positioned in the artery and 6 ml of iopamidol 300 injected slowly by hand. There is a 3 cm moderately vascular rounded adrenal tumour (phaeochromocytoma).

the assessment of symptomatic arterial stenosis and occlusion, congenital and acquired vascular malformation, arterial trauma, aneurysm, and pelvic haemorrhage. Although arteriography is an effective means of identifying the more vascular types of uterine and adnexal tumours, this is seldom required nowadays. Selective and super-selective arteriography is, however, an essential component of interventional vascular procedures such as arterial perfusion chemotherapy, the embolization of pelvic tumours, and embolization in the management of vascular malformations and focal haemorrhage.

While the percutaneous femoral catheter approach is preferred, left axillary catheterization is an alternative route. Translumbar cannulation of the lower abdominal aorta provides satisfactory mainstream arteriography of the pelvis without the possibility of subsequent selective arterial studies. From the femoral approach, a 50 cm 6 French gauge straight thin-walled teflon catheter with an end hole and multiple side holes, as used in abdominal aortography, is placed in the abdominal aorta with the side holes just above the bifurcation. Forty millilitres of iopamidol 370, or a similar contrast medium, is injected at a rate of 15 ml/ s. Radiography is performed in the A–P projection with additional oblique views when necessary to elucidate abnormalities which are seen or suspected in the A–P projection. Common and external iliac arteriography on the side of catheterization is easily carried out by withdrawal of the catheter to the

Table 8.4 Arteriography of the pelvis

Examination	Contrast medium	Contrast volume	Injection rate	Filming delay	Average film programme
Bilateral pelvic arteriography (injection above aortic bifurcation)	Iopamidol 370, Iohexol 350 or equivalent	40 ml	15 ml/s	0.5 s	2 films/s for 3 s 1 film/s for 3 s 1 film every 2 s for 6 s
Common iliac arteriography	Iopamidol 370, Iohexol 350 or equivalent	25 ml	10 ml/s	0.5 s	2 films/s for 3 s 1 film/s for 3 s 1 film every 2 s for 6 s
Selective internal iliac arteriography	Iopamidol 300, Iohexol 300 or equivalent	15 ml	5 ml/s	0.2 s	2 films/s for 3 s 1 film/s for 3 s 1 film every 2 s for 6 s

appropriate level, but catheter exchange is necessary for the contralateral side and for ipsilateral internal iliac arteriography. A 65 cm 6 French gauge polyethylene or polyurethane catheter with a single end hole and a 3 cm diameter distal J curve may be passed over the aortic bifurcation for contralateral common iliac arteriography. After passing a guide wire through this catheter and well down into the common femoral artery, the catheter can be advanced over the wire for external iliac arteriography. From that position the catheter can be gently withdrawn till its tip enters the internal iliac artery for selective arteriography of that vessel. Subsequent super-selective arteriography of internal iliac branches can usually be accomplished by advancing the catheter further over a guide wire into the internal iliac system and, if necessary, then exchanging this catheter over a guide wire for a 65 cm 6 French gauge straight thin walled polyethylene catheter. The tip of this more flexible straight catheter may then be directed by a guide wire with torque control and a slightly curved tip (Hawkins & Melichar, 1977). If manipulation is unusually difficult, the left axillary approach provides improved manoeuvrability in the internal iliac system although it requires a longer catheter.

Internal iliac arteriography from the ipsilateral femoral approach can be carried out with a 60 cm 6 French gauge polyethylene or polyurethane catheter with a single end hole and a 1 cm diameter distal J curve which enters the internal iliac origin. Super-selective studies of the internal iliac branch arteries require catheterization from the contralateral femoral or axillary approach (Fig. 8.20).

COMPLICATIONS OF ARTERIOGRAPHY

The principal complications of arteriography relate to the contrast medium and to the mechanical effects of the procedure.

Contrast media may cause allergic reactions and toxic effects. Allergic reactions are less common following arterial than venous injection, but they are mostly unpredictable and are not closely related to dose. Toxic effects are related to the type and quantity of contrast medium used, but may also be aggravated by other factors such as ischaemia and dehydration. Neurological, cardiac and renal tissues are most sensitive to the toxic effects of contrast media and it is particularly important that an appropriate contrast medium should be chosen and its quantity restricted in cerebral, coronary and renal arteriography. Care must be taken to avoid the inadvertent excessive injection of contrast medium into spinal arteries during thoracic and abdominal arteriography and translumbar aortography. Side effects and complications of contrast media are considered in more detail in Chapter 25.

Mechanical complications of catheter arteriography can occur at the puncture site or beyond this point. Excess bleeding and haematoma, false aneurysm and arterio-venous fistula, arterial spasm, thrombosis, dissection, and damage to adjacent structures can arise at the puncture site.

Excessive bleeding from the arterial puncture site and haematoma formation are the commonest technical complications of arteriography, but the incidence can be kept to a minimum by careful attention to technique. The use of large diameter catheters, prolonged examinations, excessive manipulation and catheter changes, bleeding dyscrasias, anti-coagulation, hypertension, diseased arteries and inadequate compression of the puncture site following the procedure, all increase the risk of subsequent haemorrhage and haematoma formation. Persistence or recurrence of bleeding from the arterial puncture occasionally leads to the formation of a false aneurysm. Arterio-

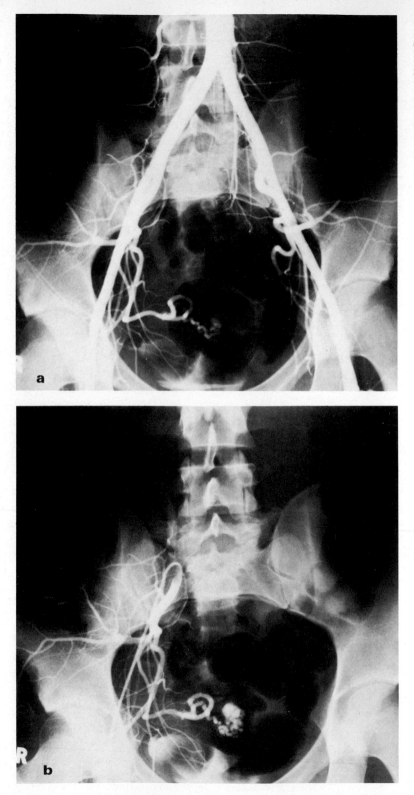

Fig. 8.20 Pelvic, right internal iliac and right uterine arteriography.
(a) Pelvic arteriography. 40 ml of iopamidol 370 has been injected at 15 ml/s into the lower abdominal aorta through a 50 cm 6F straight teflon catheter with end hole and ten side holes, introduced from the right femoral artery.

(b) Selective right internal iliac arteriography. 15 ml of iopamidol 300 is injected through a 6F polyethylene catheter with 1.5 cm diameter J curve positioned in the internal iliac artery from an ipsilateral femoral approach. The right uterine artery is enlarged and supplies a uterine vascular malformation.

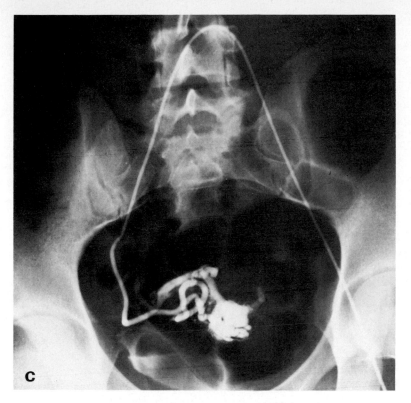

(c) Superselective right uterine arteriogram. A 65 cm 6F polyethylene catheter with 3 cm diameter J curve has been introduced via the contralateral femoral artery and passed over the aortic bifurcation. With the assistance of standard flexible-tipped and torque control guide wires it has been advanced via the internal iliac artery into the enlarged right uterine artery. A hand injection of 10 ml of iopamidol 300 outlines the congenital uterine arterio-venous malformation (examination prior to therapeutic embolization).

venous fistula is a rare complication. Single anterior wall arterial puncture, careful catheter technique and after-care reduces the incidence of these problems.

Arterial spasm at the site of catheterization in children and young adults is aggravated by patient discomfort and fear, as well as the use of unnecessarily large catheters. It should be recognized as soon as possible and is treated by the intra- or peri-arterial injection of a vasodilator such as papaverine.

Thrombosis at the catheterization site may follow arterial spasm, catheterization of a narrow diseased artery, or be associated with polycythaemia. The use of large size catheters, multiple punctures of the artery, numerous catheter changes, excess manipulation of the catheter, or over-enthusiastic compression of the puncture site following catheterization, increase the incidence of this complication. Platelet aggregation and thrombus formation on catheters may lead to distal embolization or occlusion at the catheter site during catheter withdrawal. Large calibre and long catheters provide a greater surface area for platelet aggregation. The problem is seldom evident in abdominal and peripheral arteriography with short 6 French gauge catheters. Low-grade systemic heparinization is advisable when larger and longer catheters and lengthy procedures are required, particularly in cardiac and cerebral angiography. The establishment

of patients on anti-platelet drugs, such as aspirin and dipyridamole, prior to arteriography may also reduce the incidence of this problem. Bonded heparin coating of catheters also reduces thrombus formation but makes it more difficult to pre-shape the catheter. Guide wires, however, may be effectively coated in this way to deter thrombus formation (Amplatz, 1971). It is important that arterial thrombosis at the puncture site should be recognized immediately because early surgical thrombectomy is indicated and is usually a simple and successful operation.

Damage to structures adjacent to the arterial puncture site can be serious, particularly in the axillary region. Meticulous technique is important to avoid direct damage to nerves or compression by haematoma.

Complications which can arise beyond the catheterization site include embolization, arterial dissection, catheter knotting and guide wire fractures. Thrombus stripped from the catheter surface during withdrawal is usually retained in the region of the puncture site, but peripheral embolization of thrombus from the catheter surface or puncture site is sometimes identified although seldom important. Embolization of dislodged atheroma can be serious, particularly when it occurs into the cerebral or mesenteric circulation or peripherally into an area with an already precarious arterial supply. The incidence of this complication is reduced by careful technique, the avoidance of catheterization via severely diseased arteries, particularly in the brachio-cephalic regions from which cerebral embolization can occur, the use of flexible J-tipped guide wires as a routine in patients over the age of 40 years, and discretion by the operator in not persisting with difficult selective arteriography in the presence of severe atheroma. Cotton fibre embolization is avoided by ensuring that perfusion liquids are kept away from swabs, drapes and other sources of particulate contamination, preferably by using a closed catheter perfusing system, and by using plastic sponge rather than swabs for wiping guide wires (Adams *et al.*, 1965). Air embolization can be a serious complication, particularly in the cerebral and coronary circulations, and it is important to ensure that air is excluded from all catheters and syringes before injection. During high pressure injection, it is possible for air to be drawn in from a loose connection between the syringe nozzle and the connecting tube or catheter. Connections must therefore be tight before pressure injections.

Arterial dissection occurs when the guide wire, catheter tip or contrast medium enters the subintimal region. This may occur at the site of catheter entry, but more frequently occurs at the site of the advancing guide wire, catheter tip or contrast medium injection. While atherosclerotic arterial disease predisposes to dissection, its incidence and severity is minimized by the use of soft J-tipped guide wires, gentle fluoroscopically controlled manipulation with immediate recognition of increased resistance and the avoidance of force to overcome any resistance. Small test injections of contrast medium should be made by hand under fluoroscopic control to ensure that the catheter tip and side holes are free from the vessel wall before pressure injections are made.

Catheter knotting is an uncommon complication which occurs particularly during cardiac or brachio-cephalic catheterization. The knot may be untied by manipulation of the catheter, assisted by the introduction through the knot of a second catheter which has been inserted from the opposite femoral artery (Thomas & Sievers, 1979).

Fracture of the guide wire with loss of the distal fragment has been reported in the past but is extremely rare with modern guide wire design.

Translumbar aortography may be associated with complications similar to those of catheter arteriography. Some bleeding and haematoma formation at the puncture site is inevitable because direct compression is not possible. The danger of injecting a large volume of contrast medium inadvertently into a branch vessel such as a renal, mesenteric, coeliac or lumbar artery must be avoided by the fluoroscopic visualization of a small test injection. The extravascular injection of contrast medium or needle damage to the pancreas, thoracic duct, cysterna chyli or spinal cord can result from incorrect needle insertion. Puncture of the pleura or heart can lead to pneumothorax and cardiac tamponade respectively. Careful introduction and positioning of the needle and plastic cannula under fluoroscopic control and a gentle test injection of contrast medium to confirm its position are essential before carrying out the main pressure injection.

INTERVENTIONAL VASCULAR RADIOLOGY

Interventional radiology is a term now used to encompass a wide range of techniques in which modification and extension of diagnostic radiological procedures permits the treatment of patients. Most interventional procedures are alternatives to surgery and are inherently simpler, safer, cheaper and often quicker than the conventional treatment that they replace. In other circumstances, interventional radiological procedures supplement or simplify subsequent surgery.

Interventional vascular procedures have developed directly from diagnostic angiographic techniques, require angiographic facilities and apparatus for their conduct, and fall naturally into the field of the vascular radiologist. These percutaneous procedures include the selective intra-arterial perfusion of drugs, selective vascular embolization, embolectomy, the extraction of intravascular foreign bodies, and transluminal angioplasty.

The percutaneous intra-arterial perfusion of drugs through selectively situated catheters may be used to introduce vasodilator substances in the treatment of ischaemia, vasoconstrictor drugs for the control of haemorrhage, haemolytic agents in thromboembolic disease, and cytotoxic drugs in the treatment of tumours.

Percutaneous embolization is now carried out with a wide variety of occlusive materials which are introduced through selective arterial catheters for the management of focal haemorrhage, congenital and acquired vascular malformations, and tumours. Ablation of function of the spleen, kidney, adrenal and parathyroid glands can also be performed by this technique.

Percutaneous transluminal angioplasty, using specially designed balloon dilatation catheters, is already a well-established procedure for the treatment of selected cases of arterial stenosis or occlusion.

Although beyond the scope of this chapter, these techniques now constitute an important part of the work in angiographic sections of radiology departments and should be carried out by radiologists who have already acquired expertise and experience in diagnostic angiography.

REFERENCES

Adams D. F., Olin T. B. & Kosek J. (1965) Cotton fibre embolisation during arteriography. *Radiology*, **84**, 678–81.

Amplatz K. (1971) A simple nonthrombogenic coating. *Invest. Radiol.*, **6**, 280–9.

Hawkins I. F. & Melichar F. A. (1977) Application of a new torque wire in visceral, extremity and neuro-angiography. *Radiology*, **125**, 821–2.

Hinck J., Judkins M. & Paxton H. (1967) Simplified selective femorocerebral angiography. *Radiology*, **89**, 1048–52.

Kahn P. C. (1965) The epinephrine effect in selective renal arteriography. *Radiology*, **85**, 301–5.

Legge D. A. (1977) The use of prostaglandin F2 alpha in selective visceral angiography. *Brit. J. Radiol.*, **50**, 251–5.

Levin D. C. & Dunham L. (1982) New equipment considerations for angiographic laboratories. *Amer. J. Roentgenol.*, **139**, 775–80.

Rosch J. & Grollman J. H. (1969) Superselective arteriography in the diagnosis of abdominal pathology: technical considerations. *Radiology*, **92**, 1008–13.

Rossi P. (1968) Arteriography in adrenal tumours. *Brit. J. Radiol.*, **41**, 81–98.

Seldinger S. (1953) Catheter replacement of needle in percutaneous arteriography: a new technique. *Acta Radiol.*, **39**, 368–76.

Simmons C. R., Tsao E. C. & Thompson J. R. (1973) Angiographic approach to the difficult aortic arch: a new technique for transfemoral cerebral angiography in the aged. *Amer. J. Roentgenol.*, **119**, 605–12.

Stocks L. O., Halpern M. & Turner A. F. (1969) Complete translumbar aortography. The teflon sleeve technique. *Amer. J. Roentgenol.*, **107**, 835–9.

Thomas H. A. & Sievers R. E. (1979) Nonsurgical reduction of arterial catheter knots. *Amer. J. Roentgenol.*, **132**, 1018–19.

Wallace S., Medellin H., Dejongh D. & Gianturco C. (1972) Systemic heparinization for angiography. *Amer. J. Roentgenol.*, **116**, 204–9.

FURTHER READING

Hanafee W. N. (Ed) (1972) Selective angiography; Section 18. In *Golden's Diagnostic Radiology*. Williams and Wilkins, Baltimore.

Johnsrude I. S. & Jackson D. C. (1979) *A Practical Approach to Angiography*. Little, Brown and Co., Boston.

Kadir S., Kaufman S. L., Barth K. H. & White R. I. (1982) *Selected Techniques in Interventional Radiology*, W. B. Saunders, Philadelphia.

Reuter S. R. & Redman H. C. (1977) *Gastrointestinal Angiography*, 2e. W. B. Saunders, Philadelphia.

Wilkins R. A. & Viamonte M. (Eds) (1982) *Intervention Radiology*. Blackwell Scientific Publications, London.

The Venous System
H. L. WALTERS

LOWER LIMB PHLEBOGRAPHY

From the time when phlebography achieved a wide acceptance as a result of the work of Dos Santos (1938), the techniques of ascending lower limb phlebography have been developed and refined to attain a level of accuracy and reproducibility such that contrast phlebography is the standard by which other diagnostic techniques are assessed in the evaluation of venous diseases. It remains the only examination which provides direct evidence of the pathological process, its extent and chronicity.

During phlebography contrast medium is injected into one of the tributaries of the venous system and a variety of special techniques may be required to demonstrate veins in different regions. The main variations in technique are in the method of introducing the contrast medium and in the postural and other manoeuvres designed to obtain uniform or selective venous filling. No single method can encompass all the clinical indications and provide the required specific information in each case. The basic technique for lower limb phlebography described below is, however, appropriate in the vast majority of cases. Variations of this technique, according to the clinical situation, are discussed on p. 133.

Indications

The clinical situations where lower limb phlebography may be of value can be summarized as follows:

1. The investigation of suspected deep vein thrombosis: confirmation of the diagnosis and information regarding the site, extent and nature of the thrombus which helps to determine the best management of the disease.
2. In establishing the source of pulmonary embolism and the demonstration of any residual thrombus.
3. The assessment of the deep venous system and demonstration of incompetent communicating veins prior to surgery of the superficial veins. The procedure may also be of value following surgery in cases of recurrent varicosities.
4. The investigation of venous ulceration or oedema following deep vein thrombosis—the post thrombotic syndrome. Examination evaluates the pat-

ency or otherwise of the deep veins, any damage to the venous valves and the localization of incompetent communicating veins.
5. The evaluation of the integrity of the venous system in patients with lower limb oedema of unknown cause.
6. The investigation of venous dysplasias.

Contra-indications

A known previous severe reaction to contrast medium requires a reappraisal of the need for the examination, and discussion with the referring clinician as to possible alternative means of obtaining the desired information.

Although anticoagulant therapy is not a contra-indication, special care must be taken to achieve haemostasis at the completion of the procedure.

The basic technique of ascending phlebography

Equipment

The basic requirement is a radiographic tilting table equipped for fluoroscopy and with a spot film capability. This enables the flow of contrast medium to be monitored and exposures made only when there is optimal filling of the veins.

Patient preparation

The patient is fasted for 4–6 hours prior to the examination, thus anticipating any nausea or vomiting related to the use of contrast media. In-patients with severe leg oedema should have the affected limb elevated to facilitate venepuncture.

The procedure

The patient is examined supine with a 20–40° foot-down table tilt. The provision of hand grips on the table enables the patient to steady himself and avoid any weight-bearing on the leg under examination (Fig. 9.1). This semi-upright position combined with the use of tourniquets gives maximal venous filling without flow artefacts, layering of the hyperbaric

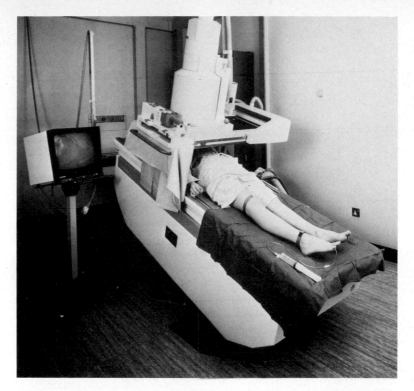

Fig. 9.1 The radiographic table has a 30° foot-down tilt. Hand grips provide support for this non weight-bearing position. Tourniquets have been positioned just before starting the procedure.

contrast medium occurring unless there is a uniform mixing with blood.

A tourniquet is applied above the ankle to distend the foot veins. The skin on the dorsum of the foot is cleaned. A 21 gauge butterfly needle is then inserted into a distal vein on the dorsum of the foot. If the needle is too proximal, the contrast medium may bypass the deep plantar veins and produce artefacts which give the false appearance of a deep venous occlusion. Whilst any of these distal veins is acceptable, the most suitable vein is the medial digital vein of the great toe which has the advantage that it communicates directly with the plantar plexus through the first inter-osseous space. In this way, injected contrast medium flows preferentially into the deep veins. The butterfly needle is secured with adhesive strapping and is attached via a polyvinyl connection to a 10 ml syringe of saline, which allows the venepuncture to be checked by injecting saline under direct vision.

The presence of oedema may make venepuncture difficult, although a vein can usually be displayed if the area is locally massaged to disperse overlying oedema fluid. After an unsuccessful venepuncture, the needle should be left *in situ* and haemostasis achieved with firm local pressure. Possible leakage of contrast medium from the original failed venepuncture is thus reduced when there is a subsequent successful attempt

at another site. Only rarely is it necessary to cut down on to a vein.

A second tourniquet is now applied above the knee in order to delay the flow of contrast medium from the calf veins, thus promoting adequate and more uniform filling of all the deep distal veins. The alternative to the self fastening Velcro tourniquet is a specially constructed pneumatic tourniquet consisting of two narrow cuffs connected by tubing to a manometer and an inflating hand bellows (Fig. 9.2). Separate control of each cuff by means of a stop-cock permits independent alteration of pressure in the cuffs (Craig, 1972).

The saline syringe is replaced by a syringe containing 60 ml of contrast medium (meglumine iothalamate 60%). The volume of contrast medium required varies between patients, reflecting the differing venous capacity of legs. Optimal venous opacification is determined by the appearance at fluoroscopy.

With the table tilted 20–40° in the foot-down position, and the leg under examination, internally rotated to separate the images of the tibia and fibula (Fig. 9.2), contrast medium is injected by hand under screen control. An injection flow rate of approximately 0.5–1 ml/s should be employed. The venepuncture site is checked to exclude extravasation. Progress of the contrast medium is observed to ensure that it passes into the tibial veins, the ankle tourniquet pressure

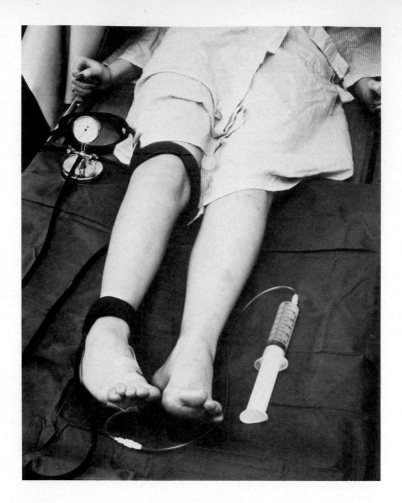

Fig. 9.2 Pneumatic tourniquets in position. The leg under examination is internally rotated to separate the images of the tibia and fibula.

perhaps requiring adjustment at this stage to ensure deep venous filling. The posterior tibial veins are normally the first to fill, followed by the fibular and anterior tibial veins. The muscular venous arcades draining the soleus and gastrocnemius often fill later than the main stem veins of the calf.

Films are exposed in the P–A position when there is uniform filling of the deep veins of the calf. Three exposures are made on a 35 cm × 35 cm radiograph, subdivided into three, to include the veins from the ankle to the knee (Fig. 9.3). Contrast filling of the popliteal venous segment is enhanced by employing gentle pressure of the deep calf veins just above the ankle. The leg is next externally rotated to obtain a lateral view of the deep calf veins, three similar exposures being made to include the veins from the foot to the knee (Fig. 9.4). These lateral views are important in demonstrating the posterior tibial and soleal veins without superimposition of other veins. Whilst the majority of thrombi begin in these calf veins, some originate in the plantar veins and so a

view of the foot should always be included in the lateral series (Lea Thomas & O'Dwyer, 1978).

The leg is then repositioned P–A and the above-knee tourniquet removed to allow contrast filling of the superficial and common femoral veins. Two exposures are made of the deep veins in the thigh. The explorator is now positioned to include the area of the groin and pelvis. A third exposure is then made, following release of the ankle tourniquet and the application of firm pressure on the calf to propel contrast medium as a bolus, in order to outline the iliac veins and lower inferior vena cava (Fig. 9.5). A Valsalva manoeuvre performed when the common femoral and external iliac veins are filled with contrast medium demonstrates the proximal segment of the deep femoral vein.

Following the procedure, and while the films are being processed, the veins are cleared of contrast medium by elevation of the leg and injecting normal saline. Some workers routinely use heparinized saline. Once the diagnostic adequacy of the films is confirmed,

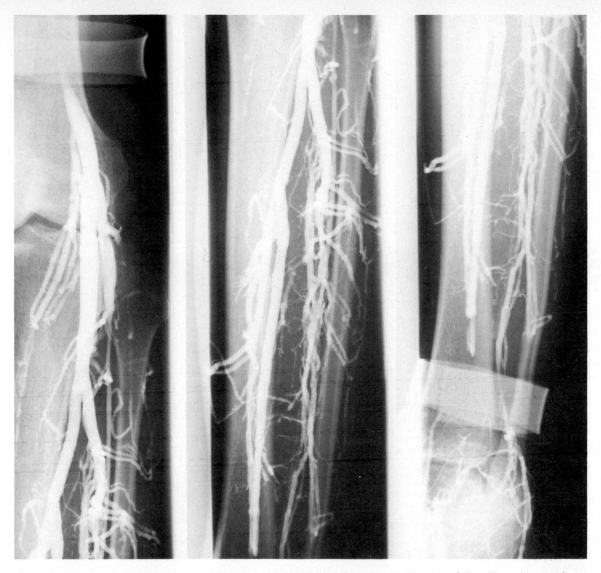

Fig. 9.3 Uniform filling of the deep calf veins exposed in the P–A position on a divided 35 cm² film. The ankle tourniquet directs contrast into the deep veins; the above knee tourniquet delays emptying of the calf veins.

early ambulation of the patient is encouraged. Active leg movements should be performed when this is not possible. Possible thrombotic complications from stasis of the contrast medium are reduced in this way.

While this technique delineates the deep veins from the foot to the lower inferior vena cava, some segments of the venous system are difficult to demonstrate fully. The main difficulties arise in the following situations:

1. The anterior tibial vein may be occluded by the ankle tourniquet. A limited repeat examination after reducing the ankle tourniquet pressure, or dispensing with the tourniquet, demonstrates the patency or otherwise of the anterior tibial vein.
2. Even employing a non weight-bearing technique, it is not possible to demonstrate the entire vast network of muscle veins in the calf (Cotton & Clark, 1965).
3. The deep femoral vein fills in only 50% of patients, either as a result of a loop connection with the superficial femoral vein or retrogradely during the Valsalva manoeuvre.
3. The internal iliac vein may fill during a Valsalva manoeuvre, but only as far as its valves will allow.

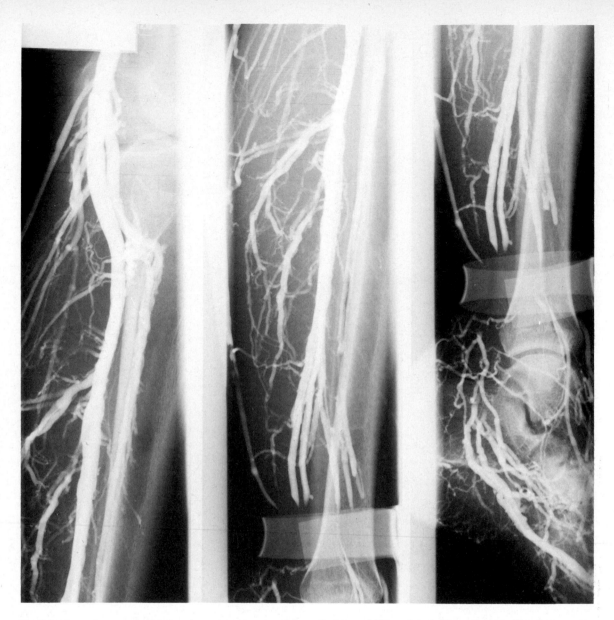

Fig. 9.4 Lateral exposures showing the main stem veins of the calf with good filling of the calf muscle veins. The plantar veins have been included on the first exposure.

5. Occasionally the iliac veins and lower inferior vena cava are not adequately demonstrated by the technique of calf compression at the completion of the standard technique. When it is necessary to show these venous segments in this situation, as in the delineation of the upper extent of a thrombus, a repeat examination with the following modification will demonstrate these veins in the majority of patients. An above knee tourniquet is applied to each thigh, in order to delay calf emptying, and 50 ml of contrast medium are injected simultaneously into each leg. With the explorator centred over the pelvis and loaded with a 35 cm × 35 cm radiograph, an exposure is made immediately after the release of the tourniquets and the application of firm pressure to both calves. This bolus technique is a valuable method of demonstrating the ilio-caval venous segment (Lea Thomas & Macdonald, 1977).

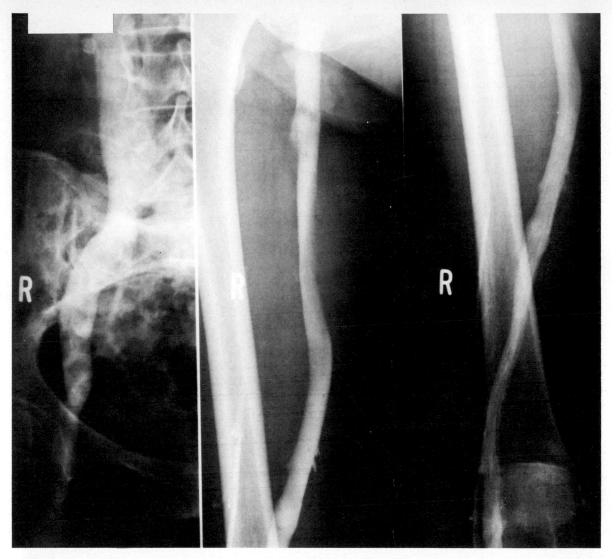

Fig. 9.5 Popliteal and superficial femoral veins demonstrated after tourniquet release. The final exposure to outline the iliac veins and lower inferior vena cava is made using the bolus technique following calf compression. The profunda femoris vein has not filled on this study.

Variations of the basic technique

The objectives of ascending phlebography in defined clinical situations must be clearly understood. In many instances the basic technique will require little modification, merely particular attention directed to achieve those objectives. The aims of phlebography may be summarized in the following venous disorders:

Deep vein thrombosis

Recent advances in treating venous thrombosis require more than simply the documentation of the presence of a thrombus. The phlebogram must aim to give an indication of the age of a thrombus, its extent and, as far as possible, its liability to embolize. The objectives are thus:

1. To show that a filling defect in a vein is persistent and constant in shape on more than one film, thus excluding various artefacts (Lea Thomas & Carty, 1975).
2. To fill as many of the deep veins as possible, including established collateral vessels around occluded veins.

3. To demonstrate the upper extent of the thrombus or occluded vein.

Retrograde phlebography or intra-osseous phlebography may be indicated when ascending phlebography, including the bolus technique, fails to demonstrate the ilio-caval segment.

Varicose veins and incompetent communicating veins

Incompetent communicating veins allow the retrograde flow of blood from the deep to the superficial veins. Whilst most of these incompetent veins are recognized clinically and have a fairly constant position, some arise in an inconstant position. Phlebography shows their location and, further, confirms the integrity of the deep veins if there is doubt on clinical grounds prior to a radical stripping procedure.

An ankle tourniquet is applied sufficiently tightly to ensure that there is no superficial venous filling. The pneumatic cuffs, as described by Craig (1972) and referred to in the basic technique, are particularly useful in this context. The presence of ulceration around the ankle, or the suspicion of an incompetent communicating vein below the malleolus, may require the placement of a cuff around the forefoot.

The flow of the injected contrast medium is monitored and an exposure is made when retrograde flow through the incompetent communicating vein is seen. These early films are valuable since the varicosities may subsequently flood with contrast medium, making identification of the level of the incompetent vein difficult.

The precise level of these veins can be measured by means of a ruler with 1 cm radio-opaque markers. This allows for magnification and the level is determined by reference to the malleoli (Fig. 9.6).

Venous dysplasias

The venous dysplasias form part of a wide clinical spectrum of congenital vascular malformations. There is frequently involvement of the arterial, venous and lymphatic systems in these malformations. (Kinmonth *et al.*, 1976). The investigation of each case must therefore be planned on an individual basis.

The demonstration of the presence or absence of a normal deep venous system is vital to the investigation of the mainly venous malformations. This information is essential if surgery is contemplated. The phlebographic technique employed is similar to the modified approach in the investigation of incompetent communicating veins. It may occasionally be difficult to occlude the superficial venous system, especially if there are coexisting varicose veins, skin ulceration

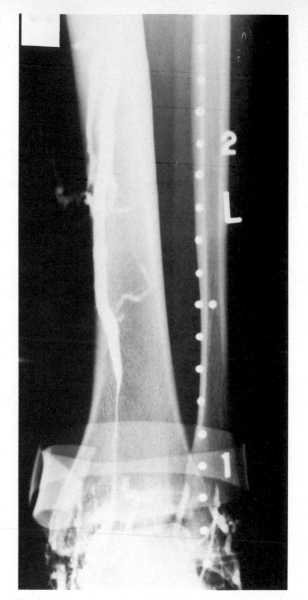

Fig. 9.6 An early exposure has been made to demonstrate this medial incompetent vein which, with the aid of the 1 cm marked ruler, is accurately measured as situated 11 cm above the tip of the medial malleolus.

and soft tissue hypertrophy. Intra-osseous phlebography may be required to demonstrate the integrity of the deep venous system in these cases.

Having demonstrated the state of the deep veins and the presence of any incompetent communicating veins, the central connections of any superficial anomalous venous channel can best be evaluated by direct injection into the anomaly. Contrast medium then delineates the extent of the lesion and its central ramification.

Small localized venous anomalies are similarly dealt with by the direct injection of contrast medium into the dysplastic veins, using a 21 gauge butterfly needle.

More extensive dysplasias may best be demonstrated by arteriography. Here the film sequence is continued through into the venous phase following an arterial injection of contrast medium.

PELVIC PHLEBOGRAPHY

In those cases where the iliac veins and lower inferior vena cava have been inadequately demonstrated by the above technique, percutaneous perfemoral injections of contrast medium can demonstrate the iliocaval segments when the femoral vein is intact.

Indications

1. The demonstration of the upper extent of venous thrombosis.
2. In establishing the source of pulmonary embolism. Iliac vein thrombosis carries a high risk of embolization.
3. The development of successful surgical procedures for the treatment of post thrombotic states involving the iliac veins requires a precise anatomical demonstration of the pelvic veins and the venous collateral pathways.

Contra-indications

As with ascending lower limb phlebography, a previous severe contrast medium reaction is a contra-indication and special care is required in patients receiving anticoagulant therapy in pelvic phlebography.

PERCUTANEOUS PERFEMORAL PELVIC PHLEBOGRAPHY

The femoral vein, if patent, is the preferred approach to demonstrate the ilio-femoral veins and lower inferior vena cava.

Technique

Equipment A fluoroscopy unit with an overcouch tube and a rapid film changer are required.

Patient preparation The patient is fasted for 4–6 h prior to the procedure and both groins must be shaved.

The procedure The patient is examined in the supine position. A control film of the pelvis, to include the area from the ischial tuberosities to the upper border of L4, checks the radiographic exposure and position.

At the groin, the femoral vein lies medial to the femoral artery. Following aseptic skin preparation, local anaesthetic is infiltrated at a point 1 cm medial to the arterial pulsation and 2–3 cm below the inguinal ligament. Care is taken with the deeper subcutaneous infiltration to avoid intravascular injection by aspiration of the syringe before injecting local anaesthetic. A small 5 mm skin incision is made prior to femoral vein puncture.

A large bore needle, such as a disposable Potts–Cournand needle,* is used to puncture the femoral vein. The stylet is removed and the needle is connected to a syringe containing saline via a polyvinyl connection. The needle is slowly withdrawn while, at the same time, applying gentle aspiration to the syringe. After a successful puncture, venous blood is aspirated and a small test injection of contrast medium is then made to confirm correct placement. The needle is then advanced a few centimeters over a flexible guide wire to ensure that it will not dislodge during the procedure. Venepuncture may be facilitated in difficult cases by asking the patient to perform a Valsalva manoeuvre, which distends the femoral vein.

The same procedure is now performed on the other femoral vein.

The saline syringes are replaced by syringes which each contain 40 ml of contrast medium (sodium iothalamate 70%). Simultaneous hand injections are then made by two operators. The injection must be forceful enough to deliver the volume in four seconds, in order to obtain a large bolus with uniform mixing with blood. The injection and filming sequence are started at the same time, eight exposures being made at the rate of one per second using the serial film changer (Fig. 9.7).

Whilst a single spot film may be adequate for demonstrating an occlusion, a series of exposures as described more adequately displays any altered anatomy, shows the extent and direction of flow through venous collaterals, and obviates the need for repeat examinations.

When the diagnostic adequacy of the films has been confirmed, the needles are removed and firm pressure applied to each venepuncture site until haemostasis is achieved.

Where the femoral vein is occluded, the proximal

* Becton–Dickinson, Rutherford, New Jersey.

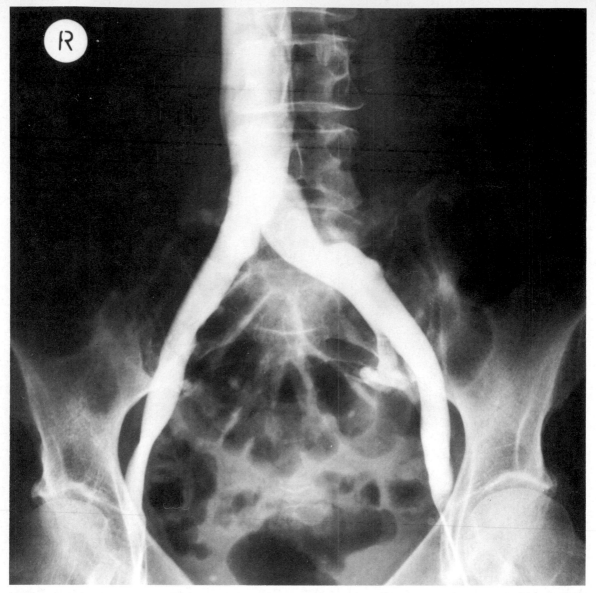

Fig. 9.7 Normal pelvic phlebogram showing external and common iliac veins and the lower inferior vena cava. There is slight filling of the left internal iliac vein and the left common iliac vein shows an indentation due to the right common iliac artery.

extent of the occlusion can be defined by one of three approaches:

1. Descending retrograde iliocavography.
2. Retrograde iliac phlebography, where the contra-lateral femoral vein is patent.
3. Pertrochanteric intraosseous phlebography, p. 141.

DESCENDING RETROGRADE ILIOCAVOGRAPHY

This technique demonstrates the level of venous occlusion in the inferior vena cava, or more distally down to the external iliac veins, when a femoral approach is not possible or has provided insufficient anatomic detail. The technique also allows the internal iliac system to be examined and can be combined with pulmonary angiography (Dow, 1973).

The usual approach is via a catheter introduced into the median antecubital vein. Alternatively, a subclavian or jugular venous approach may be made. The jugular approach allows the subsequent insertion of a caval 'umbrella filter' as one of the management options in patients with, or at high risk of developing, pulmonary embolism in the presence of a loose venous thrombus.

The procedure involves the insertion of a 7F catheter with side holes into the median antecubital vein at the elbow. The catheter is then advanced through the superior vena cava and, via the right atrium, into the inferior vena cava. As the catheter is slowly advanced down the inferior vena cava under screen control, test injections of contrast medium enable the catheter tip to be placed about 3 cm above the occlusion. The risk of dislodging any fresh thrombus or tumour is minimized in this way. The level of the occlusion is then recorded with an exposure following the injection of contrast medium. A hand injection of contrast medium is sufficient when the caval flow is low as a result of the occlusion. Where flow is little impeded, a higher rate of injection is required.

RETROGRADE ILIAC PHLEBOGRAPHY

The upper extent of an iliofemoral occlusion can be demonstrated if the contralateral femoral and iliac veins have been shown to be patent on ascending phlebography of the lower limb.

The femoral vein is cannulated as described above and a curved arterial catheter, for example a 7F renal catheter with side holes, is introduced using the Seldinger technique (see Arteriography, p. 100). The catheter is then positioned in the contralateral common iliac vein. Care is taken before placement of the catheter to ensure that there is no thrombus projecting from the common iliac vein and that the catheter tip does not reach and dislodge any thrombus in this vein. The level and nature of the upper extent of the occlusion can thus be accurately defined. A hand injection of 20 ml contrast medium is sufficient to demonstrate an obstruction, because of the reduction in iliac venous flow.

The third approach, employing the technique of pertrochanteric intraosseous phlebography (described below), will demonstrate the pelvic veins and inferior vena cava but requires a general anaesthetic. The above techniques require only local anaesthesia.

Pelvic phlebography, when indicated, supplements ascending phlebography and enables the extent of the venous thrombosis to be assessed, particularly in the iliofemoral segment and inferior vena cava, by determining the upper extent of the disease, which is an important factor in case management.

INFERIOR VENA CAVOGRAPHY

Indications

The main indications for inferior vena cavography are:

1. Inferior vena caval obstruction due to pathology arising within the vein; namely venous thrombosis, web obstruction, primary tumour or secondary tumour invasion. The examination must provide information of the extent of the obstruction and its upper limit.
2. Obstruction of the inferior vena cava (IVC) due to pathology arising outside the vein, as with compression and displacement by tumour or retroperitoneal disease.
3. As a preliminary to confirm caval patency in suspected renal or hepatic vein thrombosis. Having excluded thrombus or tumour propagation into the IVC, selective examination of these veins can then be undertaken.
4. The complex embryological development of the IVC is reflected in the variety of congenital caval anomalies which may require investigation and interpretation by inferior vena cavography. The percutaneous bifemoral approach is the method of choice for their evaluation.

Technique

The approaches and techniques for inferior vena cavography are the same as those employed in pelvic phlebography. Cavography by a percutaneous bifemoral approach is the method of choice when both iliofemoral segments are patent.

Radiographs in both the A–P and lateral projections are required for a full evaluation of the IVC. The two projections can be obtained with the one injection if equipment providing biplane rapid serial radiography is available; otherwise two separate injections are required.

The control radiographs are centred on the region of interest. Suspected disease at the origin of the IVC requires a centring point at L5, while disease near its termination must include the right atrium on the radiograph.

An injection of 40 ml of contrast medium (sodium iothalamate 70%) is made on both sides, using a pump injector and a flow rate of 15 ml per second. The filming sequence is set for two per second for three seconds and then one per second for four seconds, the programme commencing 0.5 seconds after the start of the injection. A delay may be incorporated for the last few films if there is significant obstruction. In the absence of unilateral occlusive disease, such as an iliac vein block, a Y connector joining both needles may be used and connected to a single injector. Unilateral obstruction causes preferential flow through the unobstructed side.

When the patient has to be turned into a lateral position, in the absence of a biplane facility, it is safer to insert a 7F catheter with side holes into each femoral vein using the Seldinger technique. The risk of displacing a cannula on turning the patient is thus avoided.

The IVC may alternatively be examined by introducing a catheter from the femoral vein by the Seldinger technique and advancing it to the required level in the IVC. This is the method of choice in examining the suprarenal segment of the IVC in cases of suspected obstruction. The catheter must have side holes to allow uniform opacification of the IVC. With a catheter technique, 60 ml of contrast medium is injected with a flow rate of 20 ml per second.

COMPLICATIONS OF PHLEBOGRAPHY

Complications which may arise during a phlebographic procedure may be due to the contrast medium or related to the technique.

Complications due to contrast media

Adverse reactions

These reactions are common to all situations where contrast media are injected into the vascular system and are not specific to phlebography. Adverse reactions, often of a minor nature, are more frequently seen after intravenous injection of contrast medium than following an intra-arterial injection (Shehadi, 1975).

These adverse reactions may be classified as toxic, idiosyncratic and allergic. Toxic reactions are dose related and it is probable that many of these reactions may be related to the hyperosmolar load imposed by conventionally used contrast media. The recent introduction of contrast media of low osmolality may significantly reduce these reactions.

Phlebography is contra-indicated when there is a history of a previous severe reaction to contrast medium, unless there is an urgent need for information which the phlebogram can provide but which cannot be obtained by any other method. These high risk patients may benefit from pretreatment with steroids (see Intravenous Urography, p. 223). Emergency resuscitation equipment and drugs, a standard requirement in all radiology departments, should be immediately available.

Local reactions

Pain Pain is the most frequent complication of phlebography. It is not usually severe and is experienced locally in the foot and/or calf. The pain is related primarily to the hyperosmolality of the contrast medium but also to the sodium content of the media. Dilution of the contrast medium (Bettman & Paulin, 1977) and the use of sodium-free media reduces the incidence of pain and discomfort. There is, however, a limit to which any contrast medium can be diluted before the diagnostic adequacy of the phlebogram becomes adversely affected.

The advent of the low osmolality contrast media has significantly improved patient acceptance of the examination. A comparative study, in which a conventional contrast medium (meglumine iothalamate 280) was injected into one leg, and a low osmolality medium (metrizamide 280) used to examine the other leg, showed an incidence of leg pain of 68% when the conventional medium was used and only 15% when the non-ionic medium was employed (Lea Thomas & Walters, 1979).

Thrombosis Thrombotic complications of phlebography, although well recognized, have been considered to be an uncommon or rare occurrence. This thrombogenic effect is due to the high osmolality of conventional contrast media. The incidence is minimized by clearing contrast medium from the veins at the completion of the examination by flushing with saline and encouraging early ambulation. Some workers routinely use heparin in the saline infusion. The aim in all cases is to allow contrast medium to remain in contact with veins for as short a time as possible.

Fibrinogen uptake tests, to monitor prospectively the incidence of thrombosis, show a significantly higher incidence of thrombotic complications than was previously thought. Similarly studies comparing conventional media with the low osmolality media have shown that the use of these new media virtually eliminates thrombotic complications (Walters *et al.*, 1980). Initially these media were prohibitively expensive for routine use, but recently introduced preparations are less costly and are therefore routinely used for most phlebographic procedures.

Complications due to the technique

Local complications

Local extravasation   Although rare, serious complications may arise if contrast medium extravasates into the soft tissues during the injection. The extravasated contrast medium provokes a chemical cellulitis which may progress to a bullous eruption, skin ulceration and soft tissue necrosis; gangrene having been described in extreme cases. Soft tissue necrosis is more commonly seen in patients with peripheral ischaemia (Berge *et al.*, 1978).

Extreme care is therefore necessary with the venepuncture technique. The needle should be tested for its correct placement within the vein both by injecting saline under direct vision and by checking the flow of contrast medium on fluoroscopy as the injection is made. If the patient experiences severe local pain in the foot during the examination, extravasation may have occurred as a result of either needle dislodgement or bursting of the injected vein. The injection must then be stopped and the locally extravasated contrast medium diluted by injecting normal saline.

This complication, when it occurs in the groin during pelvic phlebography using a femoral vein puncture, does not appear to have such serious sequelae as in the foot. This is presumably because contrast medium is more readily dissipated and absorbed from the bulkier soft tissues of this region.

Haemorrhage and haematoma formation   Firm local pressure at the completion of the procedure is indicated and avoids this complication. Special care is required in patients receiving anticoagulant therapy to ensure haemostasis is achieved.

Catheterization difficulties   Complications are rare. When catheterization techniques are required, providing that the Seldinger technique is carefully undertaken and neither the guide wire nor the catheter are forced into the vein.

Distant complications

Pulmonary thrombo-embolism   The exact frequency of pulmonary embolism occurring in patients when phlebography has been performed in the presence of deep vein thrombosis cannot be accurately defined because of the difficulties of diagnosing subclinical embolism. The complication has been described in a few cases, but the experience of several authors suggests that this is a rare event.

Calf compression, employed in ascending lower limb phlebography to demonstrate the iliofemoral venous segment, it has been suggested, is likely to provoke detachment of loose thrombus. This has not, however, been encountered in several large series.

Particular care, however, is required in the technique of descending phlebography to demonstrate the upper extent of thrombus occlusion in the inferior vena cava or iliac vein.

Air embolism   This is prevented by careful attention to detail to ensure that all connectors are tight, syringes are air-free, always aspirating when a new syringe is connected, and by holding the syringe in a vertical position (plunger uppermost) when an injection is made.

RELATIONSHIP TO OTHER IMAGING MODALITIES AND INVESTIGATIVE TECHNIQUES

Disorders of the venous system, in particular the immediate and delayed complications associated with deep vein thrombosis, are the cause of a significant morbidity and mortality. Recent advances in treating venous thrombosis and in the surgical management of the post-thrombotic syndrome have stimulated the development of a number of new investigative procedures. The aims of these tests are the earliest diagnosis of thrombosis, when more often effective treatment can be instituted, and a functional assessment of the venous system to provide information of the underlying pathophysiology in veins of patients with chronic venous insufficiency.

These techniques enable the venous system to be evaluated in a less invasive way than contrast phlebography. The accuracy of the contrast phlebogram, however, remains the baseline by which these newer screening techniques are assessed in terms of sensitivity and specificity.

The availability of some of these tests vary between departments, and only the principles of the techniques are discussed. Kakkar (1980) has provided a detailed account of these techniques and a critical appraisal of their current status.

Doppler ultrasonic technique

The frequency of an ultrasound beam is altered when it is reflected by a moving object, the change in frequency being related to the velocity of the object due to the Doppler effect. The corpuscles in blood vessels act as the reflectors and, in this way, ultrasound frequency changes with the rate of blood flow. This frequency change can either be translated through an amplifier into an audible signal or recorded on paper.

The normal venous flow signal in the legs of a patient lying supine varies with respiration, decreasing on inspiration and increasing with expiration. The velocity of flow in a patent vein can briefly be increased by compression of the extremity to produce an augmented flow signal.

There is thus a phasic flow signal which, in the presence of venous obstruction when the probe is placed distal to the obstruction, is lost and is replaced by a more or less continuous character signal. Augmented flow signals similarly become dampened. No signal is obtained when there is total occlusion.

The technique has a high degree of accuracy in detecting occlusions of the femoral, popliteal or iliac veins. Its main limitations arise in its failure to accurately detect non-occlusive thrombi in the proximal veins. Confusion and inaccuracy may also arise in the presence of an established collateral venous system which may simulate flow in a patent major vein. The major limitation is related to operator experience.

Radioisotope tests

Fibrinogen uptake test

Fibrinogen labelled with radioactive iodine follows the same pathways as endogenous fibrinogen and is converted to fibrin under the action of thrombin. A forming thrombus thus incorporates ^{125}I-labelled fibrinogen which is then detected by external counting over the limb.

The levels of radioactivity are measured at marked positions on the legs. The criterion for the diagnosis of thrombosis is a count rate 15–20% greater than at adjacent points on the leg or the same point on the other leg, when compared with the reading at the same position on the previous day and provided this increase persists for more then 24 hours. Counting is repeated daily for up to 7 to 8 days.

The fibrinogen uptake test has found several clinical applications. Its most important contribution has been in the prospective surveillance of patients at high risk of developing venous thrombosis, for instance patients undergoing hip surgery. The technique also enables the natural history of venous thrombosis to be monitored, the rate of dissolution of the thrombus to be followed, and an assessment of the efficacy of prophylactic agents in preventing venous thrombosis. A positive test is obtained in established venous thrombosis provided that a thrombus is still forming.

The important limitation of the fibrinogen test is its inability to detect iliac vein thrombosis and, to a lesser extent, thrombosis in the upper thigh because of the high background activity in the bladder and other vascular structures. False positive results may be obtained in the presence of a haematoma, skin wound or inflammatory swelling.

Radionuclide phlebography

The technique of radionuclide phlebography is based on the principle that macro-aggregates of albumin labelled with ^{99m}Tc, when injected into a superficial vein of the foot, may be trapped proximal to an occluding thrombus or adhere to its surface. This particle entrapment results in an area of increased activity which is detected by a gamma camera as a hot spot. The transit of the isotope is recorded and the resulting gamma camera images resemble phlebograms, although they lack the definition of contrast phlebography.

The technique produces a significant number of false positives and does not demonstrate the true extent of the disease. Its accuracy is however better for the thigh and pelvic region. The major advantage of this technique is that it can be incorporated with lung scanning procedures for the detection of pulmonary embolism.

Venous occlusion plethysmography

The technique is based on the principle of inflating a pressure cuff around the thigh to completely occlude the distal draining veins while not impeding the arterial supply to the leg distal to the cuff. The resulting increase in volume of the leg during venous occlusion can be determined by a plethysmograph. Sudden release of the cuff pressure causes a decrease in calf volume by venous emptying. Blood flow can be calculated, as a function of time, from the volume changes measured by the plethysmograph. The method thus provides functional information about venous flow.

The presence of a deep vein thrombosis reduces the maximum venous volume of the calf and, when the cuff is released, delay venous emptying. Thus thrombi which obstruct the venous outflow will be detected. The main limitation of the technique is in the detection of most calf vein thrombi since the main venous outflow tract is not obstructed. In the same way, small non-occlusive thrombi in the popliteal and femoral veins may be missed, as also may a venous occlusion which has a well-established venous collateral system.

Thermography

Thermography is, in the real sense, a non-invasive test which has recently been used to detect deep vein thrombosis. Although the clinical diagnosis of deep venous thrombosis is inaccurate, the technique of thermography is based on one of the signs used in clinical diagnosis—the increased temperature or delayed cooling of a leg containing thrombosed veins. Whilst the temperature change may be subclinical and not apparent on palpation, a sensitive infra-red camera accurately detects these abnormalities.

Exposure of the legs before recording any temperature change allows equilibration of the skin of the lower limbs at room temperature. The heat radiated from the legs is reflected by a mirror, so that the radiation strikes the lens of the infra red camera at right angles and thus prevents picture distortion.

Thermography has not been widely adopted, although studies have shown the technique to have a good accuracy when compared with phlebography and the ^{125}I fibrinogen uptake test. Its main limitation is its inability to detect thrombi in the pelvic veins and inferior vena cava. False positives are produced when there is a haematoma or in the presence of various inflammatory conditions.

The ideal non-invasive technique for detecting deep vein thrombosis does not exist. Contrast phlebography remains the standard by which these tests are assessed.

The ^{123}I fibrinogen uptake test is the most sensitive method and detects calf vein thrombosis in its earliest stage. It is therefore the technique of choice for a prospective surveillance. Its main limitation is the incidence of false positives, so that a positive test may require verification.

Techniques based on venous flow—venous occlusion plethysmography and Doppler ultrasound—are comparable in terms of their sensitivity and specificity in detecting major deep vein thrombosis in the popliteal vein and above. Their limitation is in the failure to accurately detect thrombosis of the calf veins.

Generally, the contrast phlebogram may be omitted where two, or occasionally one, of these non-invasive tests are unequivocally normal.

INTRA-OSSEOUS PHLEBOGRAPHY

Intra-osseous phlebography may be used when conventional phlebographic techniques are not possible because of venous occlusion or inaccessible veins. The technique is based on the observation that contrast medium injected into the bone marrow passes into the local venous drainage. This technique supplements conventional phlebography.

The application of the technique in various regions of the body has been widely studied by Schobinger (1966). The most frequent application of intra-osseous phlebography has been to demonstrate the iliac veins and inferior vena cava in the presence of femoral vein occlusion. A combined approach may be made to examine the pelvic veins, and inferior vena cava when lower limb phlebography will have revealed patency of the femoral vein on one side and occlusive disease on the contralateral side. The patent femoral vein is examined by percutaneous perfemoral injection and the occluded side examined by pertrochanteric injection (Fig. 9.8). Intra-osseous phlebography may occasionally be indicated to demonstrate the veins of the lower limb when intravenous access is not possible because of oedema.

The procedure is painful and requires a general anaesthetic.

Indications

The only indication for intra-osseous phlebography is failure of conventional i.v. phlebographic techniques, due either to venous occlusion or inacessibility of veins. The technique has been largely supplanted with the advent of venous catheterization techniques but it remains a useful method in some situations.

Contra-indications

1. The presence of local infection at the proposed puncture site is an absolute contra-indication because of attendant risk of osteomyelitis.
2. A known history of a bleeding diathesis, in particular haemophilia.
3. The technique is not undertaken in patients whose epiphyses are not fused because of the danger of impairing growth.
4. Previous severe contrast medium reaction.

Pertrochanteric intra-osseous phlebography

Technique

Equipment A fluoroscopy unit with an overcouch tube and rapid serial film changer is required.

Patient preparation The patient is prepared for a general anaesthetic.

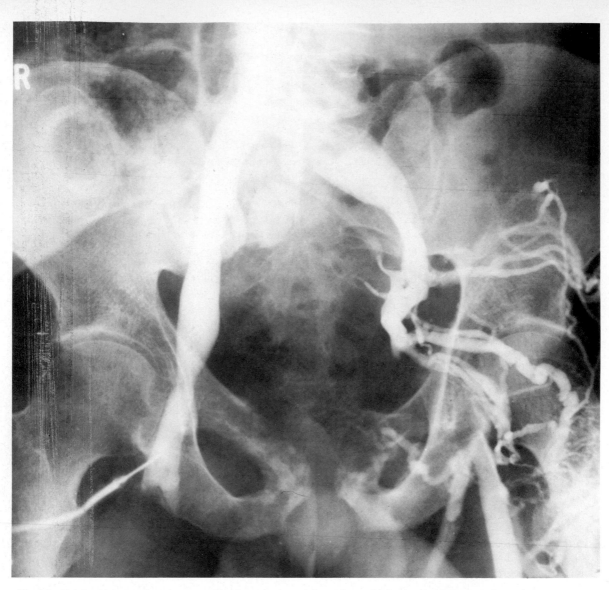

Fig. 9.8 Pelvic phlebography using a combined approach: a right perfemoral injection and left pertrochanteric intra-osseous injection in a patient with an occluded left external iliac vein. Left femoral vein was punctured but the upper extent of the occlusion could not be defined. (History of pelvic surgery followed by radiotherapy.)

Procedure A control film of the pelvis is used to check exposure and position, as described for pelvic phlebography.

The relatively slow clearance of contrast medium from the marrow cavity results in the hyperbaric contrast medium tending to gravitate to the most dependent veins. The internal iliac system is therefore preferentially demonstrated in the supine position, while the prone position better demonstrates the external and common iliac veins (Lea Thomas, 1970).

To demonstrate the iliofemoral segment, the patient is best examined in the prone position. A scrupulous aseptic technique is applied throughout the examination. Location of the greater trochanter is facilitated by an assistant who internally and externally rotates the leg while the bony prominence of the greater trochanter is located.

Puncture of the greater trochanter is undertaken with a 13 guage Lea Thomas needle which has a drill tip to allow easy penetration of the outer cortex (Lea Thomas, 1970). Correct placement of the needle is confirmed by the aspiration of marrow blood and the free clearance of a small test injection of contrast medium from the marrow into the local drainage veins. Following an unsuccessful puncture, the needle is left *in situ*, and a second needle is inserted to prevent extravasation of contrast medium through the track of the first attempt.

The needle is then connected to a pump injector and 40 ml of contrast medium (sodium iothalamate 70%) is injected at the rate of 10 ml per second. Exposures are made at the rate of 1 per second for 10 seconds.

The needle is then flushed with normal saline before its removal.

Intra-osseous phlebography of the lower limb

Intra-osseous phlebography demonstrates the deep veins, when, as in the presence of gross oedema, it is not possible to locate a superficial vein. Although some workers carry out the procedure under local anaesthetic, the examination is painful and should be performed under general anaesthesia.

The most favourable access point in the lower limb is the medial malleolus. A 16 guage bone marrow needle is used and, with a strict aseptic technique, the upper part of the bony prominence of the medial malleolus is punctured with the needle tip angled cephalad to avoid entering the ankle joint. Correct placement of the needle is checked by the aspiration of marrow blood, and a small test injection of contrast medium which is screened to confirm free clearance into the local draining veins. Following an intra-osseous injection, contrast medium passes preferentially into the deep venous system.

About 30–40 ml of contrast medium (meglumine iothalamate 60%) is usually adequate to demonstrate the deep venous system, the injection being made by hand. Exposures are made on a 35 cm × 35 cm radiograph, subdivided into three, as the contrast medium ascends the deep veins. These exposures are made when the veins are seen to be optimally filled.

Following the procedure, normal saline is infused to clear residual contrast medium and the needle is then removed.

Complications of intra-osseous phlebography

Local complications

Incorrect needle position The needle tip must be placed within the medullary cavity of the bone and its position checked by the aspiration of blood and the free clearance of a test injection of contrast medium from the medullary cavity into the local draining veins. This avoids extravasation into soft tissues and subperiosteal or intra-articular injections.

Osteomyelitis Osteomyelitis is prevented by a scrupulous aseptic technique and avoiding injections at local sites of skin infection.

Bone infarction Bone infarction has been described but appears to be a rare complication.

Distant complications

Fat embolism Fat embolism represents the most serious complication and may be fatal. It has been suggested that the risk is increased when a pressure injection is made for intra-osseous phlebography (Schobinger, 1960). This complication, however, is rare.

UPPER LIMB PHLEBOGRAPHY

The most common indication for investigation of the venous drainage of the arm is oedema associated with venous thrombosis. The site of obstruction is most commonly in either the axillary or subclavian vein.

Technique

A fluoroscopy unit with a spot film capability is required. The patient is examined in the supine position on the fluoroscopy table. When the entire venous system of the arm is to be demonstrated, puncture of a peripheral vein on the dorsum of the hand is made with a 19 gauge butterfly needle which is then secured. In the absence of the postural advantage of the semi-upright position used in lower limb phlebography to retard venous return, a tourniquet is applied above the elbow to enable uniform mixing of the blood with contrast medium and thus promotes good venous opacification without artefacts. Exposures of the veins in the forearm are then made after injecting 30–40 ml of contrast medium (meglumine iothalamate 60%).

Release of the tourniquet and firm compression of the forearm allows the contrast medium to delineate the upper arm veins as a bolus, in particular the upper course of the basilic vein which becomes the axillary vein and then the subclavian vein. This technique is of value when the median antecubital vein is not easily accessible for venepuncture.

The best approach to demonstrate the axillary and

subclavian veins is via the median antecubital vein. In the presence of obstruction of the upper arm veins the more peripheral veins are engorged and either a large bore needle, such as a 16 gauge butterfly needle, or a 7F catheter with side holes is introduced into the median antecubital vein. The catheter is then advanced to a point just distal to the occlusion with the aid of small test injections of contrast medium. Spot films of the level and extent of the obstruction are then made during a hand injection of 30 ml contrast medium (meglumine iothalamate 60%).

The cephalic vein is not used because contrast medium injected via this route bypasses the basilic vein and all but the termination of the axillary vein.

Following the procedure, firm pressure is applied to the venepuncture site until haemostasis is achieved.

SUPERIOR VENA CAVOGRAPHY

Superior vena cavography is undertaken to demonstrate the veins of the thoracic inlet and superior vena cava.

Indications

Superior vena cavography may be indicated in the following situations:

1. The evaluation of mediastinal disease, the vast majority of cases being related to neoplastic involvement of the superior vena cava.
2. The evaluation of venous thrombosis in the axillary, subclavian or innominate veins; with possible central extension into the superior vena cava.
3. The investigation of a congenital anomaly of the venous system.

Technique

Equipment

A fluoroscopy unit with spot film capability is used. As with the examination of the inferior vena cava, a biplane serial radiography unit is desirable to obtain A–P and lateral projections with a single injection.

Patient preparation

If there is any oedema of the upper limb the patient is encouraged to keep the arms elevated as far as possible before leaving the ward for the examination. This expedient may obviate the need for a modified cut down procedure.

The patient is fasted for 4–6 hours prior to the examination.

Procedure

The examination is carried out with the patient lying in the supine position. Control films are taken in the A–P and lateral planes. The A–P projection should be full field, extending from the root of the neck to the diaphragm and including the lateral chest walls. The lateral projection is coned to the mediastinum.

The arm veins are usually distended in the presence of superior vena caval obstruction. A tourniquet applied to the upper arm will further engorge the veins. Using an aseptic technique, the median antecubital vein at the elbow is identified and local anaesthetic infiltrated at the proposed venepuncture site. A small skin incision is made to facilitate catheterization. The venepuncture is made with an 18 gauge needle and, using the Seldinger technique, a 7F catheter with side holes is advanced as close to the subclavian vein as the obstruction allows.

Where the vein is not amenable to percutaneous puncture, a modified cut down is performed to expose the vein. The cephalic vein is best avoided because of its acute angle of entry near the termination of the axillary vein. The median antecubital vein has an obtuse angle of entry into the deep venous system which facilitates catheter advancement.

The procedure is repeated for the other arm. Bilateral catheterization with simultaneous injections of contrast medium provides a full anatomical demonstration of the altered venous anatomy, and avoids the mixing artefacts due to the return of unopacified blood which occurs when examining only one arm.

The patient's arms are gently abducted to allow the lateral chest wall to be positioned as close as possible to the lateral film changer when a biplane facility is available. A separate injection is made into each catheter in preference to linking the catheters via a Y connector. In the presence of obstruction, preferential flow occurs through the unobstructed or least obstructed side. A simultaneous injection of 30 ml contrast medium (sodium iothalamate 70%) is made into each catheter and the film sequence is started near the beginning of the injection. The film sequence and rate of injection depends on the degree of obstruction. If test injections made during the positioning of the catheter suggest a complete obstruction, a hand injection is made and films are taken at the rate of one per second to demonstrate the level of obstruction, the collateral flow and whether or not there is any reconstitution of a main venous channel.

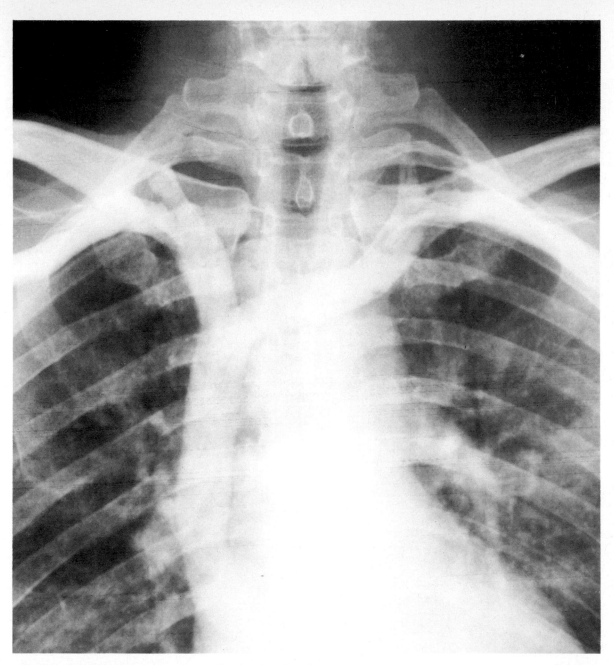

Fig. 9.9 Normal superior vena cavogram showing the subclavian and innominate veins and the superior vena cava down to the right atrium.

The film programme should be long enough to identify the venous anatomy beyond the obstruction, as well as the right atrium (Fig. 9.9). Where superior vena caval flow is less impeded, as with mediastinal deviation or compression, a more forceful injection is required, if necessary with a pump injector, to deliver contrast medium at a rate of 10 ml per second. The programme is then adjusted to take two films per second for four seconds, followed by one per second for ten seconds.

Where there is unequivocal clinical evidence of caval obstruction, for instance from involvement by a bronchial neoplasm, a large bore needle, such as a 16 gauge butterfly needle, may be used instead of catheterization since a more rapid injection, which is possible with the catheter technique, is not required in these circumstances. Both arms are examined as described in the technique above.

Having checked the diagnostic adequacy of the films, the catheters are removed and firm pressure applied to achieve haemostasis. Any sutures used when a cut down has been necessary are firmly tied.

REFERENCES

Berge T., Bergqvist D., Efsing H. O. & Hallböök T. (1978) Local complications of ascending phlebography. *Clin. Radiol.*, **29**, 691–6.

Bettman M. A. & Paulin S. (1977) Leg phlebography: the incidence, nature and modification of undesirable side effects. *Radiology*, **122**, 101–4.

Cotton L. T. & Clark C. (1965) Anatomical localization of venous thrombosis. *Ann. roy. Coll. Surg. Engl.*, **36**, 214–24.

Craig J. O. (1972) In *Practical Procedures in Diagnostic Radiology*. 2e (Eds. Saxton H. M. & Strickland B.), p. 250. H. K. Lewis, London.

Dos Santos J. C. (1938) La phlébographie directe. Conception, technique, premiers résultats. *J. int. Chir.*, **3**, 625–32.

Dow J. D. (1973) Retrograde phlebography in major pulmonary embolism. *Lancet*, **ii**, 407.

Kakkhar V. V. (1980) Diagnosis of deep vein thrombosis. *Methods of Angiography* (Ed. Verstraet M.), pp. 267–96. Martinus Nijhoff, The Hague.

Kinmonth J. B., Young A. E., O'Donnell T. F. Jr., Edwards J. M. & Lea Thomas M. (1976) Mixed vascular deformities of the lower limbs. *Brit. J. Surg.*, **63**, 899.

Lea Thomas M. (1970) Pelvic phlebography. In *Modern Trends in Diagnostic Radiology*. 4e (Ed. McLaren J. W.), pp. 201–9. Butterworths, London.

Lea Thomas M. & Carty H. (1975) The appearances of artefacts on lower limb phlebography. *Clin. Radiol.*, **26**, 527–33.

Lea Thomas M. & Macdonald L. (1977) The accuracy of bolus ascending phlebography in demonstrating the ilio-femoral segment. *Clin. Radiol.*, **28**, 165–71.

Lea Thomas M. & O'Dwyer J. A. (1978) A phlebographic study of the incidence and significance of venous thrombosis of the foot. *Amer. J. Roentgenol.*, **130**, 751–4.

Lea Thomas M. & Walters H. L. (1979) Metrizamide in ascending venography of the legs. *Brit. med. J.*, **ii**, 1036.

Schobinger R. A. (1960) *Intraosseous Venography*. Grune & Stratton, New York.

Shehadi W. H. (1975) Adverse reactions to intravascularly administered contrast media. *Amer. J. Roentgenol.*, **124**, 145–52.

Walters H. L., Clemenson J., Browse N. L. & Lea Thomas M. (1980) [125]I fibrinogen uptake following phlebography of the leg. *Radiology*, **135**, 619–21.

The Heart and Pulmonary Circulation

R. W. GALLOWAY

Angiocardiography is the radiographic visualization of the passage of contrast medium through the heart and great vessels. In venous angiocardiography, the injection is made into a leg or arm vein but the contrast medium is diluted by the blood returning to the heart and contrast is diminished. This technique has now been replaced by selective angiocardiography. The contrast medium is injected rapidly through a catheter into a selected chamber of the heart.

While Forssmann (1929) occupies the premier role of pioneers in cardiac catheterization, there is no doubt that Bleichröder (1912) was the first to pass a catheter in man and must have entered the right side of the heart from a peripheral vein on at least one occasion.

In 1931, Forssman carried the procedure further by injecting contrast medium through a catheter into the right side of the heart, but opposition from his colleagues prevented him from developing the technique. The routine introduction of catheters into the right side of the heart in man was reported in 1941 by Cournand and Ranges, who utilized the procedure to record the intra-cardiac pressures and oxygen saturations. Their technique established the safety and relative ease of the procedure.

Catheterization of the left side of the heart was developed in the following years. Seldinger (1953) described the percutaneous insertion of a catheter into an artery or vein. This technique enabled the catheter to be passed via the aorta through the aortic valve into the left ventricle. Currently, pressure injectors were developed to deliver a greater flow rate of contrast medium through a given size of catheter.

A further approach to the left side of the heart was made by Ross (1959) and Brockenbrough and Braunwald (1960), who described the technique of transseptal catheterization of the left atrium. A catheter could then be passed into the left ventricle through the mitral valve and left ventricular angiography performed.

Pulmonary angiography may be part of the investigation of congenital and acquired heart disease but may also be required in unknown pulmonary lesions as well as pulmonary embolism.

Coronary arteriography is indicated in angina pectoris which is not responding to adequate medical treatment, and is essential prior to coronary artery bypass surgery to enable correct placement of grafts and the assessment of the calibre of the distal vessels. Sones *et al.* (1959) introduced selective coronary arteriography and in 1967 Judkins described his technique using the percutaneous approach. These workers were consistently able to demonstrate the anatomy and pathology of the coronary arteries and provided the impetus for modern coronary artery surgery.

The procedures should be performed in a catheter laboratory, the patient being continuously monitored, and all resuscitation techniques must be available. The information obtained is correlated where relevant with oximetry, pressure recordings and shunt detection techniques, such as dye dilution studies, and other forms of cardiac imaging. Close collaboration of the radiologist and the cardiologist is essential to obtain the maximum data from the investigation.

BASIC REQUIREMENTS

Sterile trolley

Sterile drapes and towels, bowls and receivers, towel clips.

Skin antiseptic, e.g. 2% chlorhexidine in alcohol. Hibiscrub.

Small scalpel and blade, sponge holder, sponge and swabs.

Small Spencer Wells forceps. Fine pointed scissors.

Lignocaine 1% (plain).

Needles, 21G and 23G. 2 × 5 ml syringes, 2 × 10 ml syringes, 2 × 20 ml syringes.

Percutaneous entry needle, e.g. Vygon.

Selected catheters and guides. 3 way tap.

Catheter sheath set if catheter exchange is required, comprising sheath with seal and optional side arm for flushing.

Dextrose saline containing 5000 units of heparin to each 500 ml of solution. 5% dextrose for coronary arteriography. Cut-down set if open exposure of vessel is necessary, catgut and nylon sutures.

Sterile adhesive tape.

Catheter deflecting system including deflecting handle and wire is occasionally required.

Manometer lines. Sterile handle for spot light.

A wide choice of disposable and non-disposable catheters are available, manufactured from woven dacron, teflon, polyurethane and polyethylene, and rendered opaque by the addition of salts of barium, lead or bismuth. The catheter choice depends on the personal preference of the radiologist carrying out the procedure and on the site of injection. A length of up to 125 cm is sufficient and the size (French Gauge, F) should allow an adequate flow rate. Most adults are catheterized prior to angiography with a 7F, 8F or 9F catheter; the distal catheter having an angle of 45–90° 5 cm from the tip. End hole catheters are most suitable for recording pressure and gradients, but angiography is safer if side hole catheters are employed to diminish recoil and prevent intra-myocardial injection and even perforation of the wall of the heart. Pig-tail catheters with multiple side holes are preferred for angiography and decrease the risk of these complications. Information on the maximum flow rates of the various catheters should be available, and the pressure above which disruption of the catheter may occur must not be exceeded.

Contrast medium

All the modern intravascular contrast media in differing concentrations have been used for angiocardiography, pulmonary and coronary arteriography. A mixture of the sodium and methylglucamine salts of diatrizoic, iothalamic and metrizoic acid were employed. Cardio-conray (sodium and meglumine iothalamate, 400 mgm iodine/ml) has been widely used. Hexabrix, a mixture of the meglumine and sodium salts of ioxaglic acid in the concentration of 320 mgm iodine/ml, is a low osmolality intravascular contrast medium which has proved satisfactory in all types of angiography. Recently, iopamidol (Niopam) has been introduced as a non-ionic contrast medium of low osmolarity and, in the concentration of 370 mgm iodine/ml, is suitable for angiocardiography, as is iohexol (Omnipaque) in the concentration of 350 mg mm iodine/ml. The non-ionic media appear to be safer than conventional media.

Pressure injectors

A pressure injector is necessary to inject the contrast medium through the cardiac catheter into the heart or great vessels. The injector should be electrically safe, reliable and capable of injecting small test doses of contrast medium or larger fractionated volumes of contrast into the cardiac chambers. The pressure injector has a flow and volume control with an automatic overload protection to prevent exceeding the pre-selected pressure. The pressure injector may be attached to an ECG release attachment, enabling the injection to be made at a certain time in the cardiac cycle. Disposable syringes are usually employed and the pressure injector maintains the contrast medium at 37°C. Care must be taken to remove all bubbles of air while loading the syringe.

Radiological equipment

Tubes and generators

The X-ray tube must have high power capacity and it is desirable to have a computer controlled generator dedicated to cardiac angiography. The X-ray tubes are mounted in U or C arms capable of rotation, as well as cranial and caudal angulations. Biplane facility is necessary for the investigation of congenital heart disease.

X-ray imaging and recording

A high definition image intensifier and television system is essential. The image intensifier should have a magnification facility, the smaller field providing excellent detail. The terminology for radiographic projections must conform to the two internationally approved conventions, relating firstly to the name of the part of the body next to the imaging device and secondly by the direction of the X-ray beam (Grainger, 1981).

Videotape recording

A videotape recording facility is necessary when using cine studies. The recording can then be studied and a diagnostic assessment made immediately after the injection. Many videotape recorders now have a freeze-frame facility.

Cinefluorography

This is routinely used in the diagnosis of congenital heart disease and coronary artery abnormalities. A 35 mm camera is commonly employed with a speed of up to 150 frames per second. If, during cinefluorography, a higher frame speed than used for the reproduction is set, then fast moving processes can be studied with a slow motion effect. The cine film is processed in a specially designed unit, producing high definition and contrast. Viewing is on an analysing projector which will run forwards and backwards and has a 'still' facility. Recent analysers will make slides of the image, and also copy radiographs of each individual frame which can be used in the operating theatre or placed as a permanent record in the case sheet.

Photofluorography

The films are usually 100 mm or 105 mm in size and single exposures may be made up to a maximum speed of 8/s on a cut or roll film camera. The photofluorograms have excellent quality and detail and are replacing large format radiography. Photofluorography is used in congenital heart disease and coronary arteriography.

Radiographs

Full size radiographs (35×35 cm) may be exposed in an AOT film changer at varying rates from 1–6/s. Full size radiographs are rarely used in cardiac angiography at present, but there is a use in pulmonary angiography.

PATIENT PREPARATION

Food and fluid should not be taken for 4 h prior to the study to prevent aspiration of gastric contents. Premature infants, neonates and small babies require careful observation of their body temperature and acid base balance, which should be corrected when necessary. General anaesthesia is usually unnecessary but may be required in a very nervous or disturbed patient, and is needed if there is assisted ventilation. Children under the age of 3 months do not require any analgesia but they may be allowed to suck a teat which has been moistened in a little glycerine and perhaps a trace of brandy. Older babies and children may be given morphine and trimeprazine, according to their body weight, one hour before the angiography. Adult patients receive morphine 10–15 mg subcutaneously one hour before the procedure. If the patient becomes distressed during the catheterization and angiography, a small intravenous injection of diazepam may be given. Atropine may be required but is not given routinely.

ANGIOCARDIOGRAPHY OF THE RIGHT ATRIUM AND RIGHT VENTRICLE
(Figs. 10.1 and 10.2)

Indications

1. The demonstration of the anatomy and function of the tricuspid valve.

2. The investigation of atrial septal defect.
3. The demonstration of the anatomy and function of the pulmonary valve.
4. Pulmonary hypertension.
5. The investigation of ventricular septal defect.

Catheter insertion

A 7F, 8F or 9F catheter, with a single curve approximately 5 cm from the tip, should be used for the average adult. Ideally, a catheter should be of the side hole variety, but occasionally a combination of side holes and end hole may be used, a pig-tail catheter being preferred for angiography.

Percutaneous technique

A lower limb approach is usual. The pelvis may be elevated on a foam pad and the leg externally rotated to aid venepuncture. Under strict aseptic precautions, a small quantity of local anaesthetic is injected 2 cm below the inguinal ligament and medial to the femoral artery pulsation. A small skin incision is then made with a scalpel at the site of needle puncture and the tissues down to the vein are carefully separated with the tip of a small pair of Spencer Wells forceps. If the catheter is of end hole type, it may be introduced by the standard Seldinger technique directly into the femoral vein. If a side hole catheter is employed, or catheter exchange is planned during the procedure, it is necessary to insert a catheter exchange sheath into the femoral vein. After allowing the local anaesthetic to diffuse around the puncture site, a disposable entry needle is inserted directly into the femoral vein medial to the femoral artery. The short guide wire belonging to the catheter exchange set is then passed through the needle into the femoral vein, the needle is removed and the introducer and sheath passed using a slight rotatory movement to avoid buckling the teflon sheath as it enters the femoral vein. The central wire and introducer are removed when the teflon sheath has passed smoothly up the femoral vein, leaving the exchange sheath in the vein. The cardiac catheter, filled with heparinized dextrose saline, is then introduced through the seal at the end of the catheter exchange sheath and passed up the femoral vein and iliac vein into the inferior vena cava, having been connected to the pressure monitoring module. The ascent of the cardiac catheter should be carefully observed on the television monitor. If the progress is arrested, the catheter should be withdrawn slightly and rotated, when it will be found to pass easily up the vessel. As the catheter ascends up the inferior

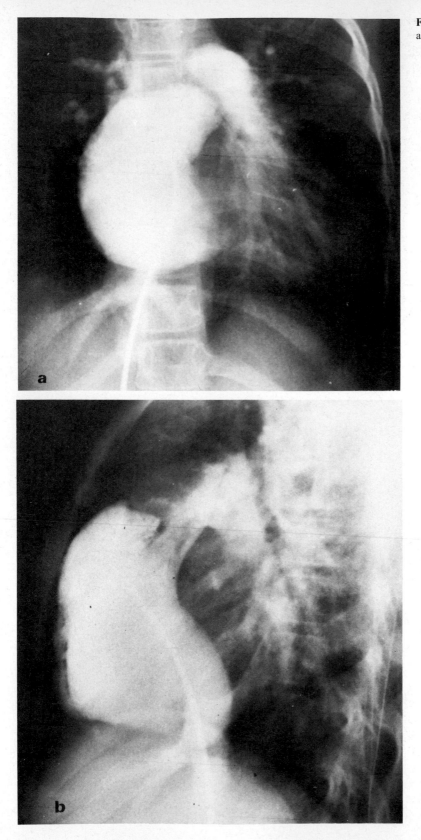

Fig. 10.1 Injection into the right atrium. A–P and lateral projections.

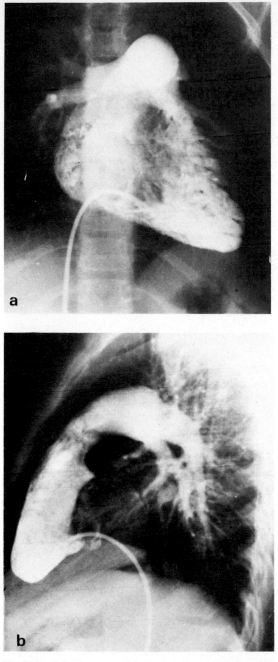

Fig. 10.2 Injection into right ventricle. A–P and lateral projections.

of blood may be taken for oximetry, and pressure recordings should be checked prior to entering the cardiac chambers. Oximetry should be performed when the catheter is in the body of the right atrium, and the catheter tip should carefully explore the atrium for evidence of atrial septal defect or of anomalous pulmonary veins draining into the right atrium. When samples of blood are taken from the cardiac catheter for oximetry, it is important that no small clots are injected back into the catheter when flushing. Similarly, care must be taken not to inject small bubbles of air into the circulation.

When right atrial angiography is to be performed, the catheter tip should be positioned in the mid-body of the right atrium. A small test injection of up to 5 ml of contrast medium confirms that the catheter lies in an optimum position and is not impinging on the wall of the right atrium. The test injection can be observed on the television monitor. Having confirmed the satisfactory position of the catheter, the pressure injector is loaded with 50 ml of contrast medium at body temperature and connected to the cardiac catheter. An extension may sometimes be required between the catheter and the pressure injector. Care must be taken not to introduce bubbles of air into the delivery system. The patient is then warned that angiography is about to be performed, advised to remain perfectly still and, when indicated, to suspend respiration. The catheter should be fixed to the skin with sterile adhesive tape prior to angiography. The passage of contrast medium is recorded on the biplane facility, using either photofluorography or cinefluorography during the injection at 25 ml/s.

The contrast medium is observed passing from the right atrium through the tricuspid valve, into the right ventricle and out into the pulmonary artery. The contrast medium subsequently passes into the pulmonary veins, the left atrium and mitral valve, and then into the left ventricle and aorta. The cardiac catheter is disconnected from the pressure injector when the injection has been completed, and is flushed through with heparinized dextrose saline. It is uncommon for any complications to arise during right atrial angiography.

Right ventricular angiography

The cardiac catheter is then advanced from the right atrium through the tricuspid valve and into the right ventricle. A ventricular trace is recorded as the catheter traverses the tricuspid valve, care being taken to ensure that the catheter, which is apparently in the right ventricle, is not lying in the coronary sinus. A

vena cava, just before it passes through the hemidiaphragm, it may become trapped in a hepatic vein. By gently withdrawing the catheter and rotating, the catheter will slip easily into the cavity of the right atrium. During the passage of the catheter, samples small test injection may be necessary to confirm the site of the cardiac tip as a dampened ventricular trace can sometimes be misleading. Difficulty may be experienced in passing the cardiac catheter through the tricuspid valve into the right ventricle, but a combination of looping the catheter in the atrium combined with rotation may enable the catheter to enter the right ventricle. The choice of catheter and catheter curve are a matter of individual preference by the radiologist, who must develop his own technique with experience. The presence of the catheter in the right ventricle often results in the production of extrasystoles, so that it is advisable to place the catheter in such a position that the extrasystoles are minimal. A small test injection of 5 ml of contrast medium is essential prior to right ventricular angiography, to ensure that the catheter tip is correctly situated in the body of the right ventricle and is not impacting in the muscular trabeculae of the ventricle. Fifty millilitres of contrast medium are injected via the pressure injector at a rate of 30 ml/s into the ventricle. The passage of the contrast medium from the right ventricle to the pulmonary artery, pulmonary veins, left atrium and left ventricle, is recorded in A–P and lateral projections. If many extrasystoles are produced, it will be noticed that reflux occurs through the tricuspid valve into the right atrium. This is not necessarily organic in nature, and is related to the abnormal contractions of the heart.

If it is impossible to pass a catheter from the lower limb up the iliac vein and inferior vena cava into the heart, there may be an obstruction to these vessels or the presence of an azygos venous system. In this case, it may be advisable to attempt to catheterize the right side of the heart via an upper limb vein. If a percutaneous technique is employed, a vein should be identified on the medial aspect of the antecubital fossa. Using a similar technique, the catheter is introduced and passed up the brachial vein, axillary vein, superior vena cava and into the right atrium. It is unwise to use a vein on the lateral aspect of the antecubital fossa, as this vein is probably the cephalic vein or its tributary, and difficulty will be experienced in passing the catheter at shoulder level into the axillary vein. A tip-deflecting catheter system is infrequently used.

Cut-down dissection techniques

With increasing skill in the use of percutaneous technique, an open cut-down into the vein is rarely

required. The cardiac catheter is normally introduced into a lower limb vein but, if this is not possible, one may use a vein on the medial aspect on the antecubital fossa. The course of the long saphenous vein is identified by drawing a line from either the pubic tubercle or the medial aspect of the pulsation of the femoral artery down to a point just lateral to the margin of the medial femoral condyle. A small quantity of local anaesthetic is injected into the skin and subcutaneous tissues, 5–6 cm below the inguinal ligament in the line of the saphenous vein. A transverse or slightly oblique incision, approximately 3 cm long, is made at this site and the subcutaneous tissues are gently dissected. If a finger is then inserted into the incision, the long saphenous vein can be palpated below the subcutaneous fat and tissue. When located, the vein is gently brought to the surface by means of a small blunt hook and the vein is dissected free of adherent tissue. After mobilization of the vein, a double loop of catgut is passed under the vein and the lower loop is firmly tied. The proximal loop of catgut is clipped to a pair of forceps and is used to exert gentle traction upon the vein. Using a pair of fine pointed scissors, a small incision is made in the wall of the vein and the catheter tip is inserted into the vein. The catheter insertion may be aided by inserting a small hook into the incision in the vein, making the orifice slightly larger, or alternatively by inserting a fine pair of curved forceps into the venous incision. The proximal loop of catgut can be loosely tied around the vein and catheter. The catheter is then advanced as previously described. The catheter is removed when angiography has been performed, and the proximal loop of catgut is firmly tied. The skin incision is then closed and a sterile dressing applied to the wound.

LEFT VENTRICULAR ANGIOGRAPHY (Fig. 10.3)

The usual approach to the left ventricle is via percutaneous catheterization of the femoral artery. If this is impossible, owing to tortuous or obstructed iliac arteries, an approach may be made through the axillary artery or, rarely, the brachial artery. If percutaneous arterial techniques cannot be used, it may be necessary to carry out transseptal puncture of the left atrium and pass the catheter from the left atrium through the mitral valve into the left ventricle. With experience and improved technique, it is rarely necessary to cut-down on a peripheral artery as a percutaneous technique is invariably successful, except occasionally in very small children.

Fig. 10.3 Injection into left ventricle. Oblique projection.

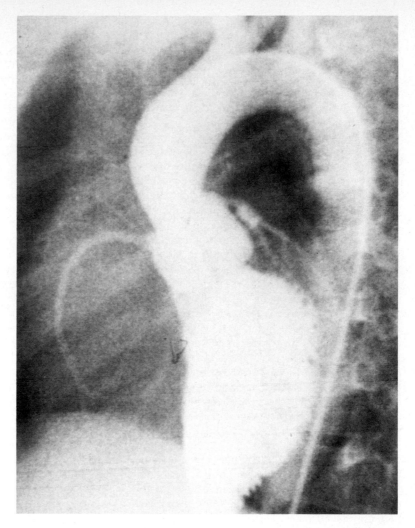

Indications

1. Congenital and acquired aortic valve disease including subvalvar and supravalvar obstructive lesions.
2. Ventricular septal defects.
3. Mitral valve lesions, including ostium primum abnormalities.
4. Cardiomyopathy.
5. Immediately before coronary arteriography.

Technique

The femoral artery is catheterized by a percutaneous Seldinger technique. A 7F, 8F or 9F pig-tail catheter is introduced into the femoral artery and, under fluoroscopic control, guided through the iliac arteries around the aortic arch into the ascending aorta. It may be necessary to use a J-guide wire to pass the catheter in those patients with tortuous iliac arteries, never using undue force. A small test injection of contrast medium visualizes the course of the artery if the iliac artery presents a severe obstruction to the passage of the catheter. Failing to pass the catheter up one iliac artery requires that femoral artery catheterization should be carried out on the other side.

A pig-tail catheter, threaded over a guide wire, passes around the aortic arch and the catheter is then ready to be passed through the aortic valve into the left ventricle. The normal aortic valve presents no difficulty to the catheter passing freely through the valve into the outflow tract of the left ventricle. If the catheter does not pass easily through the aortic valve, passage may occur if the catheter is repeatedly rotated, withdrawn and advanced again. Alternatively, the guide wire may be advanced through the catheter, so that it projects 4–5 cm beyond the catheter tip, when advancement of the catheter may enable the guide wire to pass through the valve into the outflow tract of the left ventricle. This is then followed by passage of the catheter on the guide wire through the aortic valve. The presence of the catheter in the outflow tract of the left ventricle often causes ventricular extrasystoles, whereupon it is advisable to allow the heart to settle into sinus rhythm before carrying out further manipulations. The guide wire projecting from the tip of the catheter is then withdrawn and the catheter is connected to the pressure recording apparatus. Although a pig-tail catheter is most suitable for left ventricular angiography, a curved catheter with either side holes, or end and side holes, may be most convenient for passing through the septal defect or for recording differing pressures within the body of the left ventricle. After pressure studies and oximetry have been performed prior to angiography, the catheter tip should be positioned either in the mid-body of the left ventricle or in the apex of the ventricle itself. The catheter should not be positioned close to the mitral valve in cases of suspected mitral regurgitation. The catheter tip should be free in the ventricular cavity, not impacting on or in the wall of the ventricle. A small test injection of 5–10 ml of contrast medium into the left ventricle through the catheter confirms the tip position. Prior to the left ventricular angiogram, the patient is warned of some possible discomfort during the course of injection. The pressure injector, containing 35–45 ml of contrast medium, is connected to the cardiac catheter. The injection time should be 2–4 s, depending on the suspected lesion. The passage of contrast medium is recorded in A–P and lateral planes by cinefluorography or photofluorography, the standard projections being augmented as necessary by oblique projections and by specialized axial views including the four chamber projections (see p. 157). The pressure injector is disconnected after the injection and the pressure is monitored in the left ventricle to ascertain the rise in pressure following angiography, which may be important in subvalvar and valvar lesions. Extrasystoles are common during injection but, usually, they soon cease. After scrutiny of the videotape recording, the catheter is withdrawn and haemostasis obtained on the puncture site by firm manual pressure.

When catheter exchange is planned, this may be carried out over a guide wire or rarely by the insertion of a sheath into the artery as previously described in catheterization of the femoral vein.

Upper limb arterial catheterization

Failure to pass a catheter retrogradely up the aorta, owing to tortuosity and obstruction of iliac arteries, may indicate the necessity to use an upper limb artery for the passage of the cardiac catheter. The brachial artery is liable to spasm and catheterization is not recommended unless other methods fail. The axillary artery is easier to catheterize by a percutaneous technique. Either side may be used, the arm being abducted with the hand resting alongside the head in a relaxed position. The axillary artery is punctured, using the technique previously described, at the site of maximal pulsation. The smallest catheter that will deliver the necessary flow rate is used, and is carefully passed under fluoroscopic control into the ascending aorta and down into the left ventricle. Extreme care should be taken during axillary artery catheterization to prevent haematoma formation and possible trauma to the brachial plexus.

As a general rule, arterial cut-down technique is unnecessary and undesirable in adults, being reserved for coronary arteriography by the Sones technique (see p. 159).

LEFT ATRIAL ANGIOGRAPHY

The left atrium may be visualized on follow-through angiography after injection of contrast medium into the right ventricle or pulmonary artery. A catheter may also be passed through a patent foramen ovale or via an atrial septal defect into the left atrium prior to angiography. Alternatively, transseptal puncture of the left atrium is carried out as described by Ross (1959) or Brockenbrough and Braunwald (1960). Trans-septal techniques should only be practised by an experienced cardiac radiologist. Briefly, a curved metal needle is introduced, through a pre-existing catheter, into the right atrium. The needle is then gently rotated so that the needle tip points in a postero–medial direction, i.e. towards 5 o'clock. The needle is then gently withdrawn slowly along the atrial septum and a distinct sensation is noted as the needle passes over the fossa ovalis. The needle is then advanced into the left atrium, as confirmed by the presence of the left atrial trace on the pressure recorder and by oximetry. A guide wire is passed through the needle into the left atrium. A catheter may be introduced over the guide wire for angiography. Alternatively, a pre-formed catheter can already be *in situ* on the needle and advanced over the needle into the left atrium. Transseptal catheterization and angiography is performed in obstructive lesions of the

Fig. 10.4   Injection into pulmonary artery.

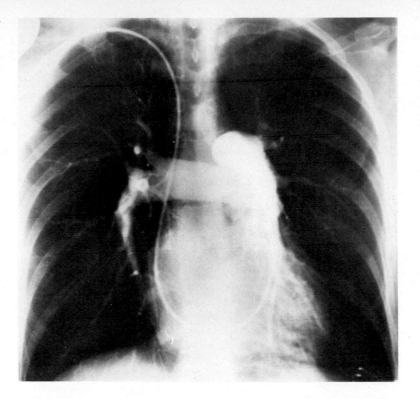

mitral valve, and in obstructive lesions of the aortic valve when it is not possible to pass a retrograde arterial catheter into the body of the left ventricle. The catheter is advanced from the left atrium into the left ventricle. Transseptal catheterization is occasionally required to record the pressure in the left atrium when the pulmonary artery wedge pressure recording is unsatisfactory. Transseptal catheterization carries a risk of perforating other cardiac chambers and the aorta. Transseptal catheterization should not be performed if the anatomy of the cardiac chambers is not clear or if there are marked anomalies of the thoracic spine, particularly kyphosis and scoliosis. The left atrium may also be entered by inserting a needle from the subclavian vein as described by Epstein and Coulshed (1971). For angiography of the left atrium, 35–40 ml of contrast medium are injected via the catheter in two seconds and the passage of contrast medium is recorded in A–P, lateral and oblique planes as required.

PULMONARY ARTERIOGRAPHY (Fig. 10.4)

Indications

1. Pulmonary embolism.
2. Pulmonary hypertension.
3. Haemoptysis of unexplained origin.
4. To opacify the left atrium where trans-septal puncture is unwise, e.g. atrial myxoma.

Technique

A 7F, 8F or 9F catheter is used, preferably of the pig-tail type, although a side hole catheter of the NIH type may be employed with a single curve approximately 5 cm from the tip. The right femoral vein is catheterized by the Seldinger technique and the catheter passed over the guide wire to the right atrium, then the right ventricle and through the pulmonary valve into the main branch of the pulmonary artery. Pressure recordings are made. The catheter tip should be positioned midway between the pulmonary valve and the bifurcation of the pulmonary artery.

The passage of the guide wire or catheter may be prevented by the presence of thrombus or obstruction, which should be recorded by contrast injection, and the lower limb approach is then discontinued. An upper limb approach may then be performed as described previously. Forty millilitres of contrast medium are injected in 1.5 s and the passage of contrast medium through the pulmonary artery, pulmonary capillaries and pulmonary veins to the left atrium is recorded by cinefluorography, photofluorography or radiographs exposed at 4/s. For study of the pulmonary vasculature, only A–P projections are required, in the lateral plane both pulmonary arteries being superimposed. After inspection of the videotape recording or large radiographs, the catheter may be advanced to the left or right pulmonary artery and a selective injection of 30 ml of contrast medium made into the pulmonary artery at 25 ml/s. The passage of contrast medium may then be recorded, not only in the A–P plane, but also in the lateral and oblique planes.

Super selective injections, combined with a magnification technique, are required for suspicious areas of embolism. At the end of the injection, the catheter is carefully withdrawn from the pulmonary artery into the right atrium because the pig-tail catheter may catch the chordae tendinae. This may be prevented by inserting a wire to straighten the pig-tail. Particular care should be exercised in carrying out pulmonary angiography in cases of pulmonary hypertension, as cardio-respiratory failure may develop.

In a recent study, Mills *et al.* (1980) have suggested that pulmonary angiography is contra-indicated if the right ventricle end diastolic pressure exceeds 20 mmHg.

The use of a pulmonary artery seeking pig-tail catheter has been recently reviewed by Grollman and Renner (1981) with a 100% success in pulmonary artery catheterization. They recommend systemic heparinization as pig-tail catheters themselves have been incriminated in thrombo-embolic problems.

Removal of pulmonary arterial clot may be performed by a suction catheter technique inserted through the femoral vein.

Balloon occlusion pulmonary angiography, using a Swan–Ganz catheter, improves image quality and may be employed at the bed-side of ill patients. The catheter is advanced into an area of the lung which is considered to be abnormal on the chest radiograph, standard pulmonary angiogram or lung scan, and the balloon is inflated. A hand injection of 10 ml of contrast medium is made during full inspiration and the image is recorded. Sequential appropriate positioning and injections are made to demonstrate all suspicious areas.

Balloon occlusion pulmonary angiography is complementary to a standard technique of injecting contrast medium into the main pulmonary artery.

PAEDIATRIC CARDIOANGIOGRAPHY

'No patient should be denied the opportunity for precise diagnosis and possible cure or improvement because he is too small, or because functional severity of his lesions appears so great that death may occur during or after catheterization.' (Sones, 1955).

Since cardiocatheterization and angiography are complimentary to each other, the data obtained must be correlated with the data from non-invasive techniques.

Technique

The patient is placed on the table in a comfortable position. The necessary monitoring leads (ECG and temperature) are connected. A reassuring nurse and slightly darkened room, coupled with the premedication, are conducive to sleep. A heating pad or gamgee jacket may be necessary to maintain body temperature. The usual site for catheter entry is the inguinal area, but occasionally it may be necessary to use the upper limbs.

The selection of catheter size and terminal curve depends on the individual preference and experience, as well as the size of the patient and the suspected abnormalities. Premature and small neonates may be catheterized with a 4F catheter on the venous side, but a 3F catheter may be adequate on the arterial side. The catheter length is reduced to around 60 cm. Specially designed paediatric catheters are now available from manufacturers, for instance the Macartney range. A balloon flow directional catheter is useful to reduce the risk of cardiac perforation in small premature infants and neonates. The contrast medium formerly employed was Cardioconray but more recently Hexabrix has been found to cause less discomfort to the baby. Use has also been made of the new non-ionic contrast medium in sick babies. The dose of contrast medium is limited by the weight of the child; 4 ml/kg of contrast medium may be injected in fractionated doses although, on occasions, we have used up to 6 ml/kg.

Radiation dosage may be reduced by the use of pulsed fluoroscopy and the grids may be removed when performing angiography on small infants.

Skin preparation with Hibiscrub is used and the catheter introduced into the femoral artery or femoral vein using a percutaneous technique. Where necessary, a paediatric catheter exchange set is inserted into the vessel. Various needles have been used to puncture the artery or vein but various sizes of Medicuts through which a guide wire can be introduced into the vessel are commonly employed. In very small children, it may be advisable to puncture the vessel with a 21 G butterfly needle; the connecting tube is cut off flush with the needle with a sharp pair of scissors when a free flow of blood is obtained and a fine guide wire is introduced through the needle into the vessel. The needle is then withdrawn leaving the fine guide wire in the vessel and a Medicut sheath is passed over the guide wire into the vessel to enlarge the puncture orifice. A larger guide wire can be inserted if necessary or the Medicut can be removed and a paediatric sheath set inserted; the appropriate catheter being introduced via the sheath into the vessel. If a sheath is not to be used, say on the arterial side, the catheter can be passed directly over the guide wire into the artery.

The cardiac chambers are then explored, pressure recordings made and samples taken for oximetry. The left and right side of the heart should be studied and angiography planned to obtain the maximum information. The left heart can be easily explored through a patent foramen ovale and there should be routine probing for the presence of a ductus arteriosus.

When the study is completed, the catheter is withdrawn and haemostasis is obtained. Complex cardiac anomalies may be difficult to interpret on the initial videotape replay. The examination should be planned in a systematic manner, in order to establish the venous–atrial connection, the atrio–ventricular connection and the ventriculo–great vessel connection. Failure to introduce a catheter by the percutaneous technique is uncommon but, if necessary, the catheter can be inserted into the vessel by a modified cut-down technique. The vessel is exposed in the normal manner and a needle and guide wire introduced as if using a percutaneous technique. Haemostasis is obtained by firm pressure after the catheter has been removed and the skin incision closed with sutures. The passage of contrast medium is recorded by bi-plane cineangiographic systems, augmented where necessary by axial cineangiography (Elliott et al., 1980). Two principles are involved: firstly axial alignment of the heart is achieved by positioning the long axis of the heart perpendicular to an X-ray beam, and secondly by rotation of the heart on this long axis so as to visualize the lesion in profile.

The projections particularly studied are the four chamber view and the long axial oblique view. These projections are now routinely performed in those units associated with the investigation of congenital heart disease, and reference should be made to the original articles by Elliott et al. (1977).

Balloon atrial septostomy

The creation of an artificial atrial septal defect is indicated where atrial mixing may improve the prognosis prior to corrective surgery. This technique is employed in transposition of the great arteries, pulmonary atresia and mitral atresia, and has also been carried out in total anomalous pulmonary venous drainage. The technique entails the passage of a catheter with a balloon at its tip through the foramen ovale into the left atrium. A single lumen or double lumen catheter may be used but it is important to make certain that the balloon lies in the left atrium. After inflation of the balloon with contrast medium, it is sharply withdrawn through the atrial septum into the right atrium. The tearing of the atrial septum creates the artificial atrial septal defect. The larger the balloon, the larger is the defect created. A balloon may be inflated with up to 5 ml of contrast medium. Care must be taken on withdrawal of the balloon catheter not to tear the inferior vena cava. Recently a blade septostomy has been introduced by a cut-down catheter insertion technique.

Umbilical vein catheterization

This may be performed within the first 7 days of life. The technique is less frequently used—the percutaneous lower limb approach being favoured. After careful cleansing of the umbilical stalk, transection of the stalk is performed by means of a sharp pair of scissors or scalpel blade, whereupon the umbilical vein is identified. A soft 5F catheter is then inserted into the vein and passed through the ductus venosus into the right atrium under fluoroscopic control. Unfortunately, in a number of patients, the ductus venosus may have undergone physiological thrombosis and the passage of the catheter is impossible. Concern has been expressed recently about the possible introduction of sepsis. Umbilical artery catheterization is now rarely undertaken.

Balloon flow directional catheters and angiography

The double lumen catheter contains a lumen for pressure recordings and injection of contrast medium with a second lumen to inflate a balloon with carbon dioxide. Originally, a Swan–Ganz catheter was popular but other similar makes are now available, for instance the Berman catheter. The catheter is introduced into a peripheral vein by a percutaneous technique and passed into the heart. The balloon is then inflated with carbon dioxide and allowed to pass by the natural flow of blood into the appropriate great vessel or chamber. Contrast medium is injected after appropriate pressure recordings and oximetry. This balloon catheter has been found to be particularly useful in investigating neonates and small children.

BRONCHIAL ARTERY CATHETERIZATION AND ANGIOGRAPHY

Indications

1. In the investigation of haemoptysis.
2. The demonstration of collateral vessels between the aortic and pulmonary circulations in congenital heart disease, particularly pulmonary atresia.
3. In space-occupying lesions of the lung.

Technique

It is helpful, if a descending aortogram is performed prior to the selective catheterization, to obtain details of the anatomy and configuration of the vessels to be selectively catheterized. After study of the descending aortogram, catheter exchange is made and the appropriate curved catheter is passed in a retrograde manner into the thoracic aorta and manipulated into the vessel to be demonstrated. The amount of contrast medium injected depends upon the weight of the patient and size of vessel. The image is recorded in A–P and the lateral planes and may be supplemented where necessary by oblique projections.

PULMONARY VENOUS WEDGE ANGIOGRAPHY

This technique is employed to demonstrate the pulmonary arterial tree in cases of pulmonary atresia, or similar conditions where it is impossible to demonstrate the pulmonary artery by right ventricular injection owing to marked obstruction.

Technique

A percutaneous retrograde catheter is passed from the femoral vein to the right atrium, then through the atrial septum into the left atrium, and is passed out into the lung field into the near wedge position. Contrast medium is then injected either by hand or by means of a pressure injector, using 0.5 ml–1 ml/kg, the injection being performed over 3–4 s. Retrograde filling of the intrapulmonary arteries and the proximal main branch is demonstrated and is recorded by cinefluorography. Extravasation of contrast medium into the lung parenchyma may occur, so that contrast

medium may enter the bronchi and cause severe coughing. Immediately after the injection, it is advisable to flush the contrast medium from the pulmonary segments.

CONTRA-INDICATIONS

There are no unequivocal contra-indications to angiocardiography and pulmonary arteriography. Care should be exercised in those patients suffering from severe pulmonary hypertension and it should be again stressed that cardioangiography should be only carried out in a catheter laboratory by experienced staff with all the facilities available for resuscitation and emergency cardiac surgery. The greatest hazard lies in the continuing failure to make an exact diagnosis upon which effective treatment may be made (Sones, 1955).

COMPLICATIONS OF CARDIOANGIOGRAPHY

Complications may be due either to the passage of the catheter into the heart or great vessel or are associated with the injection of contrast medium. Arterial spasm and thrombosis must be recognized quickly and the appropriate treatment given. Platelets may form on the outer side of catheters and on guide wires. Arterial catheter exchange should be carried out low in the abdomen to prevent platelet embolization into coronary or cerebral vessels. Pre-existing disease of the arterial wall increases the risk of arterial spasm and thrombosis. Haemorrhage from the puncture site in the artery or vein is easily controlled by firm but not extreme manual pressure at the puncture site. Infection at the site of catheter insertion is uncommon and requires treatment with the appropriate antibiotic, neonates being carefully observed for the development of systemic infection.

Catheter loops and pig-tails may proceed to knot formation unless care is taken. The knot must not be tightened when removal is attempted. Unknotting of the catheter may be performed by passing a cardiac catheter or guide wire from the opposite femoral vein, as described by Thomas and Sievers (1979).

Arrhythmias are common during cardiac catheterization and cardioangiography. The transient ectopic beats of atrial or ventricular cause are common and settle down quickly without treatment. Bradycardia needs urgent treatment as asystole may develop when external cardiac massage may be necessary to maintain circulation. Atrial flutter, fibrillation and ventricular fibrillation must be promptly treated with the appropriate counter shock technique.

Perforation of a vessel or cardiac chamber, either by manipulation or catheter recoil on pressure injection, is suspected by a change in the pressure trace or difficulty in withdrawing blood on aspiration. The injection of a small quantity of contrast medium by hand will confirm the situation of the catheter tip. If tamponade develops, prompt treatment is necessary.

An intra-mural injection of contrast medium, due to a malposition of the catheter tip, is quickly recognized during the videotape recording as myocardial staining. Manipulation of a stiff catheter with an end hole and high pressure injection and small heart chamber all contribute to this complication. The catheter tip should be seen to be moving freely at the time of test injection. Pig-tail catheters are safer.

Air embolism is a rare complication. All bubbles of air should be carefully excluded from a syringe and the syringe tilted vertically to prevent bubbles entering the catheter. The general monitoring of the patient should not be ignored; including the metabolic balance, the fluid overload and the possibility of haemorrhage.

Complications following the injection of contrast medium are described elsewhere but, in particular, hypotension, hypertension and pulmonary oedema must be recognized quickly and the appropriate treatment given.

RELATIONSHIP OF CARDIOANGIOGRAPHY AND PULMONARY ANGIOGRAPHY TO OTHER IMAGING MODALITIES

The anatomy and function of the heart may be assessed by cardiac catheterization and angiography in different planes. These techniques are invasive and carry a small but definite morbidity and mortality. M-mode (or one-dimensional echocardiography) has been supplemented by the addition of two-dimensional real time cross-sectional echocardiography, which allows temporal and spatial relationships to be displayed and provides a representation of cardiac structures in the real time mode. Accurate diagnosis and assessment of the severity of most forms of acquired heart disease may be achieved by the complimentary use of plain radiography and M-mode echocardiography (Newell et al., 1981).

Congenital heart disease lends itself particularly well to the investigation by echocardiographic techniques. A pre-catheterization and angiographic diagnosis can often be made and the investigation planned

with the appropriate cineaxial projection. Radionuclide evaluation enables the detection and quantification of shunts and flow paths, being particularly useful for the management and follow-up of patients who have a small shunt or who have had previous cardiac surgery. Radionuclide techniques are also used for measuring cardiac output, ejection fraction and movement of the ventricular wall.

Digital subtraction angiography permits intravenous angiography, combined with real time image subtraction, and has been used to study the pulmonary arteries and the motion of the ventricular wall. The technique is now being applied to paediatric cardioangiography using injections of small quantities of dilute contrast medium through the cardiac catheter. The resultant images are excellent.

Radionuclide lung scans are routinely performed in suspected cases of pulmonary thrombo-embolic disease and less pulmonary angiography is performed than previously. If, however, catheter removal of the clot is proposed, it is essential to localize the clot accurately by pulmonary angiography. Computed tomography (CT scanning) permits finer discrimination of tissues and the axial transverse tomographic plane allows for better topographic evaluation, which is particularly applicable to wedge shaped pulmonary infarcts (Sinner, 1978).

CORONARY ARTERIOGRAPHY

Basically, two techniques are employed today; the retrograde brachial approach of Sones and the percutaneous femoral technique of Judkins.

Retrograde brachial technique of Sones (Sones & Shirey, 1962)

A single Sones catheter of 7F or 8F calibre is introduced into the brachial artery by a cut-down technique, commonly in the right arm. The catheter tapers to a 5.5F diameter in the distal few centimetres, the tip being flexible and containing one end and one side hole. The right coronary artery is usually fairly easy to enter using the Sones catheter. The left coronary artery is more difficult to enter, and it may be necessary to form a loop in the end of the coronary catheter by wedging the tip of the catheter in either the aortic valve cusps or a brachio-cephalic vessel. After coronary arteriography has been performed, the same catheter is passed into the body of the left ventricle and ventriculography is carried out. The catheter is removed when the study is completed and

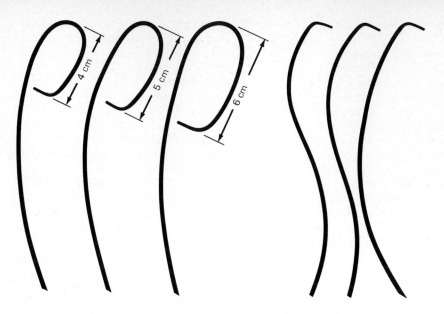

Fig. 10.5 Judkins catheters for left and right coronary arteriography.

haemostasis obtained after confirming that the brachial artery is patent and free of clots. The Sones technique is mainly employed in America, but most radiologists prefer the following technique of Judkins. Continuous ECG monitoring is vital, 5% dextrose is used for flushing.

Judkins percutaneous transfemoral technique (Fig. 10.5)

The original description in 1967 has been little altered today. It is easy to learn, carries only a small risk of local arterial complications and has become popular throughout this country. The catheters are made from either polyethylene or polyurethane reinforced to increase the torque control. There are pre-formed separate catheters for both right and left coronary arteries and each catheter is available in three sizes, approximately 6F, 7F and 8F. The tip configuration is also in three sizes, suitable for the various aortic arches that may be encountered. The catheters end in a short angle tip with a single end hole.

Indications

1. Anginal chest pain in patients in whom surgery is contemplated.
2. Chest pain of unknown aetiology.
3. To demonstrate the morphology of a coronary vessel when contemplating cardiac surgery (Conti, 1977).

Pre-medication

Atropine 0.6 mgm should be given prior to the procedure, while nervous and apprehensive patients may require 10 mg of morphine. General anaesthesia is unnecessary as a general rule.

Technique

Catheterization of the left coronary artery (Fig. 10.6)

A catheter with an appropriate tip configuration is inserted by the Seldinger percutaneous technique, the guide wire and catheter being advanced into the ascending aorta. Introduction of the Judkins catheter is facilitated by the use of a vessel dilator. The guide wire should be left in the catheter until the level of the aortic arch is reached, otherwise the loop will form prematurely in the aortic arch. The catheter tip is then passed into the sinus of Valsalva and introduced into the ostium of the coronary artery. The catheter pressure must be constantly monitored and the tip of the catheter must enter the coronary ostium but not occlude it. One or two millilitres of contrast medium are then injected and observed on the monitor to confirm the correct position of the catheter tip. Two to nine millilitres of contrast medium are then injected into the coronary ostium and the passage of contrast medium is recorded and observed on the videotape. The contrast medium should clear immediately from the coronary artery after injection and, if not, there may be partial occlusion of the coronary artery by the catheter which should be withdrawn immediately. The optimal projections for a patient can be obtained

Fig. 10.6 Left coronary arteriogram. Lateral projection.

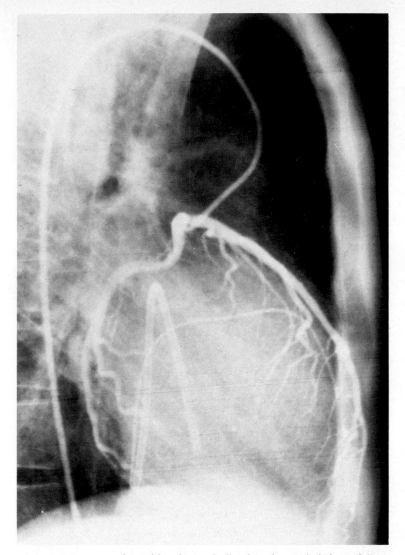

by using a C arm or U arm equipment and coronary arteriography is modified to demonstrate the specific coronary arterial pattern. In addition to P–A, lateral and oblique projections, axial oblique views may be required (Guthaner & Wexler, 1980).

The number of injections made into the left coronary artery depend on the pathology demonstrated and the skill and experience of the operator. Several injections may be made and, after completing the studies of the left coronary artery, the catheter is then withdrawn over the guide wire and catheter exchange carried out in the lower abdominal aorta, substituting the right Judkins coronary catheter for the left.

Right coronary arteriography (Fig. 10.7)
The appropriate right coronary artery catheter is advanced into the ascending aorta by withdrawing

the guide wire and allowing the angled tip to follow the contour of the arch to the aortic root. By carefully rotating the catheter tip 180° so that it projects anteriorly and to the right and withdrawing it from the aortic valve up the aorta, the catheter tip may pass into the coronary ostium. Again, the arterial pressure must be constantly monitored and care must be taken not to block the coronary ostium. A small test injection of contrast medium is made to confirm satisfactory positioning of the catheter tip. The appropriate injections are made into the right coronary artery and P–A, lateral and oblique projections taken as required to demonstrate the pathology. When the study of the right coronary artery has been completed, the catheter is withdrawn to the lower abdominal aorta, left ventricular angiography is then performed by substituting a pig-tail catheter for the coronary catheter.

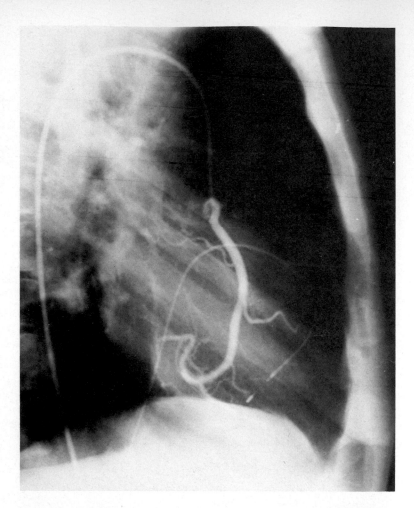

Fig. 10.7 Right coronary arteriogram. Lateral projection.

Forty-five millilitres of contrast medium are injected into the body of the left ventricle at 15 ml/s and the passage of contrast medium is recorded by cinefluorography in the oblique projection. The catheter is then withdrawn and haemostasis obtained. Rarely left ventricular angiography may be performed by the transseptal injection of contrast into the left atrium. Movement of the left ventricular wall is assessed, as well as the ejection fraction. The majority of investigators carry out left ventricular angiography immediately prior to coronary arteriography, as injections of contrast medium cause changes in myocardial contractability and diminution of the ejection fraction.

Graft angiography

This is an extension of coronary arteriography in which a catheter is introduced via the ascending aorta into the vein graft ostium. It may be necessary to carry out a supravalvar aortogram if the graft ostium cannot be entered with a selective catheter.

More recently Gamel *et al.* (1980) have developed a pre-formed single catheter for catheterization of the coronary arteries and vein bypass grafts by a percutaneous femoral technique. The catheter, of polyurethane with wire mesh, is 100 cm long and size 7F. The tip is tapered with end hole and two side holes. The tip is angled at 80° and three different tip lengths are available according to the size of the aortic root. The ostia are entered with the patient in the left anterior oblique position. A success rate of over 90% is obtained for coronary and graft catheterization. The use of a single catheter eliminates multiple insertion of guide wires and catheter changes.

Complications of coronary arteriography

Cardiac arrhythmias, ranging from asystole to ventricular fibrillation, must be promptly treated. It must be stressed again that there should be rapid disappearance of contrast medium from the coronary artery. If this does not occur, the catheter is partially occluding the ostium and should be instantly withdrawn. Embolism may occur from accumulation of thrombogenic material, either within the catheter or on the surface of the catheter or guide wire. Catheter exchange should always be made in the lower descending aorta. Local arterial complications, either thrombosis, dissection or rupture may occur and require surgical intervention. The mortality from coronary arteriography is approximately 0.2% (Pridie et al., 1976).

Percutaneous transluminal coronary angioplasty

A fine double lumen dilatation catheter with balloon is introduced into the coronary artery, using an external guiding catheter by a femoral percutaneous technique. A short soft guide wire projects beyond the balloon to direct the catheter through the stenosis for dilatation. The arterial pressure is monitored proximal and distal to the stricture. The balloon is inflated for a short period and then deflated, causing short period of blockage of the artery. Considerable success has been claimed for this new technique (Grüntzig et al., 1979), as shown by a rise in the distal pressure and confirmed by angiography. During coronary angioplasty heparin is administered and, following the procedure, aspirin and dipyridamole. Intracoronary injections of streptokinase to lyse the thrombus in acute myocardial infarction is still being evaluated.

Relations with other imaging modalities

NUCLEAR CARDIOLOGY

Myocardial imaging

When a myocardial perfusion image is viewed, the density depends on the myocardial blood flow and the myocardial tissue mass. In hot spot detection, the radio-pharmaceutical is taken up by the damaged or necrosed myocardial cells and a positive concentration gradient is achieved between the damaged and normal heart tissue. The most widely used radionuclide is 99mTc pyrophosphate. In cold spot detection, the isotope concentrates in the normal myocardial tissue proportional to the coronary blood flow, myocardial tissue mass and myocardial cellular extraction efficiency. The most satisfactory isotope used is 201Ti. When viewing the myocardial image, the picture observed is primarily of the left ventricular myocardium and to a lesser extent of the right ventricle.

Ventricular function

Radionuclide scanning of the right and left ventricular function enable a study to be made of the movement of the ventricular wall and the measurement of the cardiac ejection fraction. 99mTc labelled radiopharmaceuticals are most suitable for this study, being non-invasive, safe and applicable to a broad range of patients. They are now proving useful alternatives to the more invasive methods of investigation of the heart.

Computed tomography of cardiac structures

CT scans may be made with or without contrast enhancement and visualization of the cardiac structures and anatomy are readily demonstrated. Encouraging results have been obtained from CT scans of the cardiac chambers and other structures (Guthaner et al., 1979). With the development of more sophisticated techniques and diminishing scan times, it may be expected that computed tomography will play an increasing role in the diagnosis of cardiac lesions. A further development is the Dynamic Spatial Reconstructor, combining a high speed transaxial scanner system with 28 image intensifier chains (Robb & Ritman, 1979).

REFERENCES

Bleichröder F. (1922) Intra-arterielle Therapie. *Berl. klin. Wsch.*, **49**, 1503.

Brockenbrough E. C. & Braunwald E. (1960) New technique for left ventricular angiography and transseptal left heart catheterisation. *Amer. J. Cardiol.*, **6**, 1062.

Conti C. R. (1977) Coronary arteriography. *Circulation*, **55**, 227.

Cournand A. & Ranges M. M. (1941) Catheterisation of the right auricle in man. *Proc. Soc. exp. Biol. Med.*, **46**, 462.

Elliott L. P., Bargeron L. M., Bream P. R., Soto B. & Curry G. C. (1977). Axial cineangiography in congenital heart disease. Section II Specific lesions. *Circulation*, **56**, 1084.

Elliott L. P., Bargeron L. M., Soto B & Bream P. R. (1980) Axial cineangiography in congenital heart disease. *Radiol. Clin. N. Amer.*, **18**, 515.

Epstein E. J. & Coulshed N. (1971) Transseptal Catheterisation via right subclavian vein. *Brit. Heart J.*, **33**, 658.

Forssmann W. (1929) Die Sondierung des rechten Herzens. *Klin. Wsch.*, **8**, 2085.

Forssmann W. (1931) Ueber Kontrastdarstellung der Höhlen des lebenden rechten Herzens und der Lungenschlagader. *Münch. Med. Wsch.*, **78**, 489.

Gamal M. El., Slegers L., Bonnier H., Borsje P., Relik T., Gelder L. van, & de Vries D. (1980). Selective coronary arteriography with a pre-formed single catheter. *Amer. J. Roentgenol.*, **135**, 630.

Grainger R. G. (1981) Terminology for radiographic projections. *Brit. Heart J.*, **45**, 109.

Grollman J. H. & Renner J. W. (1981) Transfemoral pulmonary angiography: update on technique. *Amer. J. Roentgenol.*, **136**, 624.

Grüntzig A. R., Senning A. & Siegenthaler W. E. (1979) Non operative dilatation of coronary artery stenosis: Percutaneous transluminal coronary angioplasty. *New Eng. J. Med.*, **301**, 61.

Guthander D. F., Wexler L. & Harell G. (1979) CT demonstration of cardiac structures. *Amer. J. Roentgenol.*, **133**, 75.

Guthander D. F. & Wexler L. (1980) New aspects of coronary arteriography. *Radiol. Clin. N. Amer.*, **18**, 501.

Judkins M. P. (1967) Selective coronary arteriography. *Radiology*, **89**, 815.

Mills S. R., Jackson D. C., Older R. A., Heaston D. K. & Moore A. V. (1980) The incidence, etiologies and avoidance of complications of pulmonary angiography in a large series. *Radiology*, **136**, 295.

Newell J. D., Higgins C. V. & Kelley M. J. (1980) Radiographic-echocardiographic approach to acquired heart disease: diagnosis and assessment of severity. *Radiol. Clin. N. Amer.*, **18**, 387.

Pridie R. B., Booth E. & Fawzey E. (1976) Coronary angiography. Review of 1500 consecutive cases. *Brit. Heart J.*, **38**, 1200.

Robb R. A. & Ritman E. L. (1979) High speed synchronous volume computed tomography of the heart. *J. Computer Assisted Tomography*, **133**, 635.

Ross J. Jnr. (1959) Catheterisation of the left heart through the interatrial septum: a new technique and its experimental evaluation. *Surgical Forum*, **9**, 297.

Seldinger S. I. (1953) Catheter replacement of the needle in percutaneous arteriography. *Acta Radiol.*, **39**, 368.

Sinner W. N. (1978) Computed tomographic patterns of pulmonary thromboembolism and infarction. *J. Computer Assisted Tomography*, **2**, 395.

Sones F. M. (1955) Heart catheterisation in infancy. *Pediatrics*, **16**, 544.

Sones F. M., Shirey E. K., Proudfit W. C. & Westcott R. N. (1959) Cine arteriography. *Circulation*, **20**, 733.

Sones F. M. & Shirey E. K. (1962) Cine coronary arteriography. *Modern concepts in Cardiovascular Disease*, **31**, 735.

Thomas H. A. & Sievers R. E. (1979) Non surgical reduction of arterial catheter knots. *Amer. J. Roentgenol.*, **132**, 1018.

RECOMMENDED READING

Verel D. & Grainger R. G. (1977) *Cardiac Catheterization and Angiocardiography*. 3e. Churchill Livingstone, Edinburgh.

Portal and Hepatic Venous System

R. DICK

Definition of venous occlusion at different sites within the afferent and efferent venous circulation of the liver is complex and requires invasive methods.

THE PORTAL VENOUS SYSTEM

The number of methods available for introducing contrast medium into the portal venous system is matched only by their degree of ingenuity. A 'direct' portogram is easiest achieved via the splenic parenchyma (Abeatici & Campi, 1951), or liver (Lunderquist & Vang, 1974), both techniques being performed under local anaesthesia in the X-ray department. Other means of access include haemorrhoidal or jejunal veins, reopening the umbilical vein, and catheterization via the internal jugular vein and from there across the hepatic vein (Rosch & Keller, 1980). All but the last of these venous entries require surgery in an operating theatre and the more straightforward methods are desirable.

'Indirect' portography results when contrast medium, delivered during coeliac or superior mesenteric arteriography, is collected in the capillary beds of end organs and is returned to the liver by the portal venous system (Kreel & Williams, 1964).

Three methods are discussed in detail: namely percutaneous splenoportography (PSP); coeliac and superior mesenteric arterioportography (CSMAP); transhepatic portography (THP).

PERCUTANEOUS SPLENOPORTOGRAPHY (PSP)

Indications

Portal hypertension

Direct PSP remains the simplest and quickest way of delineating portal venous anatomy, the detail being superior to that obtained by arterioportography, in addition to allowing measurement of the portal pressure.

A normal splenoportogram demonstrates only the splenic and portal veins, without reflux into any of the feeding veins which convey non-opacified blood into the main channels and so dilute the contrast medium (Fig. 11.1). Reversed flow into gastric and oesophageal collateral veins in a patient with cirrhosis who has recently bled, is usually accepted as clinical evidence of portal hypertension and a probable variceal bleed. Splenic pulp pressure provides firm proof of portal hypertension, for it correlates closely with the intrahepatic or sinusoidal pressure (le Maire & Housset, 1955).

In the infant or child, an extrahepatic venous block is the most likely aetiology (Fig. 11.2), whereas portal hypertension in adults is most often due to a form of cirrhosis which has produced intrahepatic portal venous block (Fig. 11.3), and rarely an extrahepatic block or hyperdynamic (fast flow) situation. PSP immediately identifies the site of portal obstruction. Occasionally a large flow in collateral veins may result in non-opacification of a patent portal vein, thus creating a spurious appearance of portal vein thrombosis. This situation, although uncommon, is resolved either by arteriography or transhepatic portography.

A further indication in portal hypertension is the evaluation of the main veins for the surgeon considering a porto-systemic shunt. The intended vein should be of an appropriate size and position. Following surgery, PSP will show the patency of a shunt (Fig. 11.4). Some patients already have a large natural shunt.

To delineate involvement of portal venous system by adjacent pathology

The splenic and portal veins may be displaced or invaded by various processes, particularly neoplasms of the pancreas or bile ducts and primary liver cancers.

Contra-indications

1. A prothrombin time prolonged to 4 s beyond the control value.
2. A platelet count of less than 75 000 mm^3.

Both 1 and 2 are relative contra-indications in particular clinical situations. Gelfoam, compressed dry and inserted into the splenic cannula for ultimate re-expansion and sealing of the splenic tract, should be used in all patients at risk of bleeding. Splenoportography may thus be safe with a platelet level of as

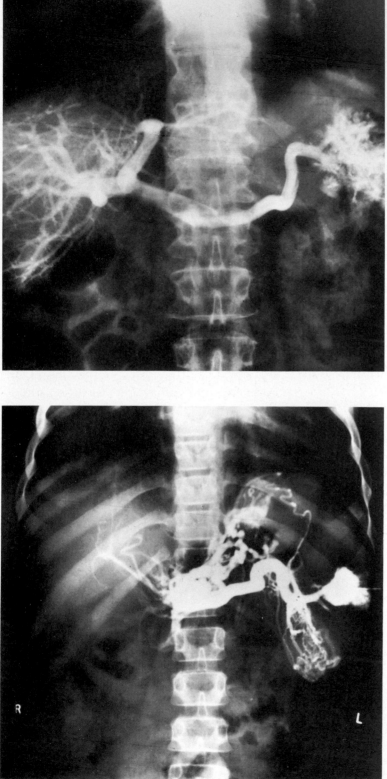

Fig. 11.1 Normal splenic portogram. Note dilution in main portal vein by superior mesenteric venous flow. Pulp pressure 10 mmHg Portal hypertension excluded.

Fig. 11.2 Splenic portogram. Portal vein block consequent to abdominal sepsis. Multiple collaterals around thrombosed vein and dilated gastric and perisplenic veins. Pulp pressure 30 mmHg.

Fig. 11.3 Splenic portogram. Late cirrhosis. Note short and left gastric and large umbilical collaterals. Small liver surrounded by ascitic fluid.

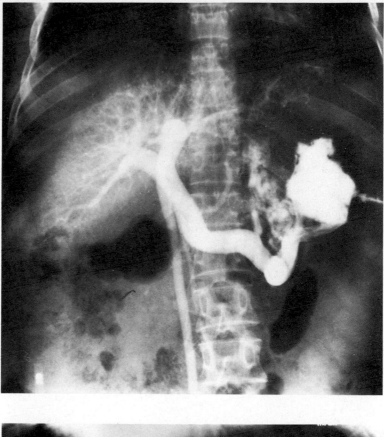

Fig. 11.4 Splenic portogram demonstrating patent portocaval shunt (surgical).

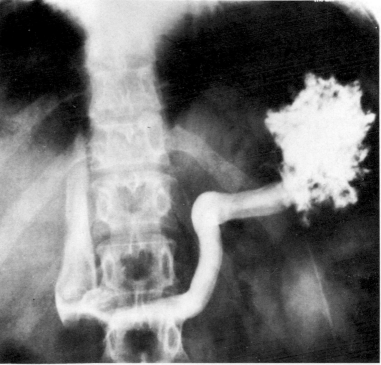

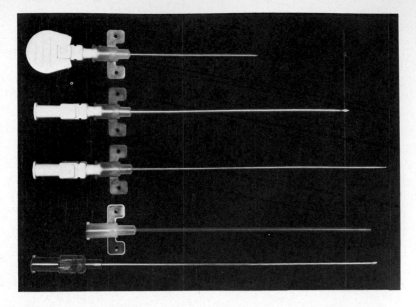

Fig. 11.5 Needle-cannulae for direct splenic portography (varying lengths and diameters). The lowest one has been disassembled.

low as 50 000 mm³ and bleeding has not been reported after Gelfoam insertion.

3. Deep jaundice.
4. Gross ascites.
5. Hypersensitivity to contrast media is a relative contra-indication if appropriate precautions are taken.

The presence of Australia antigen is not a contra-indication, although precautions are essential.

Technique

The aim is to puncture the splenic pulp, measuring the intrasplenic pressure which is equivalent to the portal venous pressure, and to delineate by contrast medium the splenic and portal veins together with the intrahepatic portal venous pattern and the 'hepatogram'. In a very few patients, the hepatic veins are seen draining towards the inferior vena cava.

Many patients have a clinical diagnosis of portal hypertension and have had a recent bleed into the alimentary tract. PSP is performed as soon as possible after basic resuscitation, although the study is elective in some patients when their liver function tests are optimal and there has been control of gross ascites.

Preparation

The procedure is explained to the patient at a preliminary examination on the ward, at which time the size of the spleen is assessed by palpation. Small children require general anaesthesia, local anaesthesia being used in all patients over 10 years of age following reassurance that the study will be neither protracted nor disagreeable. Premedication is not required on the ward, 10–20 mg 'Diazemuls' being given intravenously in the X-ray department prior to the procedure.

Method

Following a control radiograph, the left hypochondrium is examined during fluoroscopy. The patient is instructed to breathe shallowly until completion of the venogram. It is important to spend some time teaching the patient to hold their breath in shallow mid-inspiration upon request, as full respiration may dislodge the splenic cannula when it is in position. A skin marker is placed over the left lower lateral chest wall in the mid-axilliary line, opposite the middle of the visualized spleen. The numerical rib interspace selected is irrelevant, provided the puncture is along the lateral border of the spleen at the level of the hilum and well below the lower limit of the left costophrenic angle on inspiration. The actual pleural reflection may extend 2 cm below the lung seen in the costophrenic angle during screening. The skin and subcutaneous tissues are infiltrated with 5 ml of 1% lignocaine. During suspended respiration, a further 5 ml are introduced down to the splenic capsule which may either feel 'gritty' or be without resistance. A small skin incision is made with a scalpel blade. A needle-cannula (Vygon Intranule; Ecouen, France) French gauge (FG) 6 and 90 mm long (Fig. 11.5) is introduced percutaneously into the spleen under screening control during absolute suspension of respiration. It is directed 10–15° cephalad towards the hilum and slightly posterior to the horizontal plane, to a depth of 4–6 cm, in a steady movement. The needle is then quickly withdrawn and the patient resumes normal respiration. A slow flow of blood from the splenic pulp should immediately leave the cannula. If this is not the case, the cannula is gently withdrawn until blood appears. An absence of bleeding from the cannula up to its complete withdrawal indicates that the spleen has not been traversed, this being a rare event with a careful choice of puncture site.

A syringe and clear connecting tubing are attached to the cannula when venous blood appears and a 10 ml test injection of Niopam 300 (iopamidol 300 mg I/ml) is introduced via the cannula into the splenic pulp under fluoroscopic control. When the cannula is well placed, contrast medium will pool in the splenic tissue around the cannula tip before quickly entering splenic vein radicles and then the main splenic vein. If no veins are seen near the hilum, the contrast medium will have tracked under the splenic capsule or even outside the spleen. In these situations, the puncture has been misjudged and the cannula should be completely withdrawn during suspended respiration, Gelfoam fragments being injected during the cannula removal. A second cannula insertion may then be made, and is usually successful. The cannula is then taped to the skin and is supported on sterile swabs or pads during flushing with saline.

When the cannula is correctly positioned the splenic pulp pressure (normally less than 11 mmHg) is measured by linking a pressure recording line from a physiological pressure transducer, such as the Hewlett Packard 1280 series, to the *rear* of the connecting tube from the cannula.

Splenoportography is performed immediately after the pressure measurement. After disconnection of the pressure line, the table top is moved over the serial changer. The patient is informed that the main injection is imminent and will be accompanied by a sensation of central upper abdominal warmth as well as some noise from the automatic changer and injector. Assurance is given that the injection of contrast medium into the portal venous system is not painful and the patient practises holding a shallow respiration for up to 20 s. For adults, 50–60 ml Niopam 370 is injected at 8–10 ml/s. There is no need to increase the volume of contrast medium to match the degree of splenomegaly, unlike arterioportography where larger spleens require much more contrast medium to provide venous information. If the spleen is small or impalpable, percutaneous splenic puncture should be in the posterior axillary line, and the needle directed only slightly cephalad. Raising the left side by 30° may facilitate the more posterior puncture. Injection is recommended through a programmed automatic injector, set to obtain one radiograph before the contrast medium injection for later subtraction studies. The film programme is 2 films/s for 3 s, followed by 1 film/s for 3 s, and then one film every alternate second for another 7 films, giving a total of 16 films over 20 s.

The injector connection is removed following the injection, whereupon some splenic blood should leave the cannula. Normal saline is perfused through the cannula until radiographs are processed and ready for inspection (Fig. 11.1). If these are satisfactory, the cannula is withdrawn during suspended respiration and the patient is returned to the ward for 12 h bedrest and monitoring of pulse and blood pressure. The procedure should routinely take no more than 15 min from start to completion, provided all items of equipment are assembled beforehand and instantly to hand once the splenic pulp is punctured, with an ordered yet swift progression to the final venogram. Radiography has to be of high quality because there is no possibility of repeating the venogram.

Variations on basic technique

Smaller gauge needle-cannulae of variable lengths are available (FG5, 60–120 mm) for children. Both the injection rate and the volume of injected contrast medium are reduced, being 20 ml for small infants and 30–40 ml for children.

If the patient has a severe coagulopathy, Gelfoam plugs should be routinely introduced into the cannula during its final withdrawal. Zannini *et al.* (1979) have suggested injecting a vasoconstrictor, 2 units of vasopressin, into the splenic pulp at this stage and also into the splenic artery via an intra-arterial catheter in those patients with an especial likelihood of bleeding. Gelfoam embolus of the tract, however, should make the injection of vasoconstrictor unnecessary.

Complications

Severe complications are rare, with a reported incidence of 0.4–1% following many thousands of studies, and are due to massive haemorrhage and splenic rupture which require splenectomy. The incidence should be lower still with complete suspension of respiration and the use of a flexible non-metal cannula (Kogutt & Jander, 1977).

Two to four per cent of patients have local haemorrhage, which responds to blood transfusion, or pyrogenic reactions. Most other complications are avoidable and include pneumothorax, haemothorax, chemical pleuritis from an intrathoracic injection of contrast medium, puncture of perisplenic organs (kidney, liver, colon, stomach and left hemidiaphragm), the peritoneal injection of contrast medium and, rarely, the development of aneurysms or arteriovenous fistulae in the spleen.

The disrepute into which PSP fell was largely due to the risk of haemorrhage. Lande and Bard (1975), by performing coeliac arteriography *after* PSP, showed haematoma formation in 21% of cases, the cannula tracts not being plugged in this series. Surgery has confirmed that plugging the tract with Gelfoam causes immediate cessation of bleeding in fully heparinized animals and in humans (Probst *et al.*, 1978).

Relationship to other procedures

PSP gives less information about the portal venous system anatomy than transhepatic portography (PTP) (Burcharth *et al.*, 1979), but it is much easier to perform and is a convenient initial angiogram in patients with portal hypertension and a documented gastrointestinal bleed. The barium swallow has no place in the acute bleed and will obscure subsequent angiography.

Altered flow patterns in splenoportography may have to be clarified by later arterioportography or by PTP. Arteriography is necessary if a vascular lesion is suspected in the liver, primary liver cancer being a common sequel of cirrhosis, and to delineate the superior mesenteric vein prior to a mesocaval shunt. A transhepatic portogram may be urgently indicated to allow embolization of gastric oesophageal veins in acute variceal bleeding (Dick, 1981).

In summary, the advantages of splenoportography over other forms of portal angiography are its simplicity, safety, and high diagnostic yield.

COELIAC AND SUPERIOR MESENTERIC ARTERIOPORTOGRAPHY (CSMAP)

Contrast medium delivered into the territory supplied by these arteries will, in the venous phase, respectively fill the splenic/portal vein (Fig. 11.6) and the superior mesenteric/portal vein (Fig. 11.7).

Indications

1. In portal hypertension; to demonstrate anatomy when splenoportography is undesirable or impossible, for instance after splenectomy.
2. To show arterial and capillary abnormalities in the liver, spleen and viscera in patients with chronic liver disease; suspected neoplasia, aneurysms of major arteries and haemangiomas.
3. To indicate the state and position of the portal and superior mesenteric veins prior to a shunt procedure.
4. For treatment of variceal bleeding by intra-arterial vasopressin, although intravenous vasopressin may be just as effective.
5. To search for an active, non-variceal bleeding point in stomach or bowel; for instance erosion, ulceration, angiodysplasia or haemangiomas.
6. To show the patency of previous surgical portosystemic shunt (Fig. 11.8).
7. To demonstrate the presence of the portal vein prior to transhepatic portography.

Contra-indications

These are as for femoral artery catheterization (see Arteriography, p. 97).

Technique

Preparation

Preparation is generally that for arteriography. If actively bleeding, the patient requires blood replacement and possibly an inflated Sengstaken balloon catheter for transport to the hospital and angiogram suite. The patient is sedated with care using Diazemuls with Fortral or pethidine, but avoiding opiates, and the study is performed under local anaesthesia.

Method

The Cordis FG7 'Sidewinder' Type 1 or 2 catheter is the most suitable for both coeliac and subsequent superior mesenteric angiography. A side hole is required, in addition to the end hole, to stabilize the catheter position during injection.

It is best to perform coeliac axis angiography first; since the finding of malignancy, fistulae, or other lesions in the liver may alter the management of a patient who has presented with portal hypertension. In adults with spleens which are of average size or moderately enlarged, 60 ml of Niopam 370 is injected

Fig. 11.6 Coelic arteriogram. Venous phase normal study. There is significant dilution of contrast in portal vein by inflow from superior mesenteric vein (arrow).

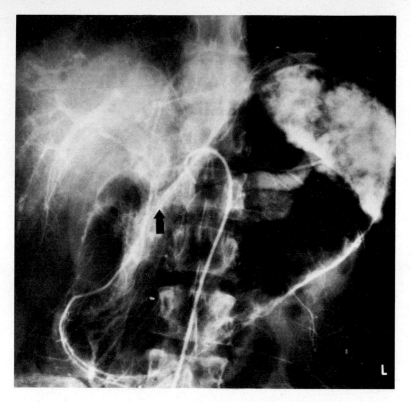

via a programmed automatic injector at the rate of 10 ml/s, the run covering 30 s in order to catch the late filling veins of the portal venous system (Russell *et al.*, 1976). A normal study is shown in Fig. 11.6. With massive splenomegaly, selective splenic arterial injection may then be required with an injection of 70 ml at 8 ml/s. A Sidewinder catheter may advance well into the splenic artery and, if not, it is exchanged for a FG7 femoro-visceral type 2 catheter. The use of gas distension of the stomach and intra-arterial vasodilators immediately before contrast is recommended, 2 mg sodium nitroprusside (Nipride) being preferable although tolazoline and prostaglandins have also been used for vasodilatation.

Despite reasonable contrast density in the splenic vein, known varices may not fill and considerable dilution of contrast medium in the portal vein may occur due to the inflow of non-opacified superior mesenteric venous blood (Fig. 11.6). For this reason, superior mesenteric arteriography is obligatory in addition to coeliac or splenic arteriography and shows the state of the superior mesenteric and portal veins (Fig. 11.7), as well as giving better delineation of gastro-oesophageal collaterals compared to splenic arterial injection. It is performed with either a Sidewinder or femoro-visceral catheter in the superior mesenteric trunk. After a trial injection to test catheter

stability, 70 ml Niopam 370 or 70 ml Urografin 370 are injected at 8 ml/s, Conray 420 being too painful. The patient practises breath holding, respiration being suspended for the duration of the run. One film is exposed every 2 s for 30 s. Subtraction (Fig. 11.9) is aided by the intravenous injection of 30 mg of Buscopan before the run to prevent bowel movement. Two milligrammes of Nipride are given intra-arterially immediately prior to connecting the catheter to the injector.

Despite the use of pharmacoangiography and high doses of contrast medium, dilution may occur and superimposition of arteries and veins sometimes cause problems. Thus, although opacification may be excellent, it is never as reliably dense as in direct portography. Smaller FG catheters and lower doses of drugs and contrast medium are used in children, compared to adults.

Variations on basic technique

Two catheters have been used to improve the contrast density in arterioportography, injecting 15 µg of epinephrine into one in the coeliac axis and 10 µg/kg of acetylcholine into the other in the superior mesenteric artery just before the injection of contrast

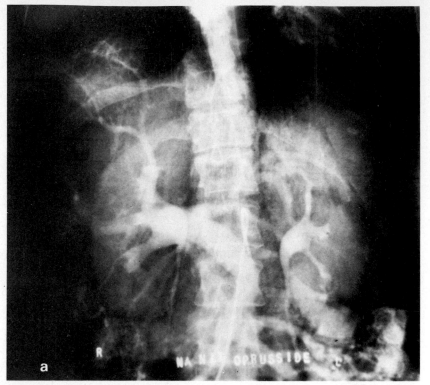

Fig. 11.7a Normal superior mesenteric and portal veins shown in the venous phase of superior mesenteric arteriogram. The patient had hepatomegaly.

medium. A further modification on the two catheter technique is to inject the splenic and superior mesenteric arteries with contrast medium simultaneously, along with vasodilators (Zannini *et al.,* 1979). Occasionally, left gastric arteriography with vasodilatation may be useful in showing oesophageal varices.

Relation to other procedures

Whether the patient has TSP or CSMAP is determined by the clinical setting. The former requires simpler equipment and less expertise, while providing the bonus of a portal pressure reading. If information is required concerning the arterial circulation as well as the portal venous system, arteriography is the method of choice. Some patients require arteriography to exclude or confirm a portal vein block which has been suggested by portography.

A great advantage of arteriography is that, if an abnormal focal area is seen within the liver, the radiologist may perform an accurately sited liver biopsy whilst the arterial catheter is *in situ*. The liver biopsy track may be plugged with Gelfoam embolus, and then checked for closure by a contrast injection through the arterial catheter. If there is evidence of haemoperitoneum complicating the biopsy, the *in situ*

catheter may be used to embolize the liver close to the site of biopsy and instantly control the bleeding.

TRANSHEPATIC PORTOGRAPHY (THP)

Lunderquist and Vang, in 1974, described the percutaneous transhepatic approach to the portal vein. Since then it has become widely used and established as a safe procedure.

Indications

Portal hypertension

THP is superior to both splenoportography and arterioportography in demonstrating the portal system, particularly the left lobe of liver. Causes of failure of these other studies to show the portal vein include portal vein thrombosis, 'stealing' collaterals preventing portal vein opacification, and hepatofugal blood flow in the portal vein diluting the incoming contrast medium. THP resolves the last two situations while ultrasonography correctly diagnoses portal vein thrombosis in 95% of patients (Webb & Berger, 1977).

By employing a tip deflecting handle and wire

Fig. 11.7b Subtraction film showing improved detail of main portal vein and its branches in left lobe.

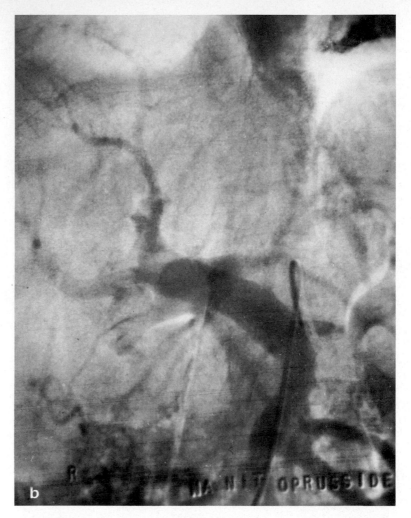

(William Cook, Europe), the catheter may be manoeuvred from the splenic or portal vein into the short and left gastric veins (Fig. 11.10), followed by injection and embolization of varices (Fig. 11.11). Variceal bleeding is arrested in 80% of cases but the rebleeding rate is 40–65%. The procedure is therefore used in patients with recent acute variceal bleeding rather than those with chronic bleeds (Smith-Laing *et al.*, 1981).

Venous sampling

Selective catheterization allows sampling of all the veins which drain into the portal system. The main application is searching for endocrine tumours of the pancreas (Fig. 11.12). In addition to the tip deflected catheter, a catheter with a short preformed curve at its tip may be exchanged over a guide wire.

Contra-indications

Defective clotting should be corrected and gross ascites reduced as much as possible. Embolization is frequently performed during bleeding, the patient being resuscitated *pari passu* with the procedure.

Lack of available expertise is a major contra-indication. Although failure to enter the portal vein occurs with experience in only 6% of cases, THP is both technically difficult and time consuming, sometimes taking longer than 1½ hours.

Technique

Following localization of the portal vein by ultrasound, and often by earlier spleno- or arterio-portography, the procedure is explained to the patient before sedation. Preliminary fluoroscopy delineates the liver

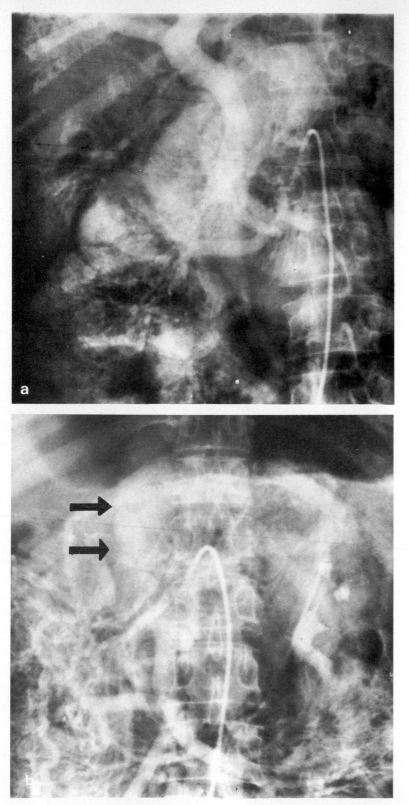

Fig. 11.8a Superior mesenteric arteriogram. Venous phase in patient with portal hypertension. Superior mesenteric and portal veins fill.

Fig. 11.8b Same patient with repeat study 9 months after successful mesocaval shunt. Contrast enters inferior vena cava (arrowed) through the patent shunt.

Fig. 11.9 Venous phase. Superior mesenteric arteriogram in patients with alcoholic cirrhosis. Subtraction film. Reflux has occurred into splenic vein demonstrating short and left gastric collaterals.

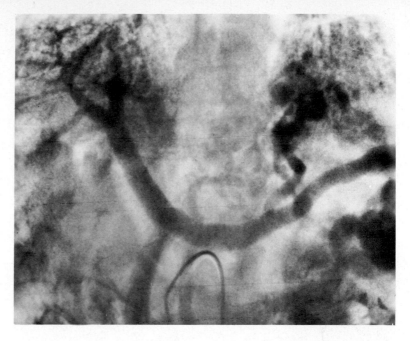

Fig. 11.10 Transhepatic portogram. Selective catheterization of left gastric vein demonstrating gastric and oesophageal collaterals. Gross splenomegaly.

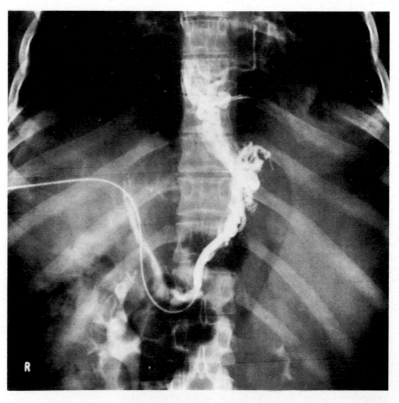

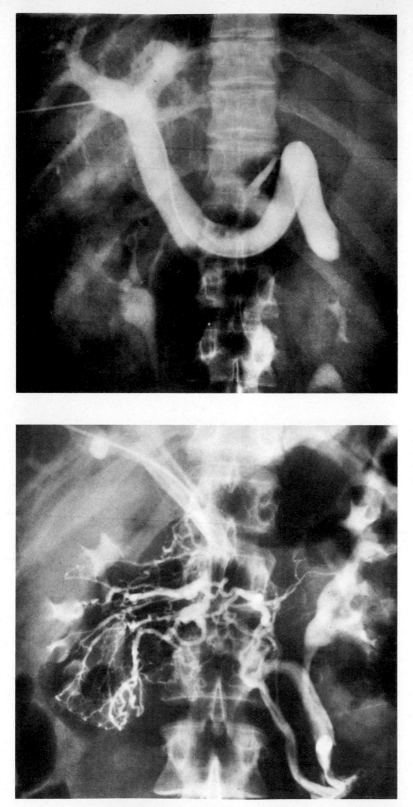

Fig. 11.11 Same patient as Fig. 11.14. Free portograms after transhepatic obliteration of varices. Note contrast 'trapped' in a short segment of left gastric vein from previous study.

Fig. 11.12 Transhepatic portogram with selective catheterization of postero-superior pancreatico-duodenal veins for sampling in patient with suspected insulinoma.

outline and helps in the selection of the entry site on the skin. This is in the mid-axillary line of the right lower thorax, well below the lower margin of the costophrenic angle, and located so that the almost horizontal needle-catheter will enter one of the major right intrahepatic branches of the portal vein.

Local anaesthesia, 10 ml of 1% lignocaine, is instilled into the skin and subcutaneous tissues down to the liver capsule during suspended respiration. The skin is incised with a scalpel blade and a FG 40 cm long trocar sheathed in a matching length polyethylene catheter (William Cook, Europe) is advanced during suspended respiration towards the anticipated site of the portal vein radicle. After withdrawal of the inner trocar, the patient resumes gentle breathing and gradual aspiration is performed during slow withdrawal of the catheter. If venous blood is obtained, 10 ml of Niopam 300 is injected through the catheter. Flow towards the spine indicates that the catheter tip is in a hepatic vein, whereupon catheter withdrawal is resumed. A central branching pattern or reflux of contrast medium into the main trunk of the portal vein indicates entry into the portal venous system. If the attempt is unsuccessful, the catheter is embolized with Gelfoam fragments in solution prior to its final withdrawal. Up to five or more attempts may be needed to enter the portal system.

Using a series of guide wires, including moveable core 'J' and rigid stainless steel 'Surgimed' types, the catheter is advanced deeply into the portal system. Two series of radiographs are then obtained, the first with the catheter in the distal part of the splenic vein and the second in the stem of the superior mesenteric vein. At each site, 30 ml of Niopam 370 is injected at 10 ml/s, exposing 15 films at a rate of 1/s. The procedure is thereafter determined by the indications. When the catheter is finally withdrawn from the liver, the extravascular hepatic and capsular tract must be sealed with Gelfoam.

Variations on basic technique

Kimura *et al.* (1981) recently carried out THP after puncturing, and thus localizing, a major portal vein branch with a fine Chiba needle (15 cm long, 0.7 mm od). By exchanging through the Chiba needle and introducing a larger catheter, THP succeeded in all 67 patients with no complications.

Complications

Transient fever is a common complication. Subcapsular and subcutaneous haematoma occur especially in patients with a bleeding tendency.

Major complications are rare. To date, two deaths have been reported worldwide, both resulting from haemoperitoneum before the sealing of tracts from the liver became routine practice. Thrombosis within the portal vein is an important sequel if embolic material intended for varices is not injected with scrupulous care but enters the portal circulation.

The volume of contrast medium must be minimized, many patients being poor risk cases and prone to develop the hepato-renal syndrome.

Relationship to other techniques

Isotope imaging, ultrasonography, and computed tomography are at present unable to show fully the major and minor vessels in the portal system. The extent of collaterals and their direction of flow requires a contrast study, PSP being the simplest and THP the most complex method. THP has both diagnostic and therapeutic possibilities and is therefore usually reserved for those requiring therapy. Accurate ultrasonographic localization of the portal vein is a prerequisite and the procedure must be meticulously performed to prevent complications.

Many physicians and surgeons prefer the non-radiological technique of endoscopic variceal injection for the treatment of bleeding oesophageal varices (Williams & Dawson, 1979).

HEPATIC VENOGRAPHY

Hepatic venography, when considered with the findings on portal venography, allows assessment of the type and stages of liver diseases and their haemodynamic consequences while permitting differentiation of diffuse diseases from tumour.

Rappaport in 1951 was the first to propose hepatic venous angiography, basing it upon a technique of hepatic vein catheterization described earlier by Warren and Bannon (1944). Historically, many methods have been tried to demonstrate the hepatic veins, with varing success. Many attempts to demonstrate the hepatic veins were crude and lacking practicality. They included the use of single and double balloon catheters in the inferior vena cava, forced retrograde filling of hepatic veins after raising intrabronchial pressure, the i.v. injection of carbon dioxide and the direct percutaneous introduction of contrast medium into the liver.

The objects are to record pressures within the hepatic venous tree, inferior vena cava and right atrium and, secondly, to obtain an angiogram following occlusion of the catheterized vein.

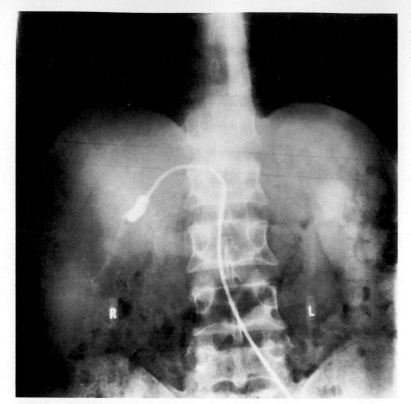

Fig. 11.13 Femoro-visceral balloon catheter in major right hepatic vein. The balloon has been inflated with contrast to occlude vein.

Ideally, hepatic venography should be simple, cause the minimal hazard and discomfort, give maximum morphological and haemodynamic information and be reproducible. All these aims can now be achieved (Nocak *et al.,* 1976).

Technique

The examination is not painful and is performed under local anaesthesia with premedication. The patient is in a fasting state, having been reassured that the procedure is neither unpleasant nor lengthy. The hepatic vein may be approached from above the diaphragm, via an antecubital or jugular vein. The first site usually requires a time consuming venous cutdown, and both methods need cardiac monitoring because the catheter traverses the heart. The recommended method is from the common femoral vein by the Seldinger technique and is straightforward unless there is gross oedema or a previous thrombosis.

Catheters available should have no side holes because of the manometry requirement. The types of catheter used are: disposable Cournand catheter FG7 100 cm (Cordis, UK); Sidewinder type occlusion balloon catheter FG7 100 cm (Cordis, UK); torque controlled occlusion balloon catheter, Cobra 11 shape.

FG7 (Cordis, UK); Meditech occlusion balloon catheter, straight yet formable at 80–90° C, FG7 65 cm (Keymed). The last two named are the most satisfactory for hepatic venography (Fig. 11.13). Straight and moveable-core 'J' wires (0.038 in, 145 cm) are used to guide the catheters up the inferior vena cava and into a selected vein. Balloon catheters are preferred when contrast is to be injected into the hepatic veins (see below), the balloon being protected during femoral vein entry by passing the catheter through a Cordis FG7 or 8 introducer. Up to three hepatic veins are usually studied, namely a major and 'middle' right hepatic vein and a large left hepatic vein. Pressures may be averaged from three sets of readings, although contrast studies are usually only performed in one vein.

To engage the right hepatic vein, both catheter and guide wire are advanced upwards to the high inferior vena cava. Following withdrawal of the guide wire into the body of the catheter, the latter is rotated to face the right side just below the right hemidiaphragm. Gentle manipulation causes the catheter to engage the hepatic vein orifice and, with help from the guide wire, is advanced into the main trunk of the vein.

After a free hepatic venous pressure is obtained, the balloon on the catheter is inflated with air or

Fig. 11.14 Occlusion balloon catheter hepatic venography. Normal study. Note filling of hepatic vein radicles (5th and 6th divisions) in a subsegment of the right lobe and free flow to other patent hepatic veins.

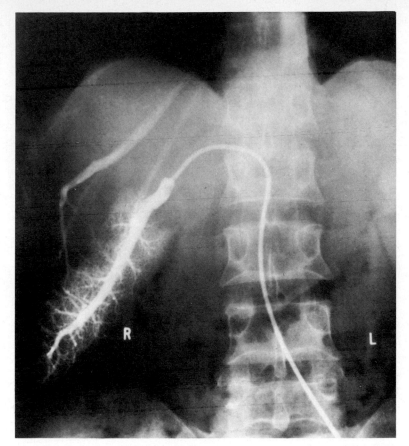

contrast medium until it completely occludes the vein, as shown by a small injection of contrast medium through the catheter. An occlusion pressure reading is obtained, corresponding to the peripheral 'wedge' pressure from the Cournand catheter. 'Occlusion hepatic venography' (Fig. 11.14) is next performed to fill the hepatic venous tree distal to the occlusion. 30 ml of Niopam 370 are injected at 5 ml/s by automatic injector, 12 films being exposed at a rate of 1/s. The balloon is then decompressed and the catheter inserted distally or into another vein, with further pressure recordings. Finally, pressures are recorded in the right atrial and at high, mid and low levels in the inferior vena cava.

Prior to the introduction of balloon catheters, peripheral wedging of a catheter was the traditional method of obtaining sinusoidal pressure (Fig. 11.15). Contrast medium thus injected has been found to cause haemorrhagic necrosis of liver cells (Jaurequi *et al.*, 1978), with subsequent pyrexia and elevation in liver enzyme levels. Occlusion balloon catheters have greatly improved the safety of 'wedge' studies, since the balloon is inflated to occlude the main hepatic vein proximal to the sinusoids, and both free and

occlusion (wedge) pressures can be obtained (Novak *et al.*, 1977).

Indications

Cirrhosis of the liver with suspected portal hypertension

The normal wedge pressure lies between 8 and 12 mmHg (Ruzicka *et al.*, 1972). If the figure does not exceed this range, in a patient being investigated for suspected portal hypertension, the diagnosis is refuted and the study is terminated at that point. When there is elevation of the wedge pressure, it is essential to obtain a 'corrected' pressure by subtracting the wedge pressure reading from the free hepatic venous pressure. This is because there are many factors which may raise the wedge pressure; including heart failure, compression of the hepatic portion of the inferior vena cava and any cause of raised intra-abdominal pressure such as ascites. The normal gradient between wedged and free hepatic vein pressure is 3–5 mmHg. Higher values indicate the degree of elevated intra-sinusoidal pressure due to disease, for instance cirrhosis, affecting the sinusoidal or post-sinusoidal

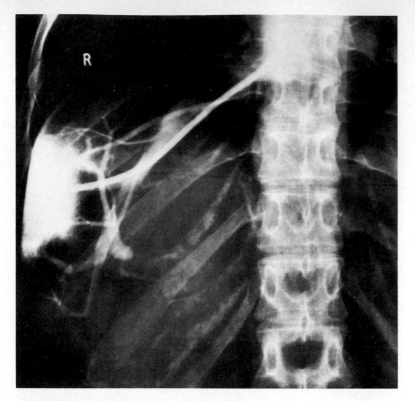

Fig. 11.15 Wedge hepatic venogram. Normal study. The catheter has been introduced from an antecubital vein and has wedged peripherally in the liver. Contrast medium demonstrates normal sinusoidogram and flow to portal vein branches as well as other hepatic veins. Direct injection of contrast medium following this type of wedge catheter study is undesirable.

territories. These patients have similar elevation of their splenic pulp pressures, in contradistinction to the group of patients with either presinusoidal portal blocks or extrahepatic portal venous obstruction who will have normal corrected hepatic venous pressures yet raised splenic pulp pressures. Therefore pressure readings taken on both sides of the liver indicate the causative level of the portal hypertension.

A 'corrected' wedge pressure of 5–10 mmHg is considered slightly elevated, 10–15 mmHg being moderately raised, while greater than 15 mmHg represents marked elevation (Cavaluzzi *et al.*, 1977).

The appearance of a main hepatic venogram with the balloon inflated in the main trunk of a vein may provide a useful assessment in cirrhosis (Novak *et al.*, 1977), the changes closely correlating with the severity of liver disease on biopsy (Smith *et al.*, 1971; Bookstein *et al.*, 1975). The appearance of the sinusoidogram after a peripheral wedge injection and the wedge pressure levels do not correlate as well with the liver biopsy as does the extent of venographic changes in the *main* hepatic veins (Cavaluzzi *et al.*, 1977).

In known cases of portal hypertension before or after a shunt operation
If only a small pressure difference exists between the corrected hepatic pressure and the pressure in an inferior vena cava compressed by a hypertrophied liver, one is able to predict that a portosystemic shunt does not function well. In patients with established surgical shunts, a hepatic venous study permits pressure measurements and shows altered haemo-dynamics, including newly developed portosplanchnic collaterals which may open up despite a perfectly functioning shunt (Novak *et al.*, 1976).

Budd Chiari syndrome
Hepatic vein obstruction is often due to thrombosis affecting either large or multiple small veins. Thrombosis may result from hypercoagulability states, from venous invasion of neoplasms, or from some unknown cause. Obstruction is occasionally due to a congenital venous 'web'. It is essential to perform pressure studies in the inferior vena cava and hepatic veins. The wedge pressure will be elevated, a corrected pressure being important because most patients have ascites. Due to technical difficulty in obtaining a true free hepatic vein pressure in some patients, Reynolds *et al.* (1957) recommend measuring this pressure in the inferior vena cava at the level of the renal veins. Thrombus in a hepatic vein allows only partial entry of a catheter. When the catheter will go no further, 20 ml of injected contrast medium shows a 'spiders web' appearance of small tortuous collateral veins and no sinusoidogram

Fig. 11.16 Wedge hepatic venogram in Budd-Chari syndrome. The catheter is unable to pass any further along the hepatic vein and injection of contrast demonstrates 'spiders web' pattern of numerous collateral hepato-portal and hepato-capsular veins.

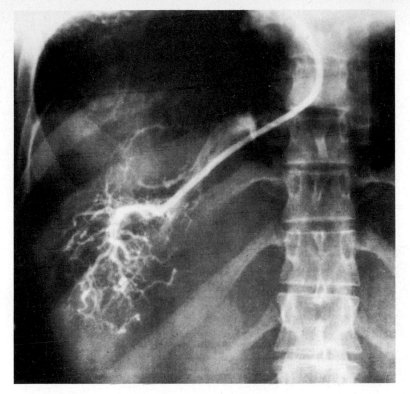

(Fig. 11.16). Thrombi may be seen as intraluminal filling defects in the hepatic veins or extending into the inferior vena cava. In complete thrombosis it may be impossible to catheterize any hepatic veins, although there may be sparing of multiple small hepatic veins draining the caudate lobe.

Inferior venacavography must be performed in both A–P and lateral projections, the first showing side to side narrowing due to hepatomegaly, while the latter demonstrates a prominent anterior shelf indenting the high hepatic portion of the inferior vena cava as a consequence of liver swelling and caudate lobe hypertrophy. Thrombus may also be demonstrated in the inferior vena cava. There are no contra-indications.

Contra-indications

There are no absolute contra-indications to hepatic venography.

Complications

None should occur provided balloon catheters are used. Contrast medium injected through simple end-hole catheters wedged into the periphery of a hepatic vein can overload the parenchyma and result in necrosis, as well as pain due to seepage of contrast medium under the liver capsule. A 'push through' effect of contrast medium from a peripheral wedge injection may cause uncontrolled filling of the portal venous system.

Relationship to other techniques

Ultrasonography and computed tomography regularly demonstrate hepatic veins, but the precise anatomy or pathology of the entire tree is best shown by catheter hepatic venography. Accurate pressure studies are generally of more clinical value than venous delineation, although there is a general agreement that cirrhosis causes severe alterations in the unsupported hepatic veins before affecting the portal vein (Smith *et al.*, 1971). A study of the hepatic venous tree is therefore worthwhile and shows obliterative changes that progress *pari passu* with the cirrhosis. The presence of reflux back into the portal vein may not be of great significance and merely indicates the opening up of hepatoportal venous shunts in cirrhosis.

Although the diagnosis of Budd Chiari syndrome is usually made by hepatic venography and inferior venacavography, the state of the hepatic veins may not be clear if none are entered. Transhepatic intraparenchymal angiography 'hepatography' is required in this case (Ruzicka *et al.*, 1972). The liver parenchyma is forced to handle 30 ml of contrast medium delivered via a percutaneously introduced catheter over 6 s. Contrast medium, and therefore blood, leaves the liver either via the portal vein, which shows reversed (hepatofugal) flow, or by a network of multiple intercommunicating collaterals which are probably of both portal and hepatic origin and drain through transcapsular vessels. In this way the suspected diagnosis of complete hepatic vein occlusion is confirmed. Earlier in the patient's course, a colloid scan of the liver may have shown pronounced isotope uptake in the caudate lobe, and a hepatic angiogram demonstrated 'pseudometastases' within the liver due to sinusoidal stasis.

REFERENCES

Abeatici S. & Campi L. (1951) La visualizzazione radiologica della porta per via splenica. *Minerva med.*, **42**, 593–605.

Bookstein J. J., Appleman H. D., Walter J. F., Foley W. D., Turcotte J. G. & Lambert M. (1975) Histological venographic correlates in portal hypertension. *Radiology*, **116**, 565–73.

Burcharth F., Mieblo N. & Anderson B. (1979) Percutaneous transhepatic portography. Comparison with splenoportography in portal hypertension. *Amer. J. Roentgenol.*, **132**, 183–5.

Casteneda Zuniga W. R., Haurequi J., Rysavy J. A., Formanek A. & Amplatz K. (1978) Complications of wedge hepatic venography. *Radiology*, **126**, 53–6.

Dick R. (1981) Interventional radiology; transhepatic injection of varices. *Brit. J. hosp. Med.*, **26**, 340–7.

Kimurak Tsuchiya Y., Ohto M., Ono T., Matsutani S., Kimura M., Ebera M., Saisho H. & Okada K. (1981) Single puncture method for percutaneous transhepatic portography using a thin needle. *Radiology*, **139**, 748–9.

Kogutt M. S. & Jander H. P. (1977) Splenoportography. A valuable diagnostic technique revisited. *South. med. J.*, **70**, 1210–12.

Kreel L. & Williams R. (1964) Arteriovenography of the portal system. *Brit. med. J.*, **2**, 1500–3.

Lande A. & Bard R. (1975) Celiac arteriography following percutaneous splenoportography. *Radiology*, **114**, 57–8.

Le Maire A. & Housset E. (1955) Le mesure de la pression portale par pontion du foie. *Presse Med.*, **63**, 1063–5.

Lunderquist A. & Vang J. (1974) Transhepatic catheterization and obliteration of the coronary vein in patients with portal hypertension and oesophageal varices. *New Eng. J. Med.*, **290**, 646–9.

Novak D., Butzow G. H. & Becker K. (1976) Hepatic occlusion venography with a balloon catheter in patients with end-to-side portacaval shunts. *Amer. J. Roentgenol.*, **127**, 949–51.

Novak D., Butzow G. H. & Becker K. (1977) Hepatic occlusion venography with a balloon catheter in portal hypertension. *Radiology*, **122**, 623–8.

Probst P., Rysavy J. A. & Amplatz K. (1978) Improved safety of splenoportography by plugging at the needle tract. *Amer. J. Roentgenol.*, **131**, 445–9.

Rappaport A. M. (1951) Hepatic venography. *Acta Radiol.*, **36**, 165–71.

Reynolds T. B. (1974) Promises, promises. Haemodynamic studies in portal hypertension. *New Engl. J. Med.*, **290**, 1484–5.

Reynolds T. B., Redecker A. G. & Geller H. M. (1957) Wedged hepatic venous pressure; a clinical evaluation. *Amer. J. Med.*, **22**, 341–50.

Russell E., Le Page J. R., Viamonte Jr. M., Levi J. U. & Meier W. L. (1976) An angiographic approach to hepatobiliary diseases. *Surg. Gynec. Obstet.*, **1431**, 414–24.

Ruzicka Jr. F. F., Carillo F. J., d'Alessandro D. & Rossi P. (1972) The hepatic wedge pressure and venogram vs. the intraparenchymal liver pressure and venogram. *Radiology*, **102**, 252–8.

Smith G. W., Westgaard T. & Bjorn-Hansen R. (1971) Hepatic venous angiography in the evaluation of cirrhosis of the liver. *Ann. Surg.*, **173**, 469–80.

Smith-Laing G., Scott J., Long R. G., Dick R. & Sherlock S. (1981) Role of percutaneous transhepatic obliteration of varices in the management of haemorrhage from gastro-oesophageal varices. *Gastroenterology*, **80**, 1031–6.

Warren J. V. & Brannon E. S. (1944) A method for obtaining blood samples directly from the hepatic vein in man. Proceedings of the Society of Experimental Biology and Medicine, **55**, 144–6.

Webb L. J., Berger L. A. & Sherlock S. (1977) Grey-scale ultrasonography of the portal vein. *Lancet*, **ii**, 675–7.

Williams K. G. D. & Dawson J. L. (1979) Fibreoptic injection of oesophageal varices. *Brit. med. J.*, **ii**, 766–7.

Zannini G., Masciariello S., Sangiulo P., Papano G. & Iarrarino V. (1979) Splenoportograhie; une technique toujours actuelle. Nouvelles perspectives. *J. Chir.*, **116**, 577–82.

The Lymphatic System

J. S. MACDONALD

The aim of lymphography is to inject radio-opaque contrast medium, usually Lipiodol, into the lymphatic system in order to delineate the lymphatic vessels and the lymph nodes. The cannulation of a peripheral lymphatic is, in miniature, similar to a venous cut down. Difficulties arise because the lymphatic vessels are small and, since lymph is colourless, are difficult to find. Kinmonth, in 1952 delineated the deep lymphatics by the subcutaneous injection of Patent Blue Violet. Subsequently, Kinmonth *et al.,* (1955) described the injection of contrast medium into these vessels and lymphangiography by radiological means then became possible. Lymphography still follows the experimental steps taken by Kinmonth, with certain modifications.

Indications

Lymphography is used in the investigation of lymphoedema (Table 12.1) and in malignant disease (Table 12.2). It should not be used indiscriminately,

Table 12.1 Lymphoedema

Primary	Secondary	
Aplasia	5%	Trauma
Hypoplasia	87%	Malignant disease
Hyperplasia	8%	Filariasis
		Infections and Inflammations

Table 12.2 Percentage of positive lymphograms at the time of diagnosis.

Hodgkin's disease	35
Non-Hodgkin lymphoma	56
Testicular tumours	49
Carcinoma cervix (1 & 2)	28
Carcinoma body of uterus	20
Carcinoma prostate (1 & 2)	38
Carcinoma bladder	23
Carcinoma ovary	23
Carcinoma kidney	21

but only in those situations where the findings are likely to influence the management of the patient.

Contra-indications

1. Severely compromised lung function.
2. Acute venous thrombosis.
3. Cardiac and pulmonary shunts.
4. Radiotherapy to any part of the lung.
5. Allergy to iodine.

The reasons for these contra-indications is discussed under Complications, p. 189.

Basic technique

Requirements

1. Automatic injection pump.
2. CSSD pack.
   6 towels, 10 in receiver, scalpel and blade, needle holder, 2 pairs of fine dissecting forceps, 2 pairs of featherweight Halstead artery forceps, 2 pairs of fine straight ophthalmic scissors, 1 yard of 4/0 Mersilk, 20 gauze swabs.
3. Skin sutures.
4. Disposable syringes. The type of syringe for the Lipiodol varies with the design of the automatic pump, and should be made of a material which does not react with the oily contrast medium, for example polypropylene. Further syringes are needed for the local anaesthetic (5 ml) and the Patent Blue Violet (2 ml).
5. Disposable giving sets, for example Macarthy's Surgical St. Thomas' Hospital pattern with a 30 swg needle.
6. Lipiodol Ultra Fluid, 2 × 10 ml ampoules. (Laboratoire Guerbet. Distributed in Great Britain by May & Baker Ltd.)
7. Patent Blue Violet 2.5%, 1 × 2 ml ampoule. (Laboratoire Guerbet. Distributed in Great Britain by May & Baker Ltd.)
8. Local anaesthetic. Two per cent lignocaine plain, 5 ml.
9. Braided silk suture 3/0.
10. Cleansing fluid.
11. Optical aid.

An automatic injection pump is necessary because Lipiodol is viscous, the needle is small, and a maximum injection rate of 10 ml/h is desirable. The system is liable to block if the rate of injection is too slow, but the patient may experience pain, probably due to distension of the lymphatics, if the rate is too fast. A small proportion of patients feel slight discomfort as the contrast medium begins to flow. Automatic injectors vary from very expensive electric pumps to injectors made in hospital workshops and driven by lead weights. At the Royal Marsden Hospital, a simple model made in the hospital workshops has proved satisfactory over 20 years. In general, the simpler the apparatus the better (Fig. 12.1).

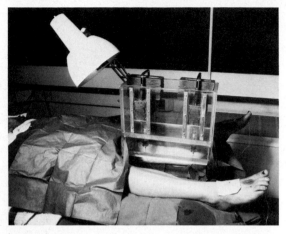

Fig. 12.1 Automatic injection pump. A single model made in the hospital workshops. The lead weights exert constant pressure on the plungers of the syringes. The weights should be adjusted to deliver about 10 ml/h.

The appropriate optical aid depends on the eyesight of the operator. Normally a pair of Bishop Harman magnifying spectacles, which give a 2 × magnification, is satisfactory. Difficult cases of lymphoedema may necessitate an operating microscope.

Method

The great majority of lymphograms are performed under local anaesthesia, and normally on out-patients. Young children require general anaesthesia to keep them still. Patients with oedematous limbs and those in whom there is doubt about their pulmonary reserve should be admitted to hospital for the investigation. It is uncomfortable for a patient to be sent home discharging oedema fluid through the incisions. Oxygen should be to hand for patients with impaired pulmonary function.

The patient is on the X-ray table for up to 1½ hours. The bladder should therefore be emptied immediately

beforehand, the patient being made as comfortable as possible and encouraged to relax. The feet are cleansed and the sterile towels from the pack are placed in position (Fig. 12.1). Local anaesthetic (0.25 ml) is mixed with 2.5% Patent Blue Violet. The dye is injected subcutaneously just proximal to the bases of the first two toes, 1 ml into each foot. The dorsum of the foot is then infiltrated with 2.5 ml of local anaesthetic. The apparatus is set up, the Lipiodol syringes being connected to the giving sets which are in turn filled with Lipiodol ready for the injection. By this time, approximately 5 min after its injection, the lymphatics have usually taken up the dye and an incision can then be made. If a lymphatic vessel is seen through the skin, the incision should be made over it. If not, an incision on the dorsum of the foot 4 cm proximal to the injection of the dye usually reveals a lymphatic vessel and there is then no need to wait until one is seen through the skin (Fig. 12.2). A 1 cm longitudinal incision in line with the lymphatic vessel is favoured because it supports the needle when this is in place and also because it heals very neatly without spoiling the field for repeat lymphography. In

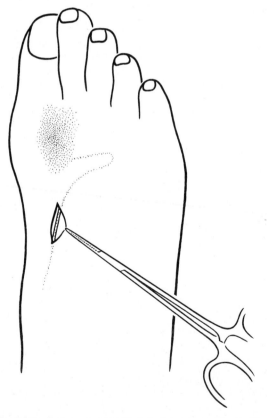

Fig. 12.2 A 1 cm longitudinal incision is made on the dorsum of the foot, exposing the blue coloured lymphatic.

some cases of Hodgkin's disease, for instance, up to seven refill lymphograms have been required during the course of the disease. When the lymphatic is located, it is brought to the surface and cleaned, and a silk tie is placed under it (Fig. 12.3). Unless the

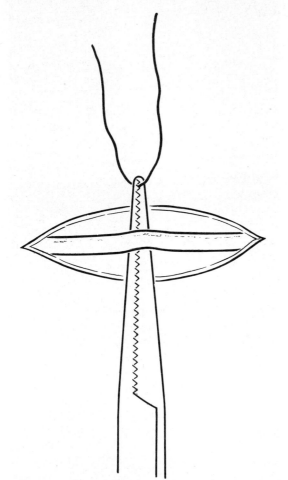

Fig. 12.3 A silk tie is drawn through below the lymphatic. The tie is cut where it is held by the forceps giving two ties, one of which is positioned proximally and the other distally.

lymphatic vessel is well cleaned, the watery dye which diffuses out of it and stains the surrounding tissues may cause two fine lymphatics lying side by side to be mistaken for one large vessel. The lymphatic vessel is then stretched by merely using the weight of a Halstead artery forceps on the proximal tie. This will also partially occlude the vessel which is then distended by gentle massage of the distal part of the foot. The lymphatic vessel is held steady with a pair of fine dissecting forceps and the needle is inserted into it (Fig. 12.4), and threaded along the lymphatic

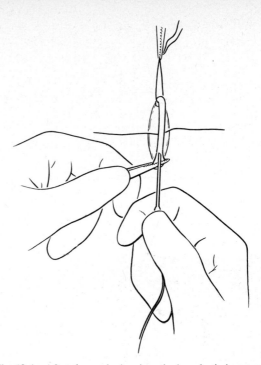

Fig. 12.4 After thorough cleaning, the lymphatic is put on the stretch by the weight of the Halstead forceps on the proximal tie and the fine dissecting forceps held in the hand on the distal tie. This firmly controls the lymphatic which is then punctured by the needle near the point where the forceps held in the hand is slightly flattening the lymphatic and holding it steady.

for approximately 0.5 cm before being firmly tied into place (Fig. 12.5). The plastic tubing of the giving set is placed between the toes, before the attached needle is inserted into the lymphatic vessel, to prevent the tubing from moving around and to help maintain the needle in position (Fig. 12.1).

Control of the injection

When the needle has been firmly tied in place, the forceps holding the proximal tie is released, pressure is exerted on the syringe and the site of the injection is inspected for any leakage. A leak is easily recognized because of the oily nature of the contrast medium. The automatic injector is then started if there is no leak. The injection site is covered with a damp swab soaked in some bland antiseptic solution, such as Savodil*, in order to protect the incision and keep the area moist, because a lymphatic vessel may cease to conduct the contrast medium as it dries out. The weight of the damp swab also helps to keep the needle

* 0.15% Chlorhexidine gluconate, 0.15% Cetrimide ICI Ltd.

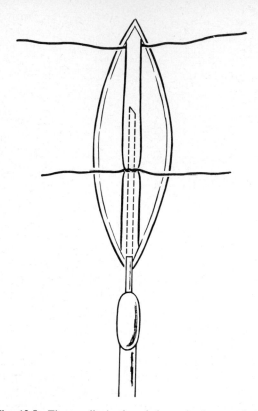

Fig. 12.5 The needle is threaded up the lumen of the lymphatic for about 0.5 cm and then tied firmly in place by the distal tie using a simple thumb knot. The proximal tie is released by the forceps allowing free flow of the contrast medium. This tie is always available for a further knot if by chance there is a leak and the needle needs to be threaded up the lymphatic further.

and attached tubing in place and, together with the tubing threaded between the toes, should be enough to obviate the need for a stitch (Fig. 12.1).

A control radiograph is taken of the foot as soon as the injection is started, to confirm there is no leak, and to show that the contrast medium is running satisfactorily through the lymphatic vessel and that the needle is actually in a lymphatic channel. The tip of the needle could be in the sheath of the vessel and, although there is no leak, there is no flow of contrast medium. Embryologically, the veins and the lymphatic vessels are closely related, the blue dye being very easily picked up by both types of vessel. It is sometimes impossible to be sure by visual inspection that the small vessel which has been cannulated is a lymphatic and not a vein, but a control radiograph always gives the answer (Figs. 12.6, 12.7 and 12.8). A lymphatic vessel appears as an unbroken line of contrast indented by the numerous valves; while the

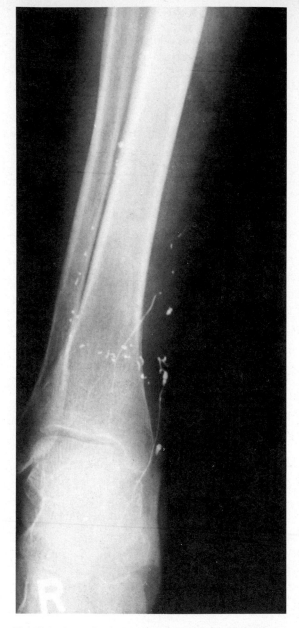

Fig. 12.6 A small vein inadvertently cannulated. Although the vein is no larger than the lymphatics in this foot (see Fig. 12.8) the check radiograph taken immediately after the beginning of the injection shows fragmentation of the column of contrast medium.

flow is faster in a vein and contrast medium globulates to produce the aptly named 'caviare sign' of Kinmonth. A further radiograph taken immediately afterwards will answer any doubts. It is safer to use control films than fluoroscopy.

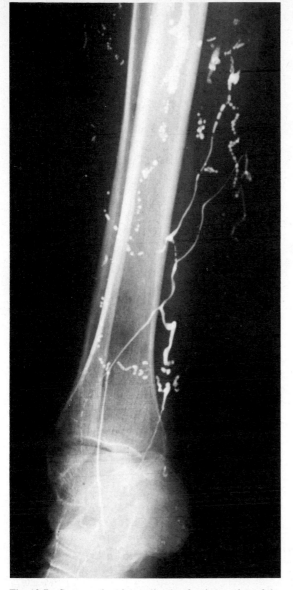

Fig. 12.7 Same patient immediately after inspection of the film shown in Fig. 12.6 and removal of the weights (stopping the pump). This now shows a typical venous injection picture with globulation of the contrast medium and the 'caviare' sign.

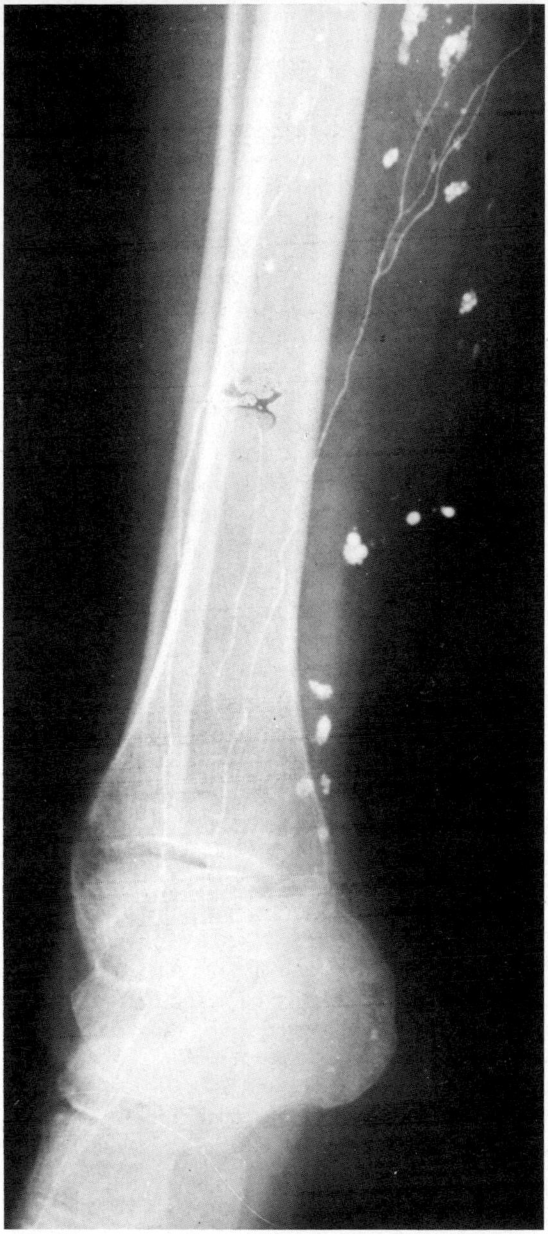

Fig. 12.8 Same patient. A lymphatic has been found and successfully cannulated. Note that these are of the same calibre as the small veins. There is still some oily contrast persisting in the veins from the first injection some 15 min previously.

The pump is adjusted to deliver the contrast medium at a rate of about 10 ml/h. If there is a palpable mass in the line of injection, or if there has been surgery of a type which may have caused disruption of the lymphatic flow, further control radiographs are taken when it is estimated that the contrast medium has reached the level in question to show if there is any marked obstruction or a lymphatico-venous commu-nication. The injection should be stopped if either of these is seen. A lymphatico-venous communication is recognized by globulation of contrast medium in the vein as described above.

The patient is used as his own control when deciding

on the volume of injected contrast medium. Even the largest patients do not require more than 8 ml of Lipiodol on each side, while a small adult may need only 5 ml and a baby less than 2 ml. The safest way to control the volume to be given is to take a control radiograph of the abdomen, stopping the injection when the contrast medium has reached the level of the fourth lumbar vertebra. The logic is that the contrast medium which is still filling the lymphatics of the legs is enough to opacify the remaining retroperitoneal area. The timing of the control radiograph of the abdomen is a question of experience, but a rough guide is that a radiograph should be taken when about two thirds of the anticipated volume for that size of patient has been injected at the recommended rate.

The needles are removed when the injection is complete. The ties are removed, leaving the lymphatic vessel intact, and the incision is then sutured. This suture is removed in about 7 days.

Radiographs to be taken

1. Preliminary assessment: chest.
2. Control (during injection): site of injection.
   Site of any possible obstruction, previous trauma or surgery which may have disrupted the lymphatic channels.
   Abdomen to control the volume of contrast medium.
3. Lymphangiogram (immediately after injection):
   Abdomen and pelvis.
   Chest to show thoracic duct, if required.
   Further films as indicated in the investigation of lymphoedema.
4. Lymphadenogram (after 24 h)
   Plain abdomen and pelvis.
   i. v. urography series to include obliques.
   Chest and penetrated view to show the mediastinum.
5. Follow-up: plain abdomen and chest.

As previously explained, the preliminary and control radiographs are for the safety of the patient. The reasons for the chest film are given in the section on Complications (p. 189). A lymphogram consists of the lymphangiogram plus the lymphadenogram. The lymphangiogram shows the contrast medium in the lymphatic vessels shortly after the completion of the injection. After the incision is sutured, the patient walks around the department for approximately 10 min to ensure that the contrast medium in the leg lymphatics is propelled into the retroperitoneal region. The lymphangiogram films are then taken (Fig. 12.9).

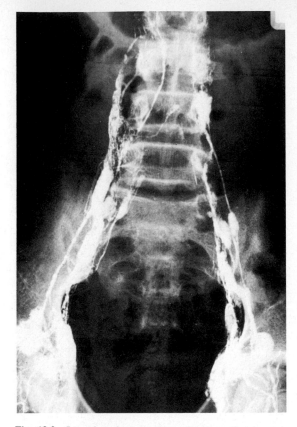

Fig. 12.9 Lymphangiogram phase. Radiograph taken on the same day as injection showing the contrast medium in the lymphatics.

After 24 hours the lymphatic vessels are clear of contrast medium. The nodes have taken up their full complement of medium by this time, the excess having been transported through the thoracic duct into the venous system and thence to the lungs. It is usually convenient to take the lymphadenogram radiographs at 24 hours (Figs. 12.10 and 12.11), but a delay of a further day or two makes no difference and does not cause any difficulty in interpretation. In practice, the 24 hour radiographs are combined with an intravenous urogram (i.v.u.). Although the overall diagnostic yield from the i.v.u. is low, extensive experience at the Royal Marsden Hospital has shown that the i.v.u. may give vital extra information in cancer cases. Oblique and A–P views allow assessment of the shape of the individual nodes, which is often a deciding factor in determining whether or not a node is likely to contain tumour (Fig. 12.11). A chest radiograph with sufficient penetration of the mediastinum is of value in showing any abnormally opacified nodes.

Lipiodol is retained in the lymph nodes in diagnostic

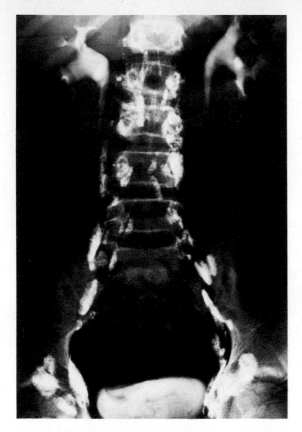

Fig. 12.10 At 24 h the contrast medium has cleared from the lymphatics and the nodes have opacified. An i.v.u. series is recommended at the time of the 24 hour films.

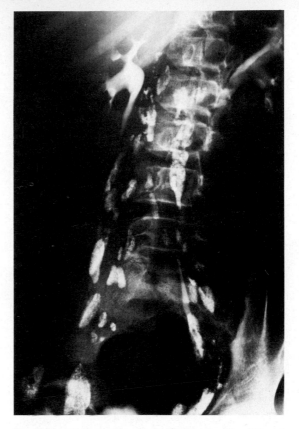

Fig. 12.11 Oblique views should also be taken, the different views show the shape of the individual nodes.

amounts for about one year in the average patient. For this reason, follow up radiographs are of great importance, particularly in malignant disease. Indeed, a lymphogram cannot be considered normal until it has been followed up. The 24 h films should be regarded as a base line and, in those patients where the nodes are abnormal, the period during which they remain opacified allows monitoring of their progress. A decision made purely on the appearances of the immediate and 24 h films, even in the most experienced hands, incurs a potential error of between 5% and 20% depending on the primary tumour type.

Variations on basic techniques

While the vast majority of lymphograms are performed via an incision on the dorsum of the foot, lymphography may be undertaken from any part where there is a lymphatic vessel suitable for injection. For instance, lymphography has been performed from the back, from the area of the mastoid process to show

the cervical chains, from the hand (Fig. 12.12) to show the lymphatics of the arm and axillary nodes, and from the spermatic cord at the time of orchidectomy. These other sites of injection are of interest, but have little practical value. It is in the evaluation of the lymphatic vessels and the retroperitoneal lymph nodes that lymphography has been of greatest value.

Variations in the technique of lymphatic cannulation are legion, but the simpler the technique the better. As in the method described above, the aims should be simplicity, reliability and safety.

Complications

The patient should be warned that the blue dye is excreted in the urine following lymphography. The blue dye stains all the body fluids and, in those of fair complexion and in small children, the skin may subsequently appear slightly blue. It is particularly important to warn the anaesthetist that this may happen in children where lymphography is performed under general anaesthesia. A blue stain will remain at

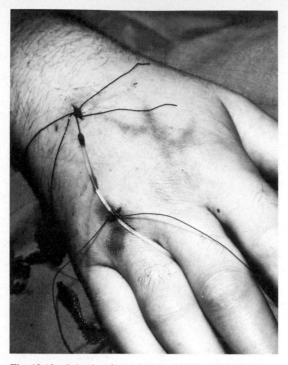

Fig. 12.12 Injection from the hand. If the patient is liable to move then a stitch can be put in the line of the catheter to hold this. Since the area injected with marker dye contains local anaesthetic there is no problem with this if needed.

days later if necessary. True pulmonary embolism following lymphography is rare. A slight blood staining of the sputum occurs after 3–10 days in approximately one fifth of patients, but seldom requires treatment and is considered to be due to a chemical reaction resulting from the splitting of the oil into its constituent fatty acids.

Again, one fifth of patients complain of mild symptoms on the night of the lymphogram; namely mild pyrexia, headache and slight nausea. This has not been satisfactorily explained, but is thought to be a CNS reaction to the oil or its breakdown products. The severest neurological complication is cerebral oil embolism, but fortunately this is rare with proper patient selection and efficient control of the procedure. The normal lung does not allow sufficiently large droplets of oil to pass into the systemic circulation to cause this complication, but patients with intracardiac shunts are not accepted for lymphography. Lymphography is also not performed in those patients who are currently having radiotherapy to any part of the lung, because there is experimental evidence that irradiated lung capillaries may fail to filter larger droplets of oil. The incidence of cerebral oil embolism at the Royal Marsden Hospital has been two in 10 000 lymphograms and both patients made a complete recovery.

If repeat lymphography is needed in patients who are known to be allergic to Patent Blue Violet, the lymphogram can often be performed without the use of a marker dye by a sufficiently experienced operator.

the site of the injected dye for many weeks following lymphography but will gradually disappear.

Allergic reactions may occur due to the marker dye or the iodized oil.

Any iodized oil which is not taken up by lymph nodes is discharged into the venous system and delivered to the lung. The normal lung is an efficient filter for the iodized oil, which is arrested in the capillaries before being absorbed and broken down into its constituent parts. There is a resultant depression of lung function which reaches its maximum at about 36 hours and this is why lymphography is dangerous in those who already have severe, compromised lung function. If the patient is suffering from the acute stage of venous thrombosis, and is therefore liable to sudden pulmonary embolism, it would also seem unwise to depress the lung function in the presence of this risk. If there is impaired pulmonary function and a lymphogram is considered to be essential, it is advisable to do the procedure as an in-patient and to inject only one side with a reduced volume of contrast medium. This often gives all the required information and, if the patient has tolerated this well, then the other side may be injected 7–10

Relationship to other imaging modalities

No other radiological method regularly shows the lymphatic vessels. Lymphography is a direct method for demonstrating the storage pattern of the iodized oil in the nodes. Other modalities at present only show abnormal masses. While a large lymph node shown on CT or ultrasound may be considered abnormal; lymphography differentiates between a secondary deposit, a lymphoma pattern or reactive hyperplasia, and shows nodal deposits which are too small to be detected by other modalities. Retention of the iodized oil in the nodes allows follow up by means of a plain radiograph which costs very little in time, trouble or money.

When a lymph node deposit has broken through the confines of the node, lymphography may be positive but becomes less accurate in assessing the extent of the disease. In these circumstances ultrasound and computed tomography (CT) become more accurate. Lymphography is also limited to those nodes which are opacified by injection of lymphatics in a few selected sites whereas ultrasound, and particularly CT, suffer no such constraints.

Lymph nodes can also be shown up by the subcutaneous injection of isotopes. This is a very easy technique and will of course, show the nodes in areas which cannot be reached by lymphogram. Detail is poor and results so far have not been of much practical use.

REFERENCES

General

Kinmonth J. B. (Ed.) (1978) *The Lymphatics*. Edward Arnold, London.

Kinmonth J. B., Kemp Harper R. A. & Taylor G. W. (1955) Lymphangiography by radiological methods. *J. Fac. Radiol.*, **6**; 217–33.

Viamonte M. & Rüttiman A. (Eds.) (1980) *Atlas of Lymphography* Georg Thieme Verlag, Stuttgart and and New York.

Lymphography in malignant disease

Macdonald J. S. & Peckham M. J. (1973) *Hodgkin's Disease.* (Ed. Smithers Sir D. W.) Ch. 18, p. 169–78. Churchill Livingstone, London.

Macdonald J. S. (1978) *Circulation of the Blood.* (Ed. James D. G.) Ch. 16, p. 303–11. Pitman Medical, London.

Turner A. G., Hendry W. F., Macdonald, J. S. & Wallace D. M. (1976) The value of lymphography in the management of bladder cancer, *Brit. J. Urol.,* **48**; 579–86.

Hendry W. F., Tyrell C. J., Macdonald J. S., McElwain T. J. & Peckham M. J. (1977), The detection and localisation of abdominal lymph node metastases from testicular teratomas, *Brit. J. Urol.,* **49**; 739–45.

Complications of lymphography

Macdonald J. S. (1976) *Complications in Diagnostic Radiology.* (Ed. Ansell G.) Ch. 13, pp. 301–17. Blackwell Scientific Publications, Oxford.

SECTION 3
THE RESPIRATORY TRACT

The Larynx 13

G. A. S. LLOYD

The radiological investigation of the larynx now comprises four techniques. These are, in the order in which they should normally be applied:

1. Plain radiography of the larynx, including a standard soft tissue lateral radiograph of the neck and four films (two A–P, two lateral) using high kilovoltage technique.
2. Conventional tomography.
3. Computed tomography.
4. Contrast laryngography.

Plain radiographic examination

The larynx is best examined in the lateral position, since the cervical spine largely obliterates the outlines of the air containing structures of the larynx in the A–P projection. The lateral radiograph is obtained by centring the incident ray at a point just behind the prominence of the thyroid cartilage. The film is placed against the shoulder and the anode film distance increased to 6 ft to minimize geometric distortion. The position is similar to that used for a lateral view of the cervical spine.

High kV technique

This may be used in both the A–P and lateral projections. The advantage of lateral high kV films over the standard soft tissue lateral radiograph is that any obscuring calcification in the thyroid cartilage is obliterated, thus allowing better visualization of the structures at glottic level (Fig. 13.1). Two high kV lateral films are obtained—one at rest and one with the patients phonating 'ee'. This helps to visualize the anterior ends of the cords and anterior commissure— an important feature which allows assessment of malignant growths of the cord and their relationship to the thyroepiglottic ligament.

A–P radiographs of the larynx using a kilovoltage of 145 kV or more with 3 mm of brass filtration give obliteration of the superimposed shadows of the cervical vertebrae, giving almost bone-free studies of the larynx. A modification which produces a totally bone-free image is the use of 5 degree zonography in addition to high kV and brass filtration. In the first

instance, high kV A–P studies are used to show cord mobility, radiographs being obtained in quiet inspiration and in phonation (Fig. 13.2a and b). This

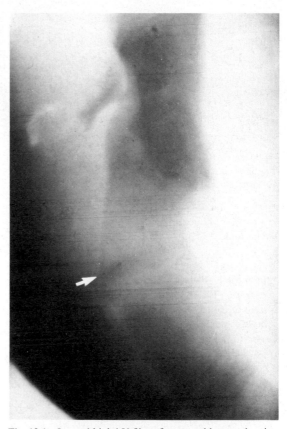

Fig. 13.1 Lateral high kV film of a normal larynx showing ventricles (arrow), with true and false cords below and above.

demonstrates cord fixation (Fig. 13.3), which is important in the pre-operative staging of a laryngeal carcinoma since it immediately classifies the tumour as T_3 or T_4 by the UICC (Union International contre le Cancer) classification.

High kV radiographs may also silhouette a tumour mass against the translucency of the air within the larynx, but conventional tomography is required for the proper demonstration of the larynx in longitudinal section.

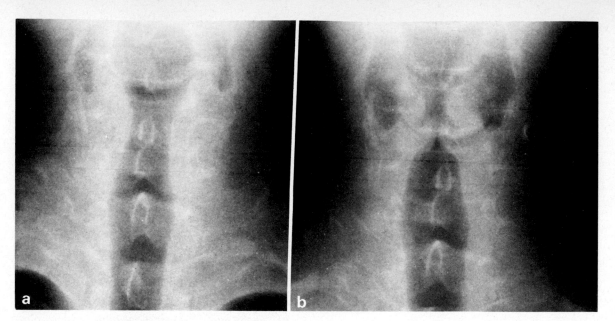

Fig. 13.2 A–P views taken by high kV technique.
(a) Film taken in inspiration with abduction of the cords.
(b) Film taken in phonation showing true and false cords, ventricles and pyriform fossae distended with air.

Tomography

Investigation of the larynx is incomplete without tomography. The technique is easy to perform and free from discomfort to the patient. It allows the outline of the laryngeal soft tissues to be seen clearly without the overlap of the bony shadows of the cervical spine, in addition to showing the lower limits of tumour extension into the subglottic space—an area difficult to examine by endoscopy.

A linear or elliptical tomographic movement of the X-ray tube in a direction longitudinal to the patient is recommended for studies of the larynx. The incomplete blurring of structures lying in the direction of tube swing, which is a feature of linear tomography, tends to enhance the definition of laryngeal structures against the contrast of the air, generally giving better results than circular or hypocycloidal movements. Accurate coning and the use of small fields are essential in the production of high quality tomography (Fig. 13.4).

Tomographic cuts are made at 0.5 cm intervals with the patient lying supine and phonating 'ee'. This causes approximation of the vocal cords, their outlines thereby being more clearly shown in relation to the surrounding air. Tomograms are obtained with both expiratory and inspiratory phonation, the latter usually producing better air distension of the ventricles

and allowing compression of the ventricle to be differentiated from infiltration.

Computed tomography (CT) of the larynx

The application of CT to the investigation of the larynx, particularly in regard to the management of carcinoma, derives from the work of Mancuso *et al.*, (1977). CT demonstrates the larynx in axial section, providing a unique view of the laryngeal structures in the horizontal plane, with the possibility of showing laryngeal cartilage invasion in addition to the soft tissue extent of a tumour. In this way CT is complimentary to conventional tomography, since it presents a cross section of the larynx as distinct from the longitudinal view provided by plain X-ray techniques and conventional tomography.

Technique and normal anatomy

The patient lies supine on the scanning table with slight extension of the head. Scanning is begun at the level of the hyoid bone, with sequential scans of 5 mm thickness and separation, in a caudal direction. Cessation of respiration is preferable but is not feasible with long scanning times, so that the scans are normally made in quiet respiration. As sequential

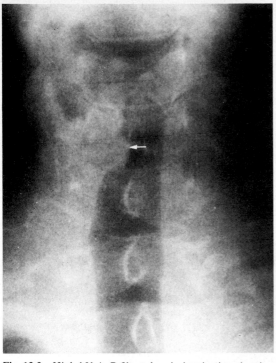

Fig. 13.3 High kV A–P film taken in inspiration showing fixation of vocal cord (arrow) due to carcinoma.

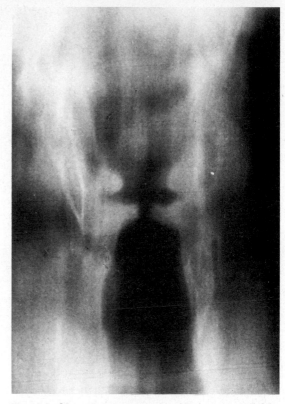

Fig. 13.4 Normal A–P tomogram showing true and false cords, ventricles and subglottic space.

Fig. 13.5 CT scan at the level of the hyoid. The crescentric epiglottis is shown within the air translucency, with the valleculae anterior to it.

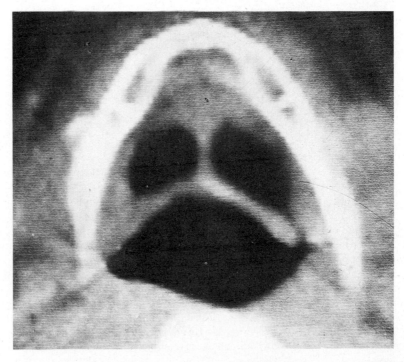

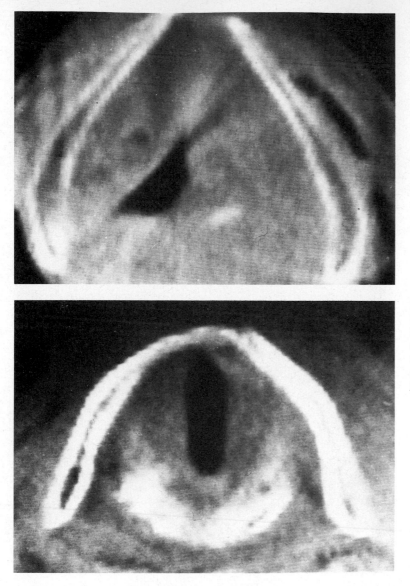

Fig. 13.6 CT scan at the level of the thyroid notch, which is shown as a gap between the thyroid laminae anteriorly.

Fig. 13.7 CT scan made at glottic level. The arch formed by the thyroid laminae is shown with the boat-shaped air gap between the cords. Note that normally there is virtually no soft tissue gap between the air space and the junction of the thyroid laminae.

scans are made from above downwards, the level is easily identified from the characteristic anatomical features of the larynx. The epiglottis and valleculae are seen at the level of the hyoid, (Fig. 13.5), while the thyroid laminae become apparent below this level. The shape of the thyroid cartilage changes in a very characteristic way on scanning at a lower level. Above the cords, the laminae do not meet in the mid-line where the thyroid notch is present and are arranged approximately 90° to one another (Fig. 13.6). The two thyroid laminae fuse just above vocal cord level and assume the shape of an arch (Fig. 13.7), which becomes more rounded at a lower level and forms the anterior portion of an oval which is completed

posteriorly by the cricoid laminae. The shape of the airway also alters on sequential scans. At the level of the hyoid, the airway is bisected by the crescentic epiglottis (Fig. 13.5), but below this level the airway assumes a triangular shape and the two pyriform sinuses are seen as two lateral appendages separated by the aryepiglottic folds. At the level of the cords the shape changes to the characteristic glottic chink or boat shape, with the sharp anterior commissure extending right up to thyroid cartilage in the mid-line (Fig. 13.6). In the subglottic area there is an even, symmetrical oval shape which changes at the level of the first tracheal ring to an oval flattened posteriorly, similar in shape to a horse-shoe.

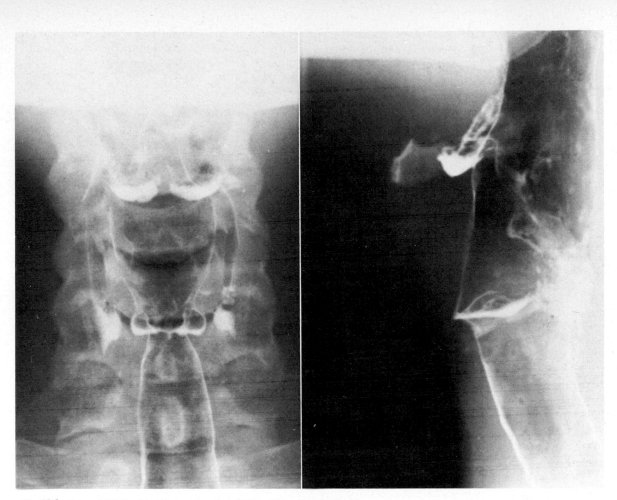

Fig. 13.8 (a) and (b) Contrast laryngography, A–P and lateral projections.

Contrast laryngography

Contrast studies of the larynx and pharynx using oily Dionosil may be used to outline the laryngeal structures. (Fig. 13.8). The technique is based on the work of Powers *et al.*, (1957).

The patient is pre-medicated with 1 mg atropine subcutaneously 30 min. prior to the examination, in order to suppress the formation of mucus. After sucking an anaesthetic lozenge, a topical spray of 1% lignocaine is used to produce local anaesthesia. Ten to twenty millilitre of oily Dionosil are then dripped slowly over the tongue from a curved laryngeal syringe during quiet inspiration.

Radiographs are obtained in A–P and lateral projections in inspiration, in phonation, and during Valsalva and reversed Valsalva manoeuvres.

For satisfactory coating of the subglottic region, it may be necessary to take films during fluoroscopy immediately after the patient has been asked to cough. This propels the contrast medium against the glottis and normally results in good delineation of the subglottic area.

Contrast studies have the advantage that the whole of the larynx and hypopharynx are visualized at one examination. The mucosal coating with contrast medium allows early changes in these structures to be seen. Hemmingson (1973), in a careful evaluation of the various modalities then available for the radiological investigation of the larynx, regarded contrast laryngography as the optimum method of investigation. The introduction of CT of the larynx, however, has radically diminished the importance of laryngography. Plain radiography with conventional tomography and CT produce an adequate preoperative investigation of most patients with laryngeal disease.

Apart from the disadvantage of being a very time consuming procedure, laryngography is only safely applicable to a proportion of patients. It is ill-advised to use the technique in patients with bulky laryngeal tumours because of the danger of producing respiratory obstruction, a complication which may also occur in patients investigated for laryngeal trauma. In conclusion, it is difficult to see the place of laryngography in the future investigation of the larynx in centres where CT is practised routinely.

Barium swallow

A preoperative barium swallow is required in patients with laryngeal cancer which has spread to the oesophagus, or which may involve the wall between the larynx and oesophagus, and with post-cricoid tumours. Barium swallow may also be required after laryngectomy to delineate the track of a post-operative fistula from the site of the anastomosis.

REFERENCES

Hemmingson A. (1972) Roentgenologic examination of the larynx. A clinical comparison. *Acta Radiol. Diag.*, **12**, 433–451.

Mancuso A., Hanafee W., Juillard J. F., Winger J. & Calcaterra T (1977) The role of computed tomography in the management of cancer of the larynx. *Radiology*, **124**, 243–4.

Powers W. E., McGee H. H. & Seaman W. B. (1957) Contrast examination of the larynx and pharynx. *Radiology*, **68**, 169.

The Bronchial Tree and Lungs—the Respiratory Tract 14

C. D. R. FLOWER

BRONCHOGRAPHY

Bronchography was first described by Sicard and Forestier in 1922 and has been widely used since that time. There is now, however, a greatly diminished demand for bronchography, the reasons for which are twofold. The advent of fibre-optic bronchoscopy has extended the range of direct vision of the bronchial tree and, coupled with the facility of biopsy, enables a tissue diagnosis to be obtained, as opposed to the purely anatomical demonstration provided by bronchography. The other reason for its decline is an increasing awareness that the limited yield of information seldom alters patient management.

Indications

Although the diagnosis of *bronchiectasis* is clinically obvious in the majority of patients, bronchography is required when contemplating surgery.

A complete demonstration of the whole bronchial tree is mandatory to provide a pre-operative 'map' for the surgeon and to ensure that no diseased segments are unrecognized prior to operation (Fig. 14.1). Occasionally the diagnosis of bronchiectasis is not evident on clinical grounds alone and a bronchogram is necessary to establish the diagnosis. Some abnormality is seen on the chest radiograph in the great majority of patients with bronchiectasis, 93% of patients in one large survey (Gudbjerg, 1957), and allows the bronchographic approach to be directed primarily at the suspicious lobe. A bilateral bronchogram is required in the minority of patients with bronchiectasis in whom the chest radiograph is normal.

In most patients with *haemopytsis*, the cause is apparent on clinical and radiographic grounds. Bronchoscopy is frequently employed and the use of the fibre-optic instrument had obviated the need for bronchography. However, there remains a group of patients with significant but unexplained haemoptysis who have a normal chest radiograph and in whom bronchography is sometimes requested to exclude a localized area of bronchiectasis or a small peripheral bronchial carcinoma (Fig. 14.2). The yield of useful information in this group of patients is very low. No occult cancers were detected in one series of 92 patients, localized bronchiectasis being seen in two patients and benign broncho-occlusive disease in another two patients. (Forrest *et al.*, 1976). It can therefore be reasonably concluded that bronchography is unlikely to yield useful information in patients, with a single haemoptysis, who have a normal chest radiograph and a normal bronchoscopy. However, the ease with which bronchography can be employed as an adjunct to fibre-optic bronchoscopy, with no significant additional hazard or discomfort to the patient, means that this small group of patients may be investigated in this way.

Bronchography is of little use in the diagnosis of *bronchial carcinoma*. Patients suspected of having a tumour require an endoscopic examination with biopsy of any bronchial occlusion or mucosal abnormality (Fig. 14.3). Tantalum bronchography has been employed in the detection of occult bronchial carcinomas and appears to be of most use in patients with a normal chest radiograph and positive sputum cytology. These early cancers, which may be missed by endoscopy, may be suspected by attention to fine morphological detail and delayed mucociliary clearance, with a 'target' being provided for subsequent bronchoscopic brushing and biopsy (Siegelman *et al.*, 1979).

Bronchography is occasionally required for the demonstration of *congenital abnormalities*, particularly in the delineation of bronchial anatomy prior to surgery. Finally, bronchography may be used to demonstrate a *bronchopleural fistula*. These fistulae are usually very small and are best delineated by the 'retrograde' route, contrast medium being instilled into the pleural space via a thin rubber catheter introduced through the chest drain. The contrast agent is usually sucked into the bronchial tree during quiet respiration.

Contra-indications

There are a small number of important contra-indications to bronchography. It should never be undertaken during an acute upper or lower respiratory tract infection. Bronchography should never be employed for the diagnosis of bronchiectasis following a pneumonia until at least three months have passed since radiographic resolution, because reversible

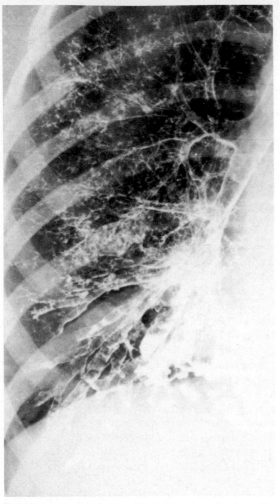

Fig. 14.1 Bronchiectasis—affecting the lower and middle lobes, but sparing the upper lobe.

bronchial dilatation is a well recognized feature of pneumonia. Asthma is a relative contra-indication because both instrumentation and the contrast agent may induce bronchospasm. Respiratory function is significantly impaired during bronchography, due to obstruction of smaller airways by the contrast medium. The examination should therefore only be undertaken with great caution in patients with a diminished respiratory reserve. It is essential that any patient with airways obstruction, or poor lung function due to any other cause, is assessed by a chest physician before being submitted for bronchography.

Technique

Although the contrast agent may be instilled into the bronchial tree indirectly by dripping it over the back of the tongue into the hypopharynx and thence through the vocal cords, it is best introduced directly into the bronchial tree via some sort of catheter. The examination should always take place under fluoroscopic control. Both local and general anaesthesia may be used, although the latter is normally only required in children.

Pre-medication and preparation

Patients with suspected bronchiectasis should have physiotherapy beforehand and nothing to eat or drink for at least 4 h before the examination. Bronchography is a disagreable experience and some form of pre-medication, is necessary and should include an agent to reduce bronchial secretions. Either omnopon and scopolamine, or pethidine and atropine, are suitable.

Intravenous diazepam can be given immediately prior to the examination if the patient is particularly apprehensive.

Local anaesthesia

The majority of examinations are performed under local anaesthesia, the most suitable agent for which is 2% lignocaine. One of the commonest hazards of bronchography is local anaesthetic overdose. No more than 200 mg of lignocaine should be used in the average adult. A satisfactory guide to dosage is to allow 1 ml of the 2% solution per 6 kg body weight.

Contrast media

The most widely used contrast agent is propyliodone (Dionosil), which is available either as a suspension in arachis oil or as an aqueous suspension containing carboxymethylcellulose. Iodinated poppyseed oil (Lipiodol), Hytrast and barium sulphate have been used in the past. Lipiodol is no longer used, being very slowly resorbed from the lung and responsible for a high incidence of iodism. Hytrast, an aqueous suspension of iopydol and iopydone, initially appeared to be a very satisfactory contrast agent but was discontinued because it induced a high incidence of chemical pneumonitis. Barium sulphate has been used in the USA but has never achieved popularity in the UK. Hypertonic contrast agents such as Gastrografin are absolutely contra-indicated, being a potent cause of pulmonary oedema.

Both the aqueous and oily solutions of propyliodone are acceptable, although neither is the ideal bronchographic agent. Aqueous Dionosil gives the better coating of the bronchial mucosa whilst oily Dionosil tends to give better filling of the small bronchial

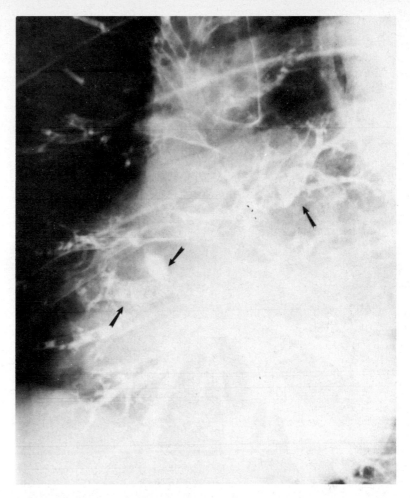

Fig. 14.2 Bronchiectasis localized to the apical and anterior segments of the lower lobe. Haemoptysis. Normal chest radiograph and bronchoscopy.

divisions. Both are absorbed by macrophages, the lungs usually being completely clear of contrast material within two days of the examination. One of the advantages of aqueous Dionosil is that it may be diluted with water and/or local anaesthetic. This dilution is important in children, where an especially viscid contrast agent causes bronchial occlusion, and is also helpful in providing good peripheral filling in adults. The aqueous solution should be warmed to body temperature, shaken vigorously, and only drawn up when the operator is ready to inject. Up to 40 ml of contrast medium may be required for the examination of both bronchial trees, but it is often possible to perform a satisfactory bilateral bronchogram with 20–30 ml.

Tantalum is a radio-dense inert metal with no known toxic effects. It is not generally available in this country, but has been used extensively in the USA. It adheres very well to the bronchial mucosa with minimal reduction in respiratory function as, unlike propyliodone, it produces no bronchial obstruc-

tion. Tantalum is introduced as a sterile dessicated powder, using an atomiser which is grounded to prevent sparking.

The time-honoured methods for bronchography have been the transnasal and cricothyroid routes. Both are described for completeness, but radiologists should be aware that these techniques are becoming obsolete since the advent of fibre-optic bronchoscopy and the ability to instill contrast material into the bronchial tree under direct vision.

Nasal route

After pre-medication, the patient is placed in a lying or sitting position with extension of the neck. Two per cent lignocaine is introduced through the most patent nostril from a nebulizer. The patient is instructed to breathe deeply and to sniff during this procedure. Approximately 4 ml of 2% lignocaine is the required amount. Although a number of manoeuvres have been described, the following method is recommended for

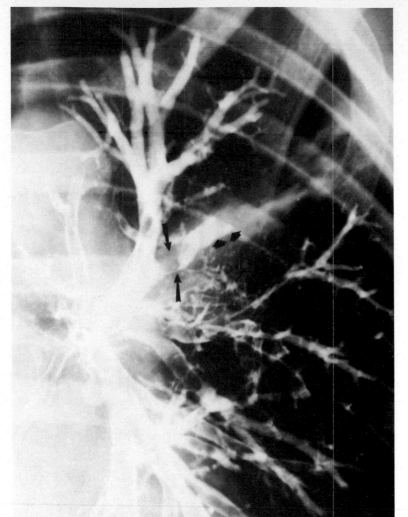

Fig. 14.3 Bronchial adenoma anterior division left upper lobe bronchus. (N.B. distal bronchiectasis—short arrows). Diagnosis established by bronchoscopic biopsy.

the introduction of a catheter through the nose into the trachea. A soft rubber catheter, FG7, is used in preference to a pre-curved catheter. A Kifa catheter, pre-curved at its distal end, is placed into the lumen in order to produce the necessary curve at the tip of the rubber catheter, to render it opaque and to allow the necessary degree of torque to manoeuvre the tip of the catheter. The catheter is introduced through the anaesthetized nostril with the patient lying on their right side. Keeping the neck extended, the catheter is initially advanced along the floor of the nose and then through the nasopharynx with the mouth open and the tongue forward. The catheter then passes readily to the vocal cords. Using carefully coned fluoroscopy, a further 2 ml of 2% lignocaine is injected when the catheter tip is seen to reach the region of the cords. The catheter is then gently manipulated between the cords under fluoroscopic control. This sometimes requires a slight rotary movement to prevent the catheter tip from lodging in one of the pyriform fossae, a situation which may not be appreciated with single plane screening. A further 2 ml of 2% lignocaine is injected immediately after the catheter enters the trachea, and the catheter then being advanced to the bronchial tree which is to be examined. Unless a selective bronchogram is required, it is best to leave the catheter tip either in the intermediate bronchus on the right or at the bifurcation of the left main bronchus. Following placement of the catheter, the inner Kifa 'guide' is withdrawn and a final 2 ml of 2% lignocaine is injected prior to the introduction of contrast medium.

Much has been written about positioning the patient during the instillation of the contrast medium in order to ensure filling of all segments of the bronchial tree. Propyliodone is mainly distributed through the bronchi by the inspiratory 'suck' which is produced by the negative pressure exerted at the periphery of the lung by each inspiration. Patient positioning is therefore only necessary to ensure that contrast medium is evenly distributed to all lobar orifices. Thus a right bronchogram is performed with the patient in the right posterior oblique position and a left bronchogram with the patient in the left posterior oblique position. It is usually advisable to have the table tilted 15–10 degrees head up to prevent flow-back of contrast medium into the trachea.

The contrast medium should always be injected under fluoroscopic control and only sufficient is delivered to allow adequate opacification. The patient is instructed to breathe normally during the instillation of contrast medium. It is now appreciated that delineation of the small peripheral bronchi is important (Trapnell, 1969) and is sometimes only achieved by deep inspiration or by asking the patient to cough, when the post-tussive inspiratory effort draws the contrast medium to the periphery.

Spot radiographs may be exposed at suitable intervals and, if necessary, complemented by overhead radiographs. The patient is given physiotherapy following the procedure.

Cricothyroid route

In experienced hands this is an acceptable and safe technique which is rapidly performed and remarkably well tolerated, but should never be attempted by an inexperienced bronchographer. It has the advantage of requiring a smaller volume of local anaesthetic.

Local anaesthetic is introduced in the mid-line down to the cricothyroid membrane, with the patient supine and the neck well-extended, and is then injected through the membrane into the trachea before immediate removal of the needle. Prior to the injection of local anaesthetic into the trachea, air must be withdrawn into the syringe to ensure that the needle tip lies within the tracheal lumen. A small incision is then made in the skin and a needle catheter assembly is introduced in a slightly caudal direction using a modified Seldinger technique. The catheter tip is placed in the bronchial tree to be examined and the subsequent procedure is as described for the transnasal route.

Modifications of basic technique

Bronchography via the fibre-optic bronchoscope

This is now the preferred technique for all bronchographic examinations in adults. Examination of the

bronchial tree prior to its opacification with contrast medium is an obvious advantage, whilst the introduction of the fibrescope under direct vision is more acceptable to the patient than the 'blind' passage of a bronchography tube. The contrast material is introduced via a fine polyethylene catheter passed through the bronchoscopy channel, the tip of which can be placed into any selected segmental bronchus under direct vision. Such localized bronchography is very useful for the demonstration of segmental bronchiectasis, which may be suspected when blood is seen to issue from a segmental orifice. The quality of the bronchographic picture is very good, except after bronchial biopsy or brushing when artefacts arise due to local haemorrhage and spasm of the traumatized airways.

Bronchography in children

General anaesthesia is required using an endotracheal tube. The contrast medium is introduced via a thin plastic catheter which is slipped through a small incision in the rubber bung at the top of the endotracheal tube, the anaesthetic gas being supplied via a side arm.

A child's bronchial tree is of small volume and may therefore be readily compromised by the use of too much or too viscid contrast medium, with subsequent respiratory embarrassment. Tracheal filling should be avoided and only the necessary minimal amount is instilled down the catheter. It is often helpful to dilute the aqueous propyliodone with sterile water. The contrast medium is dispersed along the bronchial tree by gentle insufflation during fluoroscopy and spot radiographs are obtained using the undercouch tube.

Complications

Complications may arise from poor technique, from local anaesthetic overdose or as a result of the contrast medium.

The nasal mucosa and the vocal cords may be damaged by using injudicious force during the passage of a tube via the nasogastric route. The cricothyroid route is especially fraught with hazard in inexperienced hands. Subcutaneous emphysema results from an air leak at the puncture site through the cricothyroid membrane and is only avoided by instructing the patient to press on the puncture site during coughing. Undue bleeding from the puncture may produce a cervical haematoma. Contrast medium may be inadvertently injected into the soft tissues of the neck. These complications usually occur with lack of experience and are avoided by a meticulous technique. It is of paramount importance that the operator checks that the needle is in the lumen of the trachea, by aspirating air into the syringe, before injecting local anaesthetic or contrast medium. The use of the Seldinger technique, as opposed to the direct injection of contrast medium through the cricothyroid membrane, has reduced the incidence of this complication.

Fatalities are rare during bronchography, but one of the most important causes of death is local anaesthetic overdose. Lignocaine is rapidly absorbed from the nasopharyngeal and bronchial mucosa and high blood concentrations are rapidly achieved by the administration of an excess of local anaesthetic. Furthermore, excretion of lignocaine is relatively slow. It is sometimes suggested that patients should be given a tablet of local anaesthetic to suck prior to spraying the nares. This serves little useful purpose and only increases the total absorbed dose of local anaesthetic. The amount of permissible local anaesthetic is calculated prior to the procedure, preferably according to the patient's body weight (see above). Using 2% Lignocaine, 10–12 ml may be given to the average adult, compared with 5–6 ml of the 4% solution. The toxic effects of lignocaine are manifested by depression of the respiratory and cardiovascular centres. Earlier signs of overdosage are pallor and sweating, speech disturbance, tremor, auditory hallucinations and paraesthesiae.

Respiratory function is significantly impaired during bronchography, due mainly to obstruction of the bronchi and trachea by contrast medium. This is not surprising when one considers that the total volume of the tracheo-bronchial tree in the adult is approximately 150 ml and that the contrast medium used for a bilateral bronchogram reduces this volume by as much as 20%. It is therefore a wise precaution to avoid tracheal filling whenever possible, particularly in children. Vital capacity may be reduced by a third, while measurements of diffusing capacity immediately following bronchography have shown a reduction by as much as 50%. Propyliodone tends to produce a local inflammatory reaction in the lungs and a postoperative pyrexia due to a contrast-induced 'pneumonitis' is an occasional occurrence. A general idiosyncratic reaction due to the absorption of contrast medium is a rare event; with the production of a pyrexia, rigors, headache and a rash. Bronchospasm is a well recognized complication of bronchography and may be related either to the contrast medium or to manipulation of a catheter within the sensitive bronchial tree. Bronchography should therefore only be performed on asthmatics when absolutely necessary and then only on the advice of a chest physician. Prior administration of corticosteroids and intravenous Salbutamol is usually required in asthmatics.

LUNG BIOPSY

Both localized and diffuse pulmonary disease may produce a diagnostic problem which is not resolved by clinical and radiographic means. Although the clinical history and examination of the sputum for organisms and malignant cells reduces the number of patients in this problem group, a significant number require some form of biopsy to establish the correct diagnosis. An open lung biopsy performed via a thoracotomy provides a large piece of tissue for histological examination. It is a safe procedure in experienced hands with a very low operative mortality, being the investigation of choice in some patients with chronic diffuse lung disease and in some immunosuppressed patients with diffuse pulmonary shadowing.

PERCUTANEOUS LUNG BIOPSY

Tissue may be obtained from the lung by needle aspiration, a screw biopsy needle, a cutting biopsy needle, or by the high-speed cutting drill. Each of these techniques has its proponents. Radiologists normally confine themselves to the use of one or other form of biopsy needle (Fig. 14.4). The high-speed air drill does not require any fluoroscopic control and is used to obtain a core of tissue in diffuse lung disease. The main complication of its use is a pneumothorax and it has been largely superseded by transbronchial biopsy via the flexible bronchoscope.

Needle biopsy is usually reserved for patients with localized disease. The Tru-Cut and Vim-Silverman type of cutting needles have been used to obtain tissue in diffuse disease, but the yield is not as good as with open drill or transbronchial biopsy and there is a significant associated risk of haemorrhage.

Personal preference dictates which type of needle is used to biopsy a pulmonary mass, but it is worth emphasizing the distinction between the histological 'core' obtained by cutting needle biopsy and the cytological specimen obtained by aspiration. The advantage of a histological specimen is usually outweighed by the greater hazards, namely haemorrhage and pneumothorax, which are associated with the use of cutting needles. The Rotex screw biopsy needle yields very good cytological smears and often provides small histological specimens as well, the incidence of complications being no greater than with

Fig. 14.4 Biopsy needles. (Cutting: aspiration and screw types).

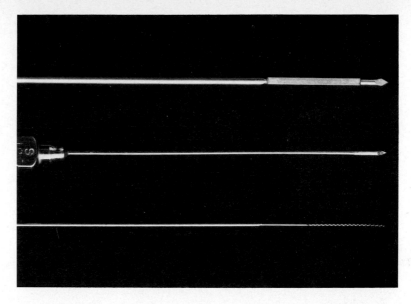

simple aspiration. The use of increasingly 'fine' needles, either a 20 or 21 gauge being optimal, has decreased both the discomfort and complications of the procedure while not diminishing the yield of diagnostic material.

Indications

The major indication for percutaneous needle biopsy is the diagnosis of localized intrapulmonary disease. In the majority of patients this means differentiating between a benign or malignant process (Fig. 14.5 and 14.6). Accuracy in the diagnosis of malignant lesions varies between centres but in experienced hands is between 90% and 95%. The 5–10% false negative rate is the major weakness of the technique. The other difficulty is the cytopathologist's frequent inability to make a specific diagnosis of a benign lesion due to the scanty amount of available material.

Biopsy should only be undertaken if the result affects the patient's management and obviates the need for a diagnostic thoracotomy. For example, in the case of a 60 year old life-long smoker whose sole abnormality is a peripheral pulmonary mass with an irregular margin, the likelihood of cancer is so high on radiographic and clinical evidence that a 'negative' biopsy will not prevent a thoracotomy and there is no point in undertaking the procedure. Biopsy is much more useful in younger patients and for masses which are likely to be due to some benign process on clinical and radiographic grounds. In patients with a presumed bronchial carcinoma, but in whom a thoracotomy is contra-indicated, biopsy gives confirmation of the diagnosis and cell typing prior to radiotherapy or chemotherapy. It also has a role in establishing the nature of a solitary intrapulmonary mass in a patient with a known extrathoracic primary malignancy when surgical excision is likely to be undertaken. Biopsy has an important role in establishing that an intrapulmonary mass is due to an inflammatory process, the diagnosis of which is usually impossible by sputum examination. This is particularly so in the immuno-suppressed patient, in some instances of tuberculosis, and in chronic lung abscess. It is obviously imperative that the smears are appropriately stained and that the correct cultures are set up.

Finally, percutaneous biopsy has an occasional role in distinguishing between multiple benign intrapulmonary masses such as Wegener's granulomata and rheumatoid nodules, and metastases.

Contra-indications

A suspected hydatid cyst is probably the only absolute contra-indication. Relative contra-indications are a bleeding diathesis, pulmonary hypertension and severe emphysema. Fear of puncturing a peripheral pulmonary artery aneurysm or vascular malformation is probably unfounded, always presuming there is a normal pulmonary arterial pressure.

Technique

The lesion to be biopsied must be localized on P–A and lateral radiographs, and tomography performed

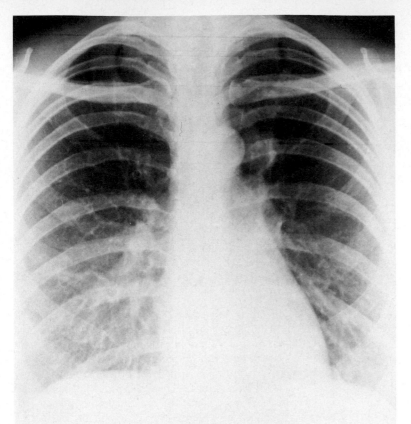

Fig. 14.5 Two centimeter mass adjacent to aortic knuckle. Tubercle bacilli identified on smear from needle biopsy.

if appropriate, prior to the procedure. Premedication is not usually required, the patient's anxiety normally being allayed by prior discussion. The procedure is ideally performed using bi-plane image intensification, but this is not often available in the UK and single plane intensification is quite acceptable. The patient is placed under the image intensifier in a prone or supine position depending upon the site of the lesion. A mark is then made on the skin under fluoroscopic control, in a position directly in line with the lesion. Local anaesthesia is injected down to the pleura. By moving the position of the arms, it is usually possible to project the lesion between the ribs and thereby obtain an unimpeded approach. Prior to its insertion, the needle is marked at the same distance from its tip as the lesion is measured radiographically to lie from the skin's surface. It is preferable to introduce the needle over, rather than under, a rib in order to avoid damage to intercostal vessels and nerves. After making a small incision in the skin, the needle is introduced vertically under fluoroscopic control in line with the lesion and central X-ray beam. It is advisable to ask the patient to suspend respiration as the needle passes through the pleura, followed by quiet respiration. The needle tip is then advanced, under fluoroscopic guidance directly to the lesion which it is often felt to enter. The position of the needle is confirmed by seeing the lesion move with the tip of the needle. For aspiration biopsies, the central stylet is removed and suction applied with a 10 ml syringe. The aspirating needle, attached to the syringe, is then withdrawn during continuous suction. A potential hazard is the introduction of air after removal of the stylet and before application of the syringe. This is avoided by instructing the patient not to breathe and placing a finger over the aspirating needle during the change-over. The performance of Tru-Cut needle biopsies follows the same approach, the needle tip being advanced to the proximal margin of the lesion prior to biopsy. Similarly, the needle screw assembly of the Rotex screw is inserted into the proximal portion of the lesion prior to advancement of the screw. The outer sheath is then extended over the screw before removal of the whole assembly.

The biopsy specimen is smeared on slides and rapidly fixed in 74% alcohol. Histological material may also be placed in formalin. Material may also be placed in sterile saline and broth for culture.

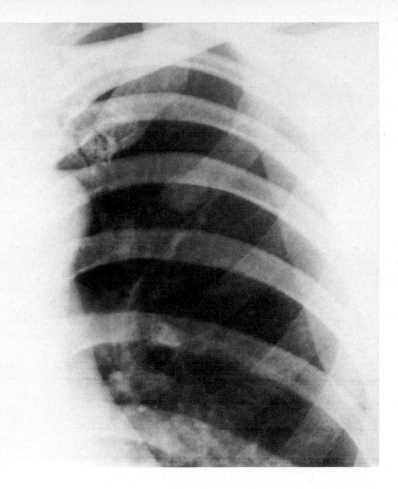

Fig. 14.6 One centimeter mass as an isolated finding on the chest radiograph. Metastasis from a renal carcinoma.

Radiographs are obtained immediately after the procedure and at 24 hours to check for a pneumothorax.

Complications

Pneumothorax is the commonest complication and occurs in 20–25% of patients, of which approximately one in six require intercostal tube drainage. The risk of a pneumothorax is higher in patients with emphysema and in the elderly. The radiologist undertaking lung biopsy must be able to deal with this complication. A rapidly developing pneumothorax is treated by inserting a No. 8 Teflon catheter with side holes, either at the site of biopsy or in the second anterior intercostal space on the affected side. The catheter assembly is attached to a Heimlich flutter valve to permit unidirectional air flow.

Haemoptysis is an infrequent complication and, although it is usually small, invariably frightens the patient. Massive pulmonary haemorrhage is extremely difficult to control and has been the major cause of death in those series where there are available mortality figures. It is most likely to occur with a cutting type needle. Treatment requires immediate bronchoscopy.

Air embolism should be prevented by a meticulous technique. The implantation of tumour cells along the needle track has provided much discussion but is extremely rare.

TRANSBRONCHIAL BIOPSY

The advent of fibre-optic bronchoscopy in the 1960s heralded a major advance in pulmonary medicine. Bidirectional tip flexion combined with a wide angle of vision permits precise guidance within the bronchial tree. A central 2 mm channel provides the opportunity for suction, the passage of a large variety of biopsy forceps and brushes, and the instillation of local anaesthetic and contrast agents. The instrument is best introduced transnasally under local anaesthesia

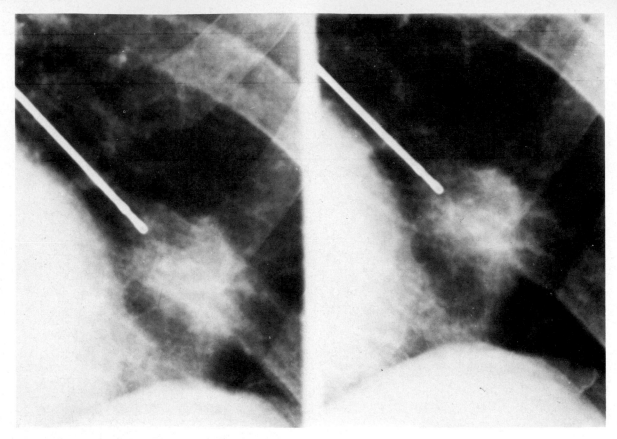

Fig. 14.7 Irregular mass—carcinoma—adjacent to heart. Unsuitable for percutaneous biopsy. Spot films obtained during bronchoscopic biopsy.

after some form of premedication. The procedure is well tolerated, remarkably safe, and may be performed on an out-patient basis. The small size of the instrument coupled with its flexibility allows visualization of the bronchial tree down to subsegmental level, which is a great advantage over the rigid bronchoscope. Whilst there are increasingly wide applications of the fibrescope, only its role in the diagnosis of localized and diffuse pulmonary disease is discussed here.

Localized disease

Localized disease in a juxtahilar position can be directly seen, and appropriate specimens obtained, without fluoroscopic control. Circumscribed peripheral opacities which are out of the direct visual range of the fibrescope may be biopsied by advancing biopsy forceps into the lesion under fluoroscopic control, after passage into the appropriate segmental bronchus

under direct vision. Nylon brushes are used in a similar fashion and specimens may be obtained for histological and cytological examination and for culture. The procedure is more time-consuming than percutaneous needle biopsy and diagnostic material is obtained from a smaller percentage of patients presenting with a peripheral pulmonary mass. However, a complete examination of the bronchial tree can be performed by this technique. Other advantages are the very low incidence of pneumothorax and the much better control of pulmonary haemorrhage. Which technique is used frequently depends upon the referring clinician's preference and is often biased by his own experience. The ideal is to have operators available who are experienced in both techniques, which can then be used in a complementary fashion. As a general rule, circumscribed lesions under 5 cm in diameter in the outer half of the lung are initially best aproached by the percutaneous method. More central, and ill-defined or cavitating lesions, are better approached via the fibrescope (Fig. 14.7).

Fig. 14.8 Sarcoidosis producing diffuse fine nodular shadowing. Diagnosis established by transbronchial biopsy.

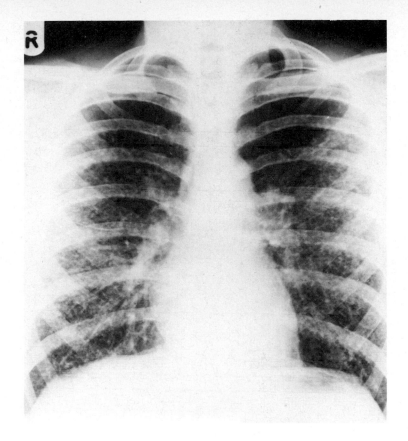

Diffuse disease

The ability to obtain representative, albeit small, histological samples in a high percentage of patients has been a major advance in the differential diagnosis of diffuse disease. Transbronchial biopsy is particularly valuable in the diagnosis of sarcoidosis, carcinomatosis, tuberculosis and opportunistic infections (Fig. 14.8). It is less useful in fibrosing alveolitis and drug-induced disease, where the distribution of histological change varies throughout the lung and the small samples obtained may be unrepresentative. If biopsy is necessary in these patients, it is often preferable to perform a trephine biopsy or an open biopsy via a limited thoracotomy.

REFERENCES

Gudbjerg C. E. (1957) Bronchiectasis: radiological diagnosis and prognosis after operative treatment. *Acta Radiol.*, (suppl) **143**.

Forrest J. V., Sagel S. S. & Onell G. H. (1976) Bronchography in patients with haemoptysis. *Amer. J. Roentgenol.* **126**, 597–600.

Siegelman S. S., Stitik F. P. & Sumner W. R. (1979) *Pulmonary System: Practical Approaches to Pulmonary Diagnosis.* Grune and Stratton, New York.

Trapnell D. H. & Gregg I. (1969) Some principles of interpretation of bronchograms. *Brit. J. Radiol.*, **42**, 125–31.

SECTION 4
THE GENITO-URINARY TRACT

The Urinary Tract

G. H. WHITEHOUSE

INTRAVENOUS UROGRAPHY

Indications

Intravenous urography is used in the investigation of a wide range of symptoms referable to the urinary tract at all ages, in determining the presence of urinary tract abnormalities in certain systemic diseases, in the investigation of renal failure, and in the assessment of abdominal trauma and of pelvic malignant disease. Kreel *et al.*, (1974) found that haematuria was the urinary symptom which was most likely to be associated with an abnormal intravenous urogram (IVU), while urographic abnormalities were found in 20% of patients who had abdominal pain other than renal colic.

The justification for performing urography in certain clinical situations has been questioned in recent years, bearing in mind that there is a definite morbidity and a small mortality associated with this investigation. For instance, it is now generally regarded that there is no need for an IVU in men with acute urinary retention or with symptoms of outflow tract obstruction who subsequently undergo prostatectomy, unless they have gross haematuria or a history of urinary disease.

The role of i.v. urography in hypertension, primarily to determine whether or not the patient has an underlying renal cause, is a more difficult problem. A change in patient management, due to the discovery of renal artery stenosis or unilateral renal disease which could account for the hypertension, is anticipated in only about 1% of hypertensive cases undergoing i.v. urography. In addition, there is a strong chance that the blood pressure will remain unchanged after the appropriate surgery. The IVU is an inaccurate method of determining the presence of renal artery stenosis. However, many clinicians share the views of Atkinson and Kellett (1974) that a small number of significant lesions are likely to be missed if i.v. urography is not performed in younger hypertensive patients, so that the IVU is considered to be a routine investigation in hypertension up to the age of 40 years.

There seems to be no indication for performing routine i.v. urography in women prior to hysterectomy for benign disease in the absence of urinary symptoms, or in asymptomatic cryptorchid patients.

Recurrent urinary tract infection is usually considered to be an indication for i.v. urography at all ages. Fair *et al.*, (1979) found urographic abnormalities in 5.5% of adult women with recurrent urinary infections but surgical intervention or a change in therapeutic approach was not required in any of these patients.

Contra-indications

Besides previous severe hypersensitivity reactions to contrast media, there are some other situations in which risks or disadvantages may outweigh the diagnostic benefits of i.v. urography.

1. Pregnancy. Irradiation to the fetus should be avoided whenever possible. Dilatation of the upper urinary tract, especially on the right, makes evaluation difficult and i.v. urography should preferably be postponed until four months after delivery, by which time there should be reversal of this effect.
2. Women of childbearing age in whom pregnancy is a possibility should have i.v. urography only within ten days of the start of the menstrual period, unless there is an overwhelming clinical indication.
3. Serious reactions to previous injections of contrast medium do not entirely preclude subsequent i.v. urography, although other imaging techniques such as ultrasonography and isotope studies should be used as an alternative whenever possible. If i.v. urography is considered essential, then steroid cover should be instituted before and after the investigation. An indwelling i.v. catheter is inserted, and resuscitation equipment must be at hand.
4. Diabetes mellitus associated with renal insufficiency is associated with a high incidence of supervening acute renal failure which may sometimes be irreversible or lead to a permanent exacerbation of renal damage. Intravenous urography should, therefore, be avoided whenever possible in this group of patients.
5. The urographic contrast medium may block the uptake of radio-isotopes of iodine which are used for the diagnosis and treatment of thyroid disease. Intra-venous urography should therefore be postponed in these cases.

Technique

Preparation It is advantageous to give a laxative prior to i.v. urography, except in the emergency situation. X-Prep liquid, which is a standard extract of senna, is generally satisfactory despite an incidence of abdominal colic, nausea and vomiting. A standard dose of X-Prep liquid (71 ml) is given on the evening before the examination, with no raw vegetables or fruit being consumed on the preceding day.

Dehydration was an important consideration when small amounts of contrast medium were routinely given to the patient, the aim being to enhance the concentration of the contrast medium in the pelvicalyceal system. The larger amounts of contrast media now injected, giving about 300 mg of iodine per kg body weight, means that effective fluid restriction for 24 hours or longer will produce a barely detectable increase in pyelographic density. Mere overnight fluid abstainence prior to i.v. urography produces no significant change in urine osmolality or opacification. It has been shown that even drinking large quantities of fluid just before the examination still produces an IVU of good diagnostic quality (Duré Smith, 1976).

Notwithstanding the insignificant effect of dehydration on the quality of the examination, it is reasonable to restrict the patient to nothing by mouth for 12 hours before i.v. urography. The empty stomach greatly reduces the chance of the patient vomiting as a reaction to the injection of contrast medium. Simplification of the instructions to the patient is another advantage of this practice.

There are some categories of patients in whom dehydration is definitely contra-indicated; namely infants, patients with renal failure, myelomatosis and diabetes mellitus. Reducing the obligatory water load in the impaired kidney leads to an exacerbation of the renal failure. Dehydration in cases of myelomatosis carries a risk of precipitating paraproteins in the kidney tubules, leading to acute renal failure. Diabetic patients, especially those with renal disease, are prone to develop acute renal failure after i.v. urography and fluid restriction is likely to exacerbate this complication.

It is important that the patient micturates as fully as possible immediately before the IVU. Residual urine dilutes the contrast medium within the bladder and thus impairs detail, as well as preventing a good mucosal coating by contrast medium on the post-micturition radiograph.

Preliminary Radiographs It is essential that the whole of the urinary tract, down to and including the symphysis pubis, is covered by the preliminary radiographs. A 35×43 cm radiograph satisfies this requirement in children and small adults. Two radiographs are often required routinely in adults to encompass all the urinary tract, a 35×43 cm film being used to include upwards from the lower border of the symphysis pubis with the exposure occurring during arrested expiration. The renal areas are then included on a 24×30 cm radiograph (30×40 cm size in larger patients) which is placed transversely with its lower border 2.5 cm below the iliac crests, with exposure again being made in arrested expiration. A low kV should be used to enhance soft tissue detail. The purpose of the preliminary radiograph is

1 to indicate correct radiographic positioning and exposure prior to contrast medium injection;
2 to demonstrate opacities which may lie within the uninary tract before they are obscured by contrast medium. If any opacities are shown to overlie the kidney, additional oblique views and/or a film in full inspiration will be required to demonstrate whether or not they lie within the urinary tract. Occasionally, a lateral radiograph is needed to this end;
3 to show whether or not obscuration of the kidneys by bowel gas or faeces necessitates tomography;
4 to visualize other abdominal organs and retroperitoneal structures, as well as delineating abdominal and pelvic mass lesions and abnormal fluid or gas collections.

It is important that the patient is in as relaxed a state as possible, which depends to a large extent on the attitude of the radiographer and the attending radiologist. There is good evidence that anxiety can influence to some extent the occurrence of reactions to contrast media. An anxious patient tends to swallow air, especially in the supine position, and the resultant bowel gas may obscure the urinary tract. Premedication is required in infants and small children. Gonad protection is applied in the male.

The contrast medium

The most commonly used urographic contrast media are excreted solely by glomerular filtration, although some tubular excretion occurs with the iodomides (Difiazio *et al*, 1978). The concentration of contrast medium in the glomerular filtrate is virtually identical to that in the plasma. The plasma level of contrast medium is itself dependent upon the dose given, the speed of injection, and the weight of the patient. The amount of contrast medium being filtered depends upon the glomerular filtration rate (GFR). Renal failure necessitates the use of a larger amount of contrast medium to offset the reduction in GFR. Larger amounts of contrast medium may be required in the elderly than in younger adults to compensate for the decrease in GFR which normally occurs in old age.

Apart from renal function, it is the amount of injected iodine which is mainly responsible for the quality of the IVU, although the particular molecular form of the contrast medium is also a factor. A dose of contrast medium which gives 300 mg of iodine per kg body weight (21G for a 70 kg person) is suitable for adults with normal renal function. Patients with renal failure require twice this standard amount of iodine.

Most of the water in the glomerular filtrate is resorbed in the proximal tubules, independent of the patient's state of hydration, along with various ions. It is the filtered contrast medium in the proximal convoluted tubules, and initially to some extent in the renal vascular spaces, which accounts for the nephrogram phase (Fig. 15.1). In summary, the maximum density of the nephrogram is dependent on the peak plasma level of contrast medium, glomerular filtration and absorption of water and sodium by the proximal tubule. The nephrographic density is independent of the degree of hydration or dehydration.

The final regulation of water content occurs in the distal convoluted tubule and collection tubules under the influence of antidiuretic hormone (ADH). It is at this site that dehydration, by causing an increase in circulatory ADH, affects the absorption of water.

The large osmotic effect of contrast media modifies the situation. A greater amount of obligatory water must be retained in the proximal tubular lumen following the filtration of contrast media, with this subsequent increase in volume being maintained throughout the tubule (Cattell *et al.*, 1967). Absorption of water from the distal tubule still occurs in the dehydrated state, with a consequent increase in concentration of contrast medium, but only to a slight extent with larger dose levels.

The sodium salts of urographic contrast media produce a higher concentration of iodine in the pelvicalyceal systems than the equivalent amounts of methylglucamine compounds. This is because methylglucamine salts are associated with a greater osmotic diuresis than their sodium counterparts. In theory this should lead to a greater distention of the pelvi-calyceal systems with methylglucamine agents, although this

Table 15.1 Commonly used urographic contrast media.

Proprietary name	Generic name		Iodine content mg/ml	Viscosity Cp at 37°C
Conray 420	Sodium iothalmate	70% w/v	420	5.4
Hypaque 65%	Meglumine diatrizoate Sodium diatrizoate	50% w/v 25% w/v	390	8.4
Urografin 370	Meglumine diatrizoate Sodium diatrizoate	52% w/v 8% w/v	370	8.5
Uromiro 380	Meglumine iodamide Sodium iodamide	70% W/v 10% w/v	380	10.7
Uromiro 420	Meglumine iodamide Sodium iodamide	41% w/v 39% w/v	420	10.3
Triosil 350	Sodium metrizoate Calcium metrizoate Magnesium metrizoate Meglumine metrizoate	60% w/v	350	3.4
Triosil 440	Sodium metrizoate Calcium metrizoate Magnesium metrizoate Meglumine metrizoate	75% w/v	440	6.6

is not in fact appreciable, while in practice there is better opacification of the pelvic-calyceal systems with sodium salts than with the equivalent methylglucamine salts for the same amount of injected iodine (Eyes *et al.*, 1981). There is, therefore, some advantage in using sodium salts.

Conray 420 has the advantage of having a high concentration of iodine in the form of a sodium salt, although the resulting high osmolality may result in some complications (see below). For an adult of normal build and good renal function, 50 ml of Conray 420 is a suitable standard dose, 80–100 ml being used when an optimal nephrotomogram is required or when abdominal compression cannot be applied to the patient. In cases of renal failure, 100 ml would be injected.

In the case of infants, methylglucamine salts are preferred to contrast media which contain sodium. A suitable regimen in neonates and infants is the injection of 2 ml of Conray 280 (methylglucamine iothalmate, 280 mg of iodine per ml) per kg body weight to a maximum of 20 ml. The recommended dose in children aged four to eight years is 20 ml of Conray 280, 40 ml being used in children aged eight to twelve years.

The contrast medium should be rapidly injected to achieve high plasma levels by a 'bolus' effect and a subsequent dense nephrogram phase, followed by an optimal urogram within 15 minutes with a prolonged peak urine concentration of contrast medium. An injection time of around half a minute should be readily achieved in most cases, although the contrast medium should be injected much slower in infants and small children—over a period of three minutes. A slower injection than normal should be used in the elderly and in those adults with a history of heart disease, to reduce the risk of inducing cardiac arrhythmias.

Radiographic procedure

The radiographic regimen may be varied to suit the particular clinical situation. The following is a routine sequence of radiographs (Fig. 15.1):

1 Nephrogram phase—a radiograph is taken immediately after the injection of contrast medium, when contrast density within the proximal renal tubules should be at its maximum;
2 Five minutes after injection—a radiograph of the renal area in full arrested inspiration. The cassette must be some 3 cm lower than for the previous renal area radiographs, to allow for descent of the kidneys.

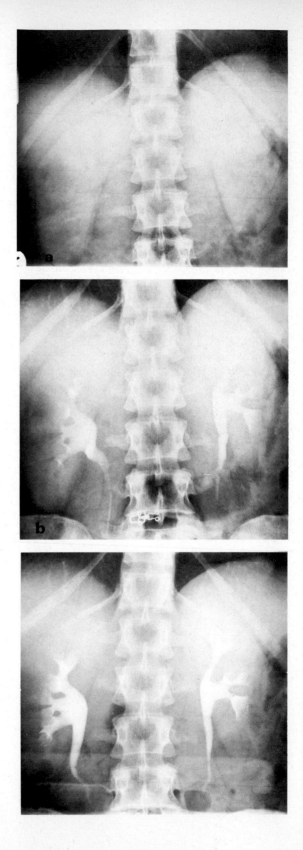

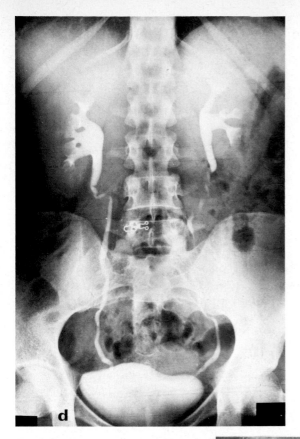

Contrast opacification of the urinary tract necessitates an increase in mA from previous values. The pelvi-calyceal systems are delineated by contrast medium at this stage.

Abdominal compression is then applied immediately after the 5 minute radiographs;

3. Fifteen minutes after injection—a further radiograph of the renal area. The pelvi-calyceal systems and proximal ureters should be well distended by contrast medium at this time;

4. A full length radiograph of the urinary tract (35 × 43 cm cassette) is taken at twenty minutes, immediately after the release of abdominal compression, with the aim of delineating the ureters and bladder.

5. Post micturition radiograph—this is taken immediately after the patient has emptied his bladder. The radiograph is of the bladder area (18 × 24 cm), the X-ray tube being angled 15° caudad and centred 2.5 cm below the anterior superior iliac spines.

Additional radiographs

1. It may be appropriate to take oblique radiographs at about 15 min, when abdominal compression has been applied to the patient, in order to demonstrate possible calyceal stem compression or to better delineate the renal outline.

2. A coned radiograph of the opacified bladder may be required ten minutes or so after the full length

Fig. 15.1 Phases of the standard IV
(a) Nephrogram
(b) 5 minute radiograph.
(c) 15 minute radiograph with abdominal compression.
(d) Full length radiograph at 20 minutes, with release of compression.
(e) Post-micturation radiograph of bladder.

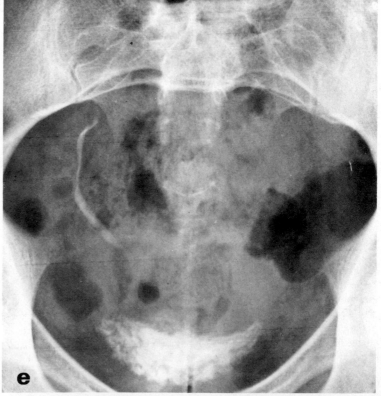

radiograph of the IVU. The radiographic positioning is usually the same as for the routine post-micturition film of the bladder area. Prostatic impingement on the bladder base may be better delineated by angling the X-ray tube 30° cephalad and centring 5 cm below the top of the symphysis pubis.

3. A full length abdominal radiograph with the patient lying prone sometimes improves the contrast delineation of the pelvi-ureteric junctions and ureters. The lower ends of the ureters are often best shown in the prone position in cases of ileal conduit.

4. A full length radiograph with the patient standing erect causes a normal but mainly extrarenal 'baggy' renal pelvis to deflate, thus distinguishing this entity from mild hydronephrosis. The renal pelvis of the ptotic kidney may become distended due to ureteric kinking in the erect position.

The limited IVU The regimen described above is recommended for all patients on their initial IVU. While it is sometimes argued that some of the radiographs in the series are unnecessary there is the chance that limiting the number of radiographs in the initial IVU will cause the overlooking of significant pathology. However, follow-up IVU's may give the required information on fewer radiographs, only a preliminary radiograph and a full length radiograph at 10 minutes after contrast injection being necessary in many cases.

Tomography Some X-ray departments routinely use tomography in i.v. urography. This is probably an overembellishment, but the presence of renal failure (see below) is a definite indication for tomography. In other instances, tomography is of assistance in i.v. urography when the renal outlines or calyceal detail are obscured by overlying bowel contents. Tomography is performed in the nephrogram phase immediately after contrast injection to show renal outlines, the presence of renal space-occupying lesions, or the opacified adrenal glands. A larger than usual dose of contrast medium is often injected prior to nephrotomography. Calyceal detail, as well as renal outlines, are usually well shown on tomography with abdominal compression 10 minutes after contrast injection.

A control tomographic cut should be taken before the injection of contrast medium. It is a widely held belief that flexing the knees, thus reducing the lumbar lordosis, will cause the long axes of the kidneys to lie at a reduced angle of inclination to the tomographic plane. This concept does not hold in practice, but elevating the chest and shoulders on pads may help to this end. The optimal level of tomographic cut depends on the A–P diameter of the abdomen at the level of the lower costal margin, and lies between 8 and 12 cm. Duré Smith and McArdle (1972) recommend a 40° arc for nephrotomography and a 25° angle for tomography of the pyelogram phase, with a minimum of three cuts being taken at the optimal level and at 2 cm above and below this level. Some consider zonography, which uses a small angle of swing to give a thick tomographic cut, to be particularly suitable for showing the kidneys. The 25° swing, however, gives a thickness of 1.5 cm in sharp focus and is considered to be superior to zonography in showing calyceal deformity and eliminating bowel shadow. A multilayer cassette is routinely used in renal tomography.

Abdominal compression

The purpose of abdominal compression is to obstruct the ureters, allowing fuller distention and delineation of the pelvi-calyceal systems, with more consistent opacification of the ureters immediately following release of compression. Small sinuses and tracts arising from the calyces are better shown, the degree of pelvi-calyceal distention itself being of pathological significance in some cases. The most effective method of compression employs an inflatable balloon supported by a rigid plastic board which is strapped to the patient by a belt (Fig. 15.2). The balloon is

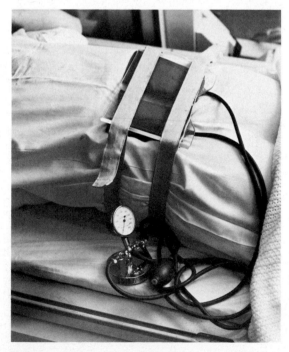

Fig. 15.2 Compression device used in i.v. urography. Two inflatable balloons lie on a plastic board and are maintained in position by two belts.

positioned midway between the anterior superior iliac spines immediately before the 5 minute radiograph, after which the straps are tightened and the balloon is inflated by a sphygmomanometer device.

For compression to be effective, it is necessary to cause tolerable discomfort. The compression is usually well-tolerated for the 15 minutes or so during which it is applied, but may occasionally result in vasovagal symptoms which are soon alleviated by releasing the compression and placing the patient in the head down position. Abdominal compression is contra-indicated following recent abdominal trauma or surgery, in cases of ureteric colic and other urinary tract obstruction, abdominal pain and tenderness, and in the presence of an abdominal mass or aortic aneurysm. There is evidence that the compression reduces the GFR, so it is advisable to avoid abdominal compression in patients with myelomatosis or renal failure. The lack of abdominal compression may be compensated by increasing the standard dose of contrast medium, for instance using 80—100 ml of Conray 420.

Modifications of basic technique

Renal failure

There must be no fluid restriction before i.v. urography is performed on patients in renal failure. Larger amounts of contrast medium are given compared to those with normal renal function and tomography is essential (Saxton, 1969). A satisfactory dose of contrast medium is one which provided 600 mg of iodine per kg body weight by a bolus injection. This amount of iodine is provided by 100 ml of Conray 420 or 100–115 ml of Urografin 370 in a 70 kg adult patient. Methylglucamine salts are often preferred to contrast media which are sodium salts in patients who have hypertension or cardiac disease, but the additional sodium load seems to have no practical importance in the absence of these complications. Tomography is routinely performed immediately after contrast injection and again 10 minutes later. In addition to tomograms, routine radiographs are taken before contrast injection and 10, 20, 30 and 60 minutes later (Sherwood et al., 1974). Further radiographs, up to 24 hours later, may be necessary to exclude urinary obstruction.

The renal size and configuration and the pelvicalyceal systems are not delineated with blood urea levels in excess of 60 mmol/l.

The risk of i.v. urography causing a further diminution of renal function is discussed under 'Complications' on p. 223.

Contrast medium is sometimes excreted into the biliary tract, and occasionally direct into the small intestine, when there is severe renal failure. This extrarenal excretion is also known to occur in the presence of acute unilateral ureteric obstruction, when it is probably related to prolonged high plasma levels of contrast medium (Sokoloff & Talner, 1973).

Non-ionic contrast media should, by having a lower osmolality than conventional contrast agents, theoretically produce better contrast density within the urinary tract in advanced renal failure. Experimental evidence suggests this is unlikely to be the case (Webb et al., 1978).

It has been claimed that dialysis prior to i.v. urography should improve the urinary concentration of contrast medium by decreasing the osmotic load on the kidneys. The general experience, however, seems to be that at best this is an inconsistent finding, enhanced contrast opacification sometimes occurring after prolonged dialysis (Becker, 1973).

Urinary obstruction

A high dose of contrast medium is indicated in cases of significant hydronephrosis. Delay in the excretion of contrast medium necessitates radiographs being taken up to 24 hours, with tomography when there is marked impairment of contrast excretion. A radiograph in the prone position is often useful, provided sufficient contrast medium has accumulated in the calyces (Saxton, 1969). As described above, a full length erect radiograph may be useful in distinguishing minor degrees of hydronephrosis. If there is still some doubt as to the diagnosis, or if the patient gives a history of loin pain after the ingestion of large amounts of fluid, a diuretic may be given to accentuate and demonstrate a low grade hydronephrosis. Frusemide, 20 mg intravenously, is given after a further injection of 50 ml Conray 420 and radiographs are taken at five minute intervals until the kidneys are 'washed out' or there is overt pelvicalyceal distention.

Acute obstruction

In the presence of ureteric colic, a preliminary radiograph is followed by a full length radiograph at 15 minutes after the injection of a fairly large amount of contrast medium (60 ml Conray 420). Suspicion of ureteric obstruction at this time probably necessitates a series of delayed radiographs up to 24 hours, especially if there is a radiolucent calculus. Very large doses of contrast medium seem to increase the risk of spontaneous peripelvic extravasation on the same side as the acute ureteric obstruction. While the vast majority of cases in which this occurs are unharmed

(Hale & Whitehouse, 1970), peripelvic cysts and abscesses have resulted on occasion (Cooke & Bartacz, 1974). Abdominal compression is not applied as it may precipitate this phenomenon.

Hypertension

The detection of renal artery stenosis and the pitfalls of i.v. urography in establishing this diagnosis are well recognized by radiologists (Saxton, 1969; Talner, 1981). With the standard doses of contrast medium that are now routinely employed, it is probably unnecessary to take radiographs every minute between the nephrogram and five minute radiographs. Intravenous frusemide was once in vogue to differentiate between normal and ischaemic kidneys on i.v. urography, but has been virtually abandoned because of the inconsistent results.

Pregnancy

When i.v. urography is deemed essential in advanced pregnancy, the investigation should consist of only two radiographs: a preliminary full length film and a full length erect film 25–30 minutes after the injection of the usual amount of contrast medium, without abdominal compression. This late radiograph allows time for the pelvi-calyceal system to be opacified, while the erect position minimizes the physiological distention of the pelvi-calyceal systems and ureters which is associated with pregnancy.

After renal transplantation

Intravenous urography is routinely performed at one to four weeks after transplant surgery but may be indicated sooner if there is a suspicion of ureteral obstruction, extravasation of urine, retroperitoneal haemorrhage, or lymphocele. Ultrasonography often gives useful information in these complications, and isotope studies are very helpful in assessing the cause of impaired function.

The standard amount of contrast medium is used, although the volume is doubled in cases of impaired renal function. A preliminary radiograph is taken in the right posterior oblique position if the renal transplant is on the right side, and a left posterior oblique for a left sided kidney. Radiographs are taken immediately after contrast injection and at 5, 10 and 30 minutes, and then after micturition. Tomography may well be required, and a pre-injection tomographic cut is therefore mandatory. The optimal levels are 13–16 cm above the table top, with a 40° angle of tube swing.

Complications

Ansell (1976) has categorized reactions to intravenous contrast media as minor, intermediate and severe.

Minor reactions (Witten *et al.*, 1973; Davies *et al.*, 1975) Some 60% of patients who undergo i.v. urography complain of trivial and transient symptoms, including a feeling of heat which is either generalized or mainly in the throat, tinnitus, a sensation of disorientation, tingling, abdominal sensations and a metallic taste. There are sometimes unpleasant perineal sensations which include a desire to empty the bladder or a spurious sensation of spontaneous micturition. The generalized sensation of warmth increases with the amount of injected contrast medium and with the speed of injection. Nausea is present in 5–8% of cases, with vomiting in a third of these patients.

Arm pain may be limited to the injection site or extends up the arm. Pain at the injection site is associated with the perivenous injection of contrast medium, often not clinically apparent, and is particularly severe following extravasation of Conray 420 or other agents containing a high concentration of sodium salts. Post-injection radiographs show stasis of contrast medium within the vein when there is pain up the arm. This upper arm pain also tends to be more severe with contrast media which have a high sodium concentration, such as Conray 420 and Triosil 440, than with other urographic agents, but is usually rapidly relieved by elevating the arm.

Intermediate reactions Syncope is uncommon, occurring either immediately after the injection of contrast medium or following abdominal compression. The Trendelenberg position and relief of compression relieves the vasovagal attack. It has been claimed that atropine relieves vasovagal attacks and reduces their incidence. Vomiting is sometimes of distressing severity, occasionally precedes a severe reaction, and may be relieved by metoclopramide.

Severe abdominal pain sometimes occurs in anaphylactoid reactions, but in most cases is associated with hypotensive collapse.

Allergic reactions occur in less than 2% of cases. Urticaria is the commonest form, but angioneurotic oedema and bronchospasm are other and more serious manifestations. Sneezing and rhinitis are other minor effects. Most cases have a clinical history suggestive of a hypersensitivity state.

Routine antihistamine prophylaxis, even in patients with an allergic history, has no significant benefit in terms of reducing the incidence and severity of allergic reactions to urographic agents. Moreover, intravenous antihistamines themselves sometimes produce severe allergic reactions. However, it seems justifiable to give routinely a prophylactic antihistamine, such as chlorpheniramine maleate (Piriton) 10 mg i.v., to patients who have a history of previous allergic reaction to contrast media. Antihistamines should not be mixed with the contrast media as they may be rendered therapeutically useless and form precipitates. Steroid prophylaxis, 150 ml prednisolone during the 18 hours preceeding the IVU and 75 mg over the succeeding 12 hours, has been suggested in those who have had a previous severe anaphylactoid reaction to contrast medium (Zweiman & Hildreth, 1974).

There is no doubt that intravenous antihistamines, 10 mg of chlorpheniramine maleate being most widely used, are of value in the treatment of allergic reactions induced by contrast media. This is sufficient to treat acute skin reactions. In cases of bronchospasm and angioneurotic oedema, oxygen plus 100–200 mg of hydrocortisone hemisuccinate i.v. and 0.5 ml of 1:1000 adrenaline are also given as first line treatment. Aminophylline, 0.25G in 10 ml slowly i.v., may also be given for severe bronchospasm. Laryngotomy or tracheotomy may be required to maintain the airway in severe laryngeal oedema.

Severe reactions Death occurs as a direct result of i.v. urography in one in 40 000 to 50 000 cases. The majority of deaths are in patients over the age of 50 years.

Hypotension, when it occurs as a severe reaction, is usually profound and is often associated with transient loss of consciousness and occasionally incontinence. The possibility of airway obstruction requires urgent attention. The patient is often clinically shocked, usually within a few minutes of contrast medium injection. Oxygen and i.v. steroids are mandatory. A vasopressor agent and correction of hypovolaemia are sometimes additional requirements. Steroids and antihistamines provide no protective benefit when repeat urography is subsequently performed, the chance of hypotension occurring again being no more than in first-time urograms. A persistently dense nephrogram with a reduction in renal size and impaired pelvi-calyceal opacification is found on radiography during the hypotensive phase.

Cardiac arrest and arrhythmias are other severe reactions to contrast agents, being especially likely to occur in older patients and those with a previous history of cardiac disease, and are attributable to the direct cardiotoxic effects of contrast media. Pulmonary oedema, a rare complication of intravascular contrast media, is most likely to be precipitated by the cardiotoxic effect in patients who are in insipient cardiac failure. The high sodium load imposed by contrast media such as Conray 420 is possibly a predisposing factor and it is sometimes considered

appropriate to use a methylglucamine salt for i.v. urography in patients with cardiac failure.

Rigors occasionally occur after the administration of i.v. contrast agents, usually when large doses of methylglucamine salts are used in patients over the age of 50 years (Ansell, 1976).

Convulsions are not common but occasionally occur with i.v. urography in patients with an epileptic tendency. Convulsions are sometimes secondary to hypotensive collapse or cardiac arrest.

It must be emphasized that pretesting with a small amount of contrast medium is a useless practice which does not give a prediction of severe adverse effects. The false sense of security engendered by negative pretesting is itself a hazard.

Salivary gland enlargement A small concentration of inorganic iodide is regularly found in contrast media. *In vivo* de-iodination occurs after i.v. injection with the production of further iodide. The salivary glands concentrate and excrete this inorganic iodide. Accumulation and excretion of iodide by the salivary glands is especially pronounced in renal failure and it is in this situation that painful swelling, or 'iodine mumps' is especially prone to occur (Talner *et al.*, 1973).

Electrocardiographic abnormalities Ischaemic changes, bundle branch block, atrial and ventricular ectopics and ventricular tachycardia sometimes occur after the i.v. injection of a contrast medium (Berg *et al.*, 1973; Stadalnik *et al.*, 1974). These ECG changes may be associated with ischaemic chest pain and are particularly likely to occur in the older age group, especially when there is a clinical history of myocardial ischaemia. These groups of patients should have a slower than usual injection of contrast medium.

Renal failure and i.v. urography Dehydration prior to i.v. urography is, as previously discussed, likely to exacerbate pre-existing renal failure. However, good hydration has failed to have a protective effect in many patients who have developed acute or chronic renal failure following urography. These patients develop a substantial rise in serum creatinine over the week following i.v. urography, accompanied by a transient oliguria in the majority. While baseline renal function is restored in most cases, some patients have a permanent deterioration. Half of the reported cases of acute renal failure after i.v. urography have occurred in diabetics with pre-existing renal insufficiency. Elderly patients in renal failure are also more at risk. A particularly large dose of contrast media (more than 600 mg/kg body weight) and repeated contrast procedures over a short period of time are additional predispositions in other patients. The likely explanation is that depression in renal blood flow due to the contrast medium results in a further depression of glomerular filtration in the already compromised kidney, particularly in those patients who have grossly diseased renal vessels. Recent reviews of this effect include Older *et al.*, (1980) and Webb *et al.*, (1981).

Relation to other imaging techniques

Inadequate delineation of the pelvi-calyceal system and ureter on i.v. urography is widely regarded as an indication for retrograde pyelo-ureterography. Ultrasonography is helpful in the detection of hydronephrosis in the non-opacified kidney and may precede antegrade pyelography, rather than retrograde studies, in these cases.

Renal mass lesions demonstrated by i.v. urography are further investigated by ultrasonography. Depending on the clinical, urographic and ultrasonographic features, renal cyst punctures or angiography are the next procedures performed to determine whether the mass is a cyst or a tumour.

Ultrasonography (Scheible & Talner, 1979)   In addition to demonstrating a hydronephrosis and helping to determine if a renal mass is a cyst or a tumour, ultrasonography may be used in the assessment of renal size and also in localization prior to percutaneous biopsy. Urinary tract obstruction or polycystic disease may be excluded by ultrasound in renal failure. Retroperitoneal extrarenal masses and perirenal fluid collections are amenable to ultrasonographic assessment. The presence of rejection as well as other complications of renal transplantation such as fluid collections and ureteric obstruction, may be demonstrated by ultrasound. The staging of bladder tumours is possible by ultrasonography and the modality shows promise in the assessment of the prostate.

Ultrasonography may, within limitations, provide an alternative to i.v. urography for demonstrating structural renal abnormalities during pregnancy and in patients who are allergic to contrast media.

Isotope studies (Maisey, 1980)   The demonstration of anatomy using radionuclide imaging does not match the quality obtained with i.v. urography. Tc^{99m} labelled radionuclides demonstrate renal mass lesions as 'cold' areas. This is usually of little practical importance, even as an alternative to i.v. urography in patients who are allergic to contrast media, because ultrasonography is likely to give more information of a morphological nature. However, isotope scanning is often more sensitive than ultrasonography in detecting small solid renal tumours. Good nephrotomography usually determines normal variants in renal format, namely 'pseudotumours' which are sometimes mistaken on i.v. urography for pathological renal masses, but isotope scanning is occasionally required to establish that a 'pseudotumour' consists of normal functioning renal tissue. An accurate assessment of the extent of renal damage from trauma is possible by isotope scanning.

Dynamic isotope studies using Tc^{99m} DTPA give an accurate indication of renal blood flow and glomerular filtration, providing a better indication of renal function than is obtained from i.v. urography.

Computed tomography (CT)   (Davidson, 1980) CT scanning, even with contrast enhancement, often produces no more information concerning renal disease than is obtainable from simpler, less expensive and more readily available techniques such as i.v. urography and ultrasonography. CT Scanning is, however, very helpful in the evaluation of extrarenal retroperitoneal mass lesions.

REFERENCES

Ansell G. (1976) *Complications in Diagnostic Radiology*. Blackwell Scientific Publications, Oxford and London.

Atkinson A. B. & Kellett R. J. (1974) Value of intravenous urography in investigating hypertension. *J. roy Coll. Phys.*, **8**, 175–8.

Becker J. A. (1973) Before and after dialysis urography. *Radiology* **109**, 271–5.

Benness G. T. (1970) Urographic contrast agents. A comparison of sodium and methylglucamine salts. *Clin. Radiol.*, **21**, 150–6.

Berg G. R., Hutter A. M. & Pfister R. C. (1973) Electrocardiographic abnormalities associated with intravenous urology. *New Engl. J. Med.*, **289**, 87–8.

Cattell W. R., Fry I. K., Spencer A. G. & Purkiss P. (1967) Excretion urography 1. Factors determining excretion of Hypaque. *Brit. J. Radiol.*, **40**, 561–70.

Cooke G. M. & Bantuvz J. P. (1974) Spontaneous extravasation of contrast medium during intravenous urography. *Clin. Radiol.*, **25**, 87–93.

Davidson A. J. (1980) In *Uroradiology*. (Ed. Sherwood T.), Blackwell Scientific Publications, Oxford.

Davies P., Roberts M. B. & Roylance J. (1975) Acute reactions to urographic contrast media. *Brit. med. J.* **ii**, 434–7.

Difazio L. T., Singhvi S. M., Heald A. F., McKinstry D. N., Brosman S. A., Gillenwater J. Y. & Williard D. A. (1978) Pharmokinetics of iodamide in normal subjects and in patients with renal impairment. *J. Clin. Pharmacol.*, **18**, 35–41.

Dure Smith P. & McArdle G. H. (1972) Tomography during excretory urography. Technical aspects. *Brit. J. Radiol.*, **45**, 896–901.

Dure Smith P. (1976) Fluid restriction before excretory urography. *Radiology*, **118**, 478–9.

Eyes B. E., Evans A. F. & Whitehouse G. H. (1981) A comparative trial of two urographic contrast media—Conray 420 and Urografin 370. *Australasian Radiol.*, **25**, 150–6.

Fair W. R., McClennan B. L. & Jost P. G. (1979) Are exretory urograms necessary in evaluating women with urinary tract infections? *J. Urol.*, **121**, 313–15.

Hale J. E. & Whitehouse G. H. (1970) Spontaneous extravasation of urine during emergency intravenous pyelography. *Brit. J. Surg.*, **57**, 302–6.

Kreel L., Elton A., Habershon R., Mason A. M. S. & Meade T. W. (1974) Use of intravenous urography. *Brit. med. J.*, **4**, 31–3.

Maisey M. (1980) *Nuclear Medicine*. A clinical introduction. Update Books, London.

Older R. A., Korobkin M., Cleeve D. M., Schaaf R. & Thompson W. (1980) Contrast induced acute renal failure. *Amer. J. Roentgenol.*, **134**, 339–42.

Saxton H. M. (1969) Urography. *Brit. J. Radiol.*, **42**, 321–45.

Scheible W. & Talner L. B. (1979) Gray scale ultrasound and the genitourinary tract: a review of clinical applications. *Radiol. Clin. N. Amer.*, **17**, 281–300.

Sherwood T., Doyle F. H., Boulton-Jones M., Joekes A. M., Peters D. K. & Sissons P. (1974) The intravenous urogram in acute renal failure. *Brit. J. Radiol.*, **47**, 368–72.

Sokoloff J. & Talner L. B. (1973) The heterotopic excretion of sodium iothalamate. *Brit. J. Radiol.*, **46**, 571–7.

Stadalnik R., Davies R., Vera Z., Hilliard G. & Da Silva O. (1974) Ventricular tachycardia during intravenous urography. *J. Amer. med. Ass.*, **229**, 686–7.

Talner L. B., Coel M. N. & Lang J. H. (1973) Salivary secretion of iodine after urography. *Radiology*, **106**, 263–8.

Talner L. B. (1981) In *Uroradiology*. (Ed. Sherwood T.), Blackwell Scientific Publications, Oxford.

Webb J. A. W., Reznek R. H., Cattell W. R. & Fry I. K. (1981) Renal function after high dose urography in patients with renal failure. *Brit. J. Radiol.*, **54**, 479–83.

Witten D. M., Hirsch F. D. & Hartman G. W. (1973) Acute reactions to urographic contrast medium. *Amer. J. Roentgenol.*, **119**, 832–40.

Zweiman B. & Hildreth E. A. (1974) An approach to contrast studies in reactive humans. *J. Allergy clin. Immunol.*, **53**, 97–103.

RETROGRADE PYELOURETEROGRAPHY

Indications

Retrograde contrast delineation of the pelvi-calyceal system and ureter is performed when insufficient information has been obtained from i.v. urography. The present practice of injecting large quantities of urographic contrast media, and to some extent the ready application of tomography, has resulted in a decline in the number of retrograde pyelo-ureterograms performed in recent years. The investigation still has an application in the evaluation of non-functioning kidneys and questionable abnormalities seen on i.v. urography. Filling defects, obstructive lesions and fistulae in the ureter may be inadequately shown on i.v. urography and optimal delineation is then sometimes obtained by retrograde contrast studies.

Contra-indications

Provided pyelorenal intravasation or prolonged stasis of contrast medium in the renal pelvis is avoided, the risks of systemic absorption are very slight. However, hypersensitivity to contrast medium should be regarded as a relative contra-indication.

The retrograde catheterization of ureters is not possible in cases of ureteric diversion.

Technique

There are two methods of performing retrograde pyelo-ureterography.

1. A catheter is inserted into the ureter so that its tip reaches, if possible, the renal pelvis. Catheter placement is performed in the operating theatre at the time of cystoscopy. A 5 French gauge radio-opaque catheter is used, with a blunt end which is unlikely to traumatize the ureter. While a 5 gauge is suitable in most cases, difficult insertion may necessitate the use of a 4 French gauge catheter. The catheter should be gently positioned under image intensifier control, thus ensuring satisfactory placement and the prevention of ureteric spasm and perforation. The patient is then taken to the X-ray Department for contrast injection. Unfortunately, there is a risk that the catheter may slip out of the ureter during this transference. The opportunity is taken to collect a sample of urine via the ureteric catheter for culture and analysis. The initial catheter position having been checked, the injection of contrast medium is made under fluoroscopic control (Fig. 15.3).

It is advantageous to employ a slightly head down position to obtain better pelvi-calyceal filling. The investigation is performed under sterile con-

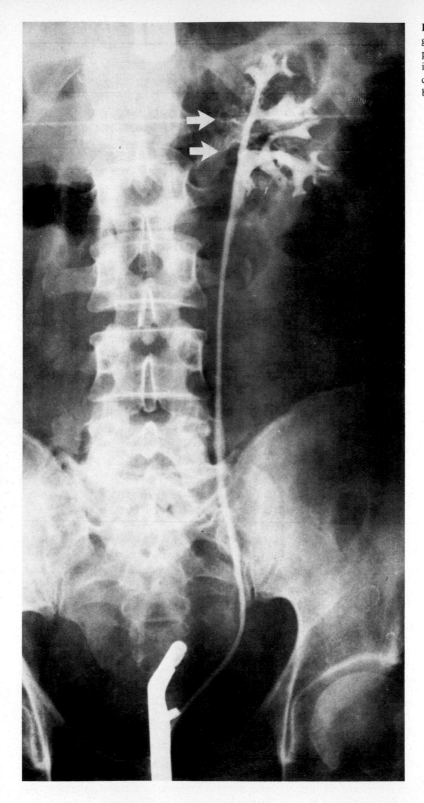

Fig. 15.3 Retrograde pyelo-uretero-gram. The catheter tip lies in the renal pelvis. Extravasated contrast medium is seen adjacent to the renal pelvis and calyces and there is also pyelolymphatic backflow (arrows).

ditions. The contrast media used are fairly dilute, for instance Urografin 150, so that small filling defects such as non-opaque calculi are not completely obscured during injection. The contrast medium, having been warmed to body temperature, is usually injected from a syringe. Air bubbles should be removed from the system. The injection should be slow, with as little applied pressure as possible. Usually 5–10 ml of contrast medium are required to delineate the pelvi-calyceal system. A modification is to infuse the contrast medium under gravity from a bottle which is elevated no more than 50 cm above the level of the kidney. Radiographs are taken to show the pelvi-calyceal system in the A–P and oblique positions with elevation of the contralateral side. After inspection of these radiographs, the catheter is then gently withdrawn some 5 cm into the ureter and the injection is continued in order to delineate the ureter. Spot radiographs are taken during injection, a 35 × 35 cm radiograph split into three being suitable, with further withdrawal of the catheter often being necessary. A disadvantage of the technique is the inconsistant demonstration of ureteric detail. Movement of the patient into the prone position may result in better delineation of the ureter. In the presence of ureteric obstruction, as much contrast medium as possible is aspirated before withdrawal of the catheter. A radiograph is then taken after withdrawal of the catheter from the ureter to show the presence of any hold-up.

2. The second method consists of the impaction of the end of an olivary tipped catheter (Kingston *et al.*, 1977) or the balloon of a Swan–Ganz catheter (Clark, 1974) into the ureteric orifice at the time of cystoscopy. The investigation may be performed in the operating theatre or in the X-ray department. The injection of 10 or 20 ml of contrast medium under fluoroscopic control results in consistent delineation of the ureter as well as the pelvicalyceal system. Movement of the patient is less likely to cause dislodgement than in the case of ureteric catheterization, Over-distention of the drainage system should be avoided, otherwise flank pain or calyceal rupture will result (Fig. 15.3).

Variations of basic technique

Ulmsten and Drehl (1975) have described the investigation of ureteric function by means of a multichannel retrograde catheter which enables intralumenal pressures to be recorded simultaneously at three levels in the ureters, Ureteropyelography is also performed via the catheter. Using the technique of inserting a button headed catheter in or just beyond the ureteric orifice, Christiansen (1970) has described a double contrast technique to show radiolucent filling defects within the renal pelvis. A total of 5 ml of Diodone 60% and 30–60 ml of carbon dioxide are used, the patient being rotated into various positions to distribute the contrast medium.

Complications

A retrograde catheter which is too rigid may damage the wall of the ureter and pelvis, while a very soft catheter may coil up on itself and even form a knot on withdrawal. Perforation of the ureter has caused retroperitoneal infection (Howards & Harrison, 1973). Acute renal failure has rarely been reported after retrograde pyelography (Alfrey *et al.*, 1967).

Urinary tract infection may occur as a result of the investigation, especially in cases of ureteric obstruction. A hydronephrosis may be converted into a pyonephrosis, especially if aspiration is not performed before withdrawal of the catheter. Prophylactic antibiotics are sometimes routinely given before retrograde pyeloureterography, although this is not a universal practice. Pre-existing urinary infection should certainly be eliminated before undertaking the investigation. It would seem reasonable to give antibiotics when ureteric obstruction is encountered or when there has been mural perforation by the catheter. Neomycin used to be routinely added to the contrast medium, but this is an invalid and dangerous practice.

Relation of other imaging techniques

Nowadays, antegrade pyelography is often preferred to the retrograde route in the further investigation of ureteric obstruction which has previously been demonstrated by i.v. urography or ultrasonography.

REFERENCES

Alfrey A. C., Rottshafer O. W. & Hutt M. P. (1967) Acute renal failure following retrograde pyelography. *Arch. intern. Med.*, 119, 214–17.

Clark P. (1974) Retrograde ureterography. *Proc. roy. Soc. Med.*, 67, 1207–10.

Christiansen J. (1970) Retrograde pyelography with double contrast. *Acta Chir. Scand.*, 136, 435–9.

Howards S. S. & Harrison J. H. (1973) Retroperitoneal phlegmon: a fatal complication of retrograde pyelography. *J. Urol.,* **109**, 92–3.

Kingston R. D., Shah K. J. & Dawson–Edwards P. (1977) Ascending uretero-pyelography in renal failure. *Clin. Radiol.,* **28**, 483–9.

Ulmsten U. & Diehl J. (1975) Investigation of ureteric function with simultaneous intraureteric pressure recordings and ureteropyelography. *Radiology,* **17**, 283–9.

ANTEGRADE PYELOGRAPHY

Antegrade pyelography is the direct percutaneous injection of contrast medium into the pelvi-calyceal system.

Indications

The combination of inadequate information from i.v. urography together with a failed retrograde pyelogram provide a prime indication for antegrade pyelography. However, antegrade pyelography may be used in preference to retrograde pyelo-ureterography, especially in obstructive urinary tract problems, to avoid the hazard of infection from retrograde studies (Sherwood & Stevenson, 1972). Another indication is where ureteric implantation into an ileal loop or the sigmoid colon makes it impossible to perform retrograde studies. The technique may also be used to define a ureteric fistula after radical cystectomy, uretero-sigmoidostomy and hysterectomy (Saafelt, 1976). Antegrade pyelography also provides a means of performing urodynamic studies on the ureter and is used to give guidance for subsequent nephrostomy and guided catheter procedures (Pfister & Newhouse, 1979).

Contra-indications

There is a reluctance to perform antegrade pyelography on both kidneys at the same sitting or where there is a single functioning kidney. Hypertension and a bleeding tendency are contra-indications.

Technique

Antegrade pyelography is performed under local anaesthesia, although children require sedation. An i.v. urogram is obtained if possible, but often the patient selected for antegrade pyelography has a poor or absent i.v. pyelogram. Fortunately, it is almost always possible to see the renal outline on a preliminary plain radiograph. The patient lies in the prone position. A metallic marker is placed under fluoroscopic control on the proposed puncture site in relation to the bony landmarks of ribs and vertebrae. Ultrasonography is also useful in providing guidance. The skin and subcutaneous tissues at the marked site are infiltrated with 1% lignocaine. A 15 cm long 20 gauge lumbar puncture needle is attached to a syringe containing a small amount of local anaesthetic for further infiltration. In the majority of cases the puncture site will lie 1–2 cm below the twelfth rib in the midclavicular line. The needle is directed towards a calyx, rather than to the renal pelvis, because the renal parenchyma provides a better seal around the needle track than the thin walled renal pelvis. A peripheral point of entry makes the inadvertant puncture of a vessel less likely.

The needle is advanced through the loin in a vertical direction, under fluoroscopic control, with continuous injection of lignocaine. There will be a characteristic 'give' as the needle tip enters the collecting system, some 7–8 cm from the surface in an adult and 2–3 cm deep in an infant. Failure to aspirate urine at the appropriate depth necessitates retraction of the needle and readvancement in a slightly different direction until there is placement of the needle tip into the collecting system. The correctly positioned needle is then connected to a flexible extension tubing which is taped to the patient's back. If desired, the hydrostatic resting pressure may be measured at this stage using a water manometer connected to the extension tubing. A urine sample is obtained for appropriate cytological, chemical and bacteriological studies. Contrast medium, for example Conray 280 or Urografin 290, is carefully and slowly injected through the needle under fluoroscopic control. In the obstructed system, no more contrast medium should be injected than the aspirated volume of urine. The site of obstruction may be better delineated by bringing the patient upright on the screening table. Appropriate radiographs are taken once the pelvi-calyceal system and ureter have been well-delineated by contrast medium (Fig. 15.4). As much contrast medium as possible should be aspirated through the needle on completion of the procedure. The patient should subsequently remain in hospital for 24 hours.

Modifications of basic technique

Pressure flow studies by antegrade pyelography are useful in establishing the diagnosis of ureteric obstruc-

Fig. 15.4 Antegrade pyelography performed on non-functioning right kidney. The grossly dilated pelvi-calyceal system proved to be a pyonephrosis, 600 ml of pus being aspirated. A fibrotic stricture was present at the pelvi-ureteric junction.

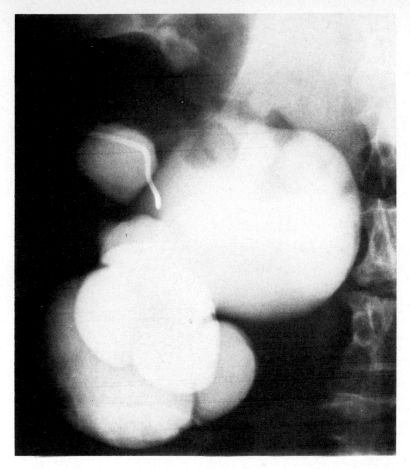

tion. A catheter which has been introduced with the needle puncturing the renal collecting system allows measurement of pressure within the system. The catheter is perfused at a rate of 10 ml per minute, with pressure in the upper urinary tract being constantly monitored through a side arm in the perfusion system (Whitaker, 1979). Any rise in renal pelvic pressure reflects the degree of ureteric obstruction. Bladder pressure is simultaneously measured via a per-urethral catheter. While this method is very useful in differentiating obstructed dilated ureters from dilated but non-obstructed ureters, it is sometimes inconsistent in differentiating the pressure of obstructive lesions in the uretero-pelvic junction from atonic failure of ureteric muscle (Sherwood, 1974).

Percutaneous catheter nephrostomy is an extension of antegrade pyelography. A catheter is usually threaded over a guide wire, which has itself been positioned in the collecting system along a needle inserted for antegrade pyelography. This method is used primarily in the management of obstructive uropathy (Fig. 15.5), but it is also useful in the conservative treatment of ureteric leaks and fistulae. In addition, stenoses may be dilated or calculi removed and brush biopsy or nephroscopy performed via the percutaneous nephrostomy. The subject has been reviewed by Barbaric (1979) and Saxton (1981).

Turner *et al.*, (1980) have described antegrade pyelography in the investigation of ureteric obstruction and leakage in the transplanted kidney. An 18 gauge lumbar puncture needle is passed from the lateral aspect of the kidney under fluoroscopic control into the drainage system.

Complications

Over-filling of the obstructed renal pelvis by contrast medium results in loin pain. The patient may also complain of pain with extravasation of contrast medium. Infection and haemorrhage have not been reported as problems with antegrade pyelography.

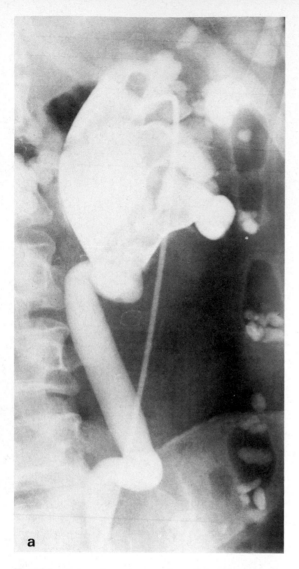

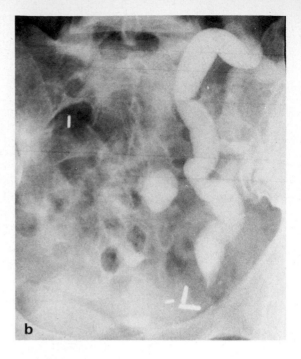

Fig. 15.5 Antegrade pyelogram via an indwelling drainage catheter. The hydronophrosis and ureteric dilatation was secondary to carcinoma of the cervix. (b) shows the site of distal ureteric obstruction.

Relationship to other imaging modalities

Antegrade pyelography should be regarded as a preferable alternative to retrograde pyelo-ureterography in cases of ureteric obstruction with poor delineation on i.v. urography. Not only does antegrade pyelography confirm the presence of obstruction, sometimes with the help of dynamic studies, but it also delineates the cause of the obstruction.

REFERENCES

Barbaric Z. L. (1979) Interventional uroradiology. *Radiol. Clin. N. Amer.,* **17,** 413–34.

Pfister R. C. & Newhouse J. H. (1979a) Interventional percutaneous pyeloureteral techniques. I. Antegrade pyelography and ureteral perfusion. *Radiol. Clin. N. Amer.,* **17,** 341–50.

Saafeld J. (1976) Antegrade pyelography. *Brit. J. Radiol.,* **48,** 155.

Saxton H. M. (1981) Percutaneous nephrostomy technique. *Urol. Radiol.,* **2,** 131–40.

Sherwood T., Doyle P. T. & Williams D. I. (1974) Antegrade pyelography in adults and children. *Proc. roy. Soc. Med.,* **67,** 1210–15.

Sherwood T. & Stevenson J. J. (1972) Antegrade pyelography: a further look at an old technique. *Brit. J. Radiol.,* **45,** 812–20.

Turner A. G., Howlett K. A., Evan R. & Williams G. B. (1980) The role of antegrade pyelography in the transplant kidney. *J. Urol.,* **123,** 812–14.

Whitaker R. H. (1979) An evaluation of 170 diagnostic pressure flow studies in the upper urinary tract. *J. Urol.,* **121,** 602–12.

RENAL CYST PUNCTURE

Indications

Cyst puncture is an important diagnostic procedure in the logical and sequential investigation of a renal mass lesion. Renal masses may be found coincidentally when i.v. urography is performed for an unrelated reason such as lower urinary tract obstruction or urinary infection. The majority of renal masses are simple cysts, renal carcinoma being a much less frequent cause. Rarely, a carcinoma is found in the wall of a simple cyst. Occasionally, renal abscesses, haematomas, metastases to the kidney from an extrarenal primary tumour, hydatid cysts and adenomas cause mass lesions which are discernable on the IVU. Most rounded mass lesions with a well-defined margin are eventually found to be simple cysts. Ultrasonography is a useful investigation following the discovery of a renal mass on i.v. urography. A well-defined mass which has ultrasonographic features consistent with a simple cyst should be punctured and aspirated at this stage. A mass which appears solid or has a mixed pattern of echoes on ultrasonography should be further investigated by renal arteriography.

Contra-indications

Contra-indications to renal puncture are an abnormal bleeding tendency and an obvious renal carcinoma on i.v. urography and ultrasonography.

Puncture of a renal hydatid cyst carries a potential risk of dissemination of the disease. Hydatid disease should be considered a possible cause of a renal mass lesion when there is curvilinear calcification in its wall on radiography, multiple septa on ultrasonography, or when the patient comes from an endemic area. The Casoni test is of diagnostic help.

A renal aneurysm, if punctured, could result in severe haemorrhage. A phaeochromocytoma should usually not be mistaken for a mass of renal origin if nephrotomography is performed, but needle puncture could result in acute severe hypertension.

Method

No premedication is required prior to cyst puncture. Initially, 50 ml of Conray 420 is injected intravenously to opacify the pelvi-calyceal system. The patient lies prone on the X-ray table. A radiolucent pad is placed under the upper part of the abdomen to restrict anterior movement of the kidney. Full sterile precautions are taken, the loin and its environs being cleansed with an antiseptic solution and the area is draped with sterile towels. A metallic marker is then placed on the skin under fluoroscopic control to immediately overlie the centre of the renal mass. A local anaesthetic agent, 1% lignocaine, is used to

infiltrate the skin and the underlying tissues down to the kidney. A small incision is made in the skin at the marker site by a scalpel blade. A 15 cm 20 gauge Greenberg needle is introduced through this site in a vertical direction. The exception is in some upper pole lesions when a cephalad inclination is appropriate (see 'Complications' below). The needle may be guided into the renal mass by an ultrasonic transducer. The patient is required to hold his breath during advancement of the needle under fluoroscopic control into the kidney. A distinct 'give' is often noted by the operator when a cyst is penetrated by the needle. The patient is then allowed to breathe again.

The stylette is removed and the needle is connected via plastic tubing to a syringe. Sometimes the needle has a Teflon sheath which is left in the cyst when the needle and stylette are withdrawn. While this results in less trauma from respiratory excursion, the Teflon sheath may be more easily dislodged from the kidney during respiratory movement than the metal needle. Gentle suction is applied, whereupon fluid will enter the syringe if the needle is in a cystic mass. Aspiration of some of the cyst fluid is followed by replacement with contrast medium (Conray 280 or Urografin 290) and an equal volume of air (Fig. 15.6). The total volume of contrast medium and air should be no more than the volume of aspirant. No attempt is made to completely empty the cyst, the quantity aspirated being sufficient for analysis and dependent to some extent on the size of the cyst. The needle is then removed during arrested respiration.

Radiographs are obtained with the patient in the prone, supine and upright positions, as well as in both lateral decubitus planes, to show each part of the cyst wall on double contrast. The radiographs are superimposed on the IVU, or nephrogram phase of a previous arteriogram, to ensure that all of the mass shown on the nephrogram is accounted for by the contrast/air filled cyst and not by a solid component to the mass (Fig. 15.7). The aspiration of too much fluid may cause buckling of the edge of a simple cyst with the spurious appearance of a filling defect.

Failure to aspirate fluid indicates a solid lesion, if A–P and lateral radiographs have confirmed that the needle tip is within the mass. A few drops of fluid may often be aspirated by brisk suction, even from a solid mass, and this is invaluable for cytological examination.

Necrosis within a tumour, giving a fluid-filled space, is associated with a thick, glairy aspirate containing altered blood. Contrast studies show the cavity to be irregular in outline and the wall to have a substantial solid component (Figs. 15.8 and 15.9). A traumatic tap of a simple cyst may initially show blood-stained

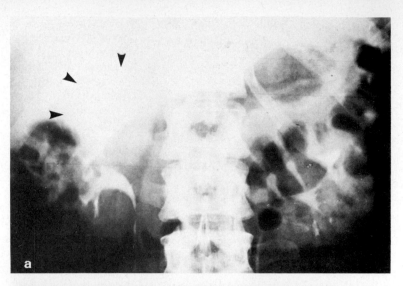

Fig. 15.6 Simple cyst in right kidney viewed by
(a) Double contrast renal cystography
(b) Shoot through prone position
(c) Erect position
(d) Decubitus position.

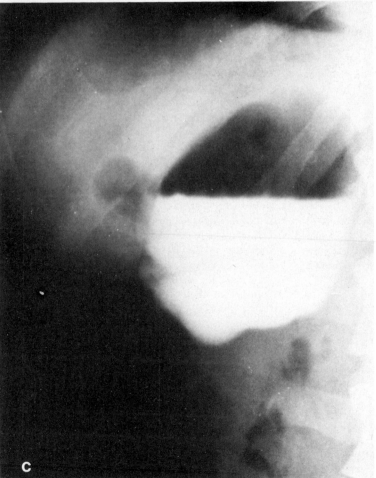

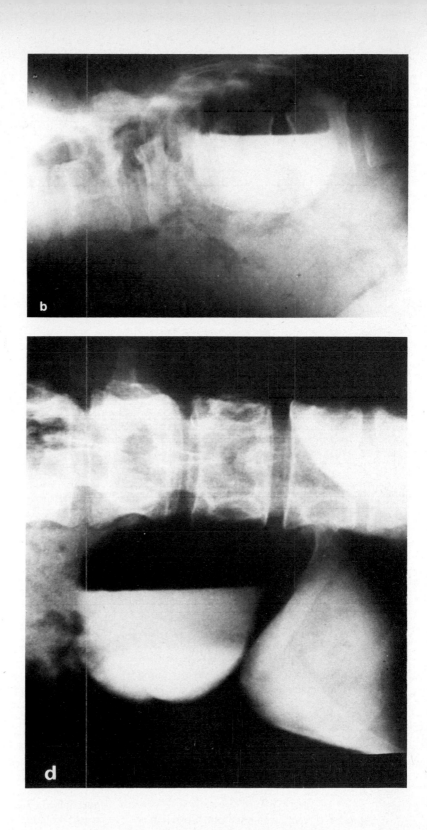

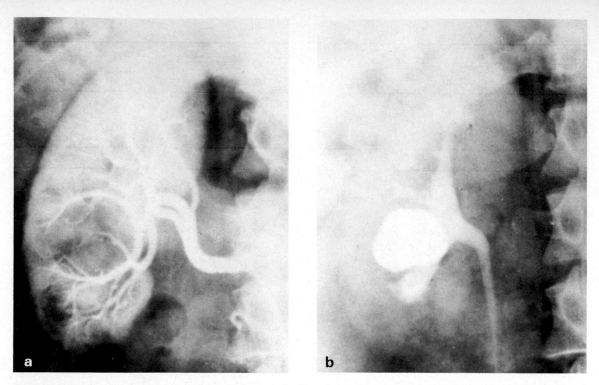

Fig. 15.7 Woman aged 72 years presented with haematuria. Rounded mass seen in right kidney on IV urography (a) renal ateriogram showed rounded mass lesion with regular border displacing surrounding arteries, (b) clear fluid aspirated on cyst puncture. Contrast delineation of cyst accounts for all defects seen on arteriogram and IVU.

fluid, although this should clear rapidly on subsequent aspiration.

Simple cysts contain a clear, slightly straw-coloured fluid which on biochemical analysis often contains a high concentration of glucose. The fat, protein and lactate dehydrogenase (LDH) levels are low. Cytology shows no abnormal cells. The blood-stained or murky fluid obtained from 'cystic' or necrotic tumours has high fat and protein levels but low LDH and glucose levels. Tumour cells should be sought on cytology. Aspirants from infected cysts or renal abscesses contain a high LDH level in fluid which is often murky. Fat and protein levels may be slightly raised and, while some cytology shows abnormality, there are no tumour cells.

A chest radiograph is taken after the procedure, to exclude a pneumothorax, and the patient is observed overnight in hospital.

Modification of basic technique

Most simple cysts recur, even after total aspiration of their fluid contents. Sclerosants have been injected,

for instance 2–3 ml of iophendylate (Myodil) into simple cysts (Sherwood & Stevenson, 1971). Any reduction in the recurrence rate following this injection is only slight. There is a resultant elevation of temperature in at least 10% of patients following injection of Myodil into a cyst (Lang, 1977).

Complications

The incidence of complications is proportional to the experience of the operator. Lang (1977) found the incidence of major complications to be about 0.75% in experienced hands. Peri-renal haemorrhage is the commonest complication and is especially likely to occur with direct aspiration through a syringe attached to a rigid needle.

Pneumothorax and haemopneumothorax is the second commonest complication, occurring exclusively during direct puncture of lesions in the upper pole of the kidney. A cephalad obliquity to the needle under fluoroscopic control, preferably using a teflon sheath, should minimize this complication.

Arteriovenous fistula, rupture of the duodenum or

Fig. 15.8 Woman aged 68 years with large right flank mass (a) IVU shows large right renal mass with medial displacement of pelvi-calyceal system, (b) viscid brown fluid aspirated from mass. Contrast injection showed irregular, loculated cavity with large solid component to mass.

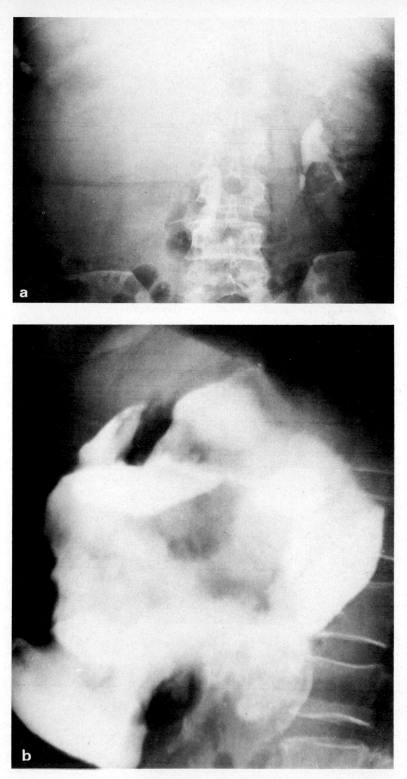

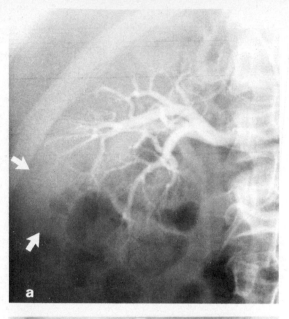

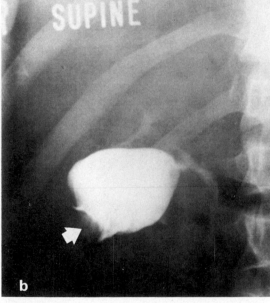

Fig. 15.9 Man aged 32 years with haematuria (a) right renal arteriogram shows avascular mass in kidney (arrows) (b) cyst puncture revealed turbid fluid and renal cystogram showed irregular filling defect on its lateral margin (arrow), the rest of the cyst outline being smooth. At operation, carcinoma in wall of cyst.

colon, and biliary peritonitis are rare complications of the needle puncture.

Infection is an uncommon hazard. Puncture of renal abscesses is usually an uncomplicated event, but requires antibiotic therapy. The aspirated pus is, of course, cultured for organisms.

Mild haematuria may occur, rarely being massive.

Peri-renal fluid collections, such as urinomas, are uncommon complications.

Seeding of tumour cells along the needle track is a hazard of some biopsy techniques, for instance in cases of bronchial carcinoma. This mode of tumour dissemination would, therefore, seem to be a theoretical possibility when needle puncture is performed on malignant renal masses. A large comparative series showed there to be no difference in five year survival between cases where renal carcinoma was needled and those in which it was not (van Schreeb *et al.*, 1967). There is, however, a recorded case of tumour spread as a result of direct needle puncture of a renal carcinoma (Bush *et al.*, 1977). The chance of this potential hazard must be regarded as being very small.

Relation to other diagnostic techniques

The alternative to cyst puncture with aspiration and contrast delineation is arteriography or surgical exploration. Arteriography itself carries risks and has some diagnostic limitations. Surgical exploration has a greater morbidity than the radiological diagnostic approach, as reviewed by Jeans *et al.* (1972), unnecessary nephrectomy being performed in 11% of cases (Plaine & Hinman, 1965). However, a cyst containing altered blood from past haemorrhage causes diagnostic uncertainty on aspiration and delineation and requires surgery. Cysts which obstruct calyces or cause pressure atrophy of renal parenchyma are other indications for surgical exploration (Sherwood, 1980).

The diagnostic pathways taken in the differentiation of a renal mass as a cyst or tumour are shown on Fig. 15.10.

Renal mass lesions over 2 cm in diameter are amenable to good resolution on ultrasonography. A simple cyst on ultrasonography has a sharply defined interface with the surrounding parenchyma and, even with increased gain, is free of intrinsic echoes. An ill-defined mass with multiple echoes indicates a solid tumour. Some tumours have some echoes interspersed with anechoic parts, a finding which is also sometimes seen with renal abscesses, haematomas, infected cysts and some cases of hydronephrosis.

McClennan *et al.* (1979) have reviewed the role of CT scanning in the investigation of renal masses. A high level of accuracy has been claimed in the diagnosis of renal cysts in this study, and the need to aspirate cysts is questioned with the application of strict diagnostic criteria. CT scanning gives useful

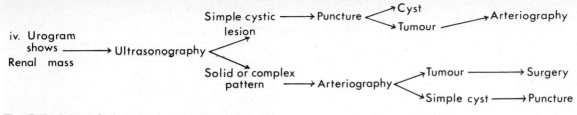

iv. Urogram
shows ⟶ Ultrasonography ⟨ Simple cystic lesion ⟶ Puncture ⟨ Cyst, Tumour ⟶ Arteriography
Renal mass ⟨ Solid or complex pattern ⟶ Arteriography ⟨ Tumour ⟶ Surgery, Simple cyst ⟶ Puncture

Fig. 15.10 Scheme for investigating a renal mass.

information on a variety of other mass lesions, including the determination of size and metastic spread of malignant tumours.

REFERENCES

Bush W. H., Burnett L. L. & Gibbons R. P. (1977) Needle tract seeding of renal cell carcinoma. *Amer. J. Roentgenol.,* **129**, 725–7.

Jeans W. D., Penry J. B. & Roylance J. (1972) Renal puncture. *Clin. Radiol.,* **23**, 298–311.

Lang E. K. (1977) Renal cyst puncture and aspiration: a survey of complications. *Amer. J. Roentgenol.,* **128**, 723–7.

McClennan B. L., Stanley R. J., Melson G. L., Levitt R. G. & Sagel S. S. (1979) CT of the renal cyst: is cyst aspiration necessary? *Amer. J. Roentgenol.,* **133**, 671–5.

Plaine L. I. & Hinman F. (1965) Malignancy in asymptomatic renal masses. *J. Urol.,* **94**, 342–7.

Sherwood T. & Stevensen J. J. (1971) The management of renal masses. *Clin. Radiol.,* **22**, 180–7.

Sherwood T. (1980) *Uroradiology.* Blackwell Scientific Publications, Oxford.

von Schreeb T., Arner O., Skovsted G. & Wikstad N. (1967) Renal adenocarcinoma—is there a risk of spreading tumour cells in diagnostic puncture? *Scand. J. Urol. Nephrol.,* **1**, 270–6.

MICTURATING CYSTOGRAPHY

Indications

1. In recurrent urinary infections in the paediatric age group, the presence of vesico-ureteric reflux is demonstrable on micturating cystography. Lower urinary tract obstruction may be found in boys with recurrent urinary infection.
2. In neurogenic voiding disorders, vesico-urethral anatomy is shown and vesico-ureteric reflux is demonstrable.
3. The demonstration of anatomical abnormalities of the bladder neck and urethra; for instance urethral valves, strictures and other causes of urethral obstruction in the male, and urethral diverticula in the female.
4. As part of the assessment of disorders of bladder and urethral function in association with pressure/flow studies.
5. Cystography is also useful in the delineation of vesico-vaginal fistula in the female when i.v. urography has provided insufficient detail.

Contra-indications

Active urinary tract infection should be eliminated before cystography is performed via a bladder catheter.

Some contrast medium is absorbed into the systemic circulation from the bladder (Currarino *et al.*, 1977), so that hypersensitivity to contrast medium is a relative contra-indication.

Technique

Following i.v. urography

The process of micturition after the bladder has been allowed to become uncomfortably full may be radiographically recorded by video, when the image quality may not be good; by cine, which necessitates a high dose of X-radiation; or by spot radiographs on full size or 100 mm format. Spot radiographs are usually adequate. The image is usually recorded in the oblique projection on order to limit the radiation dose and reduce obscuration of contrast medium by overlying bone. The information supplied by this basic technique may be sufficient to make some fundamental observations, such as the exclusion of lower urinary tract obstruction. Extension of the investigation to include voiding flow pattern is useful in the evaluation of symptoms such as frequency, urgency and nocturia (Turner–Warwick *et al.*, 1979). The demonstration of vesico-ureteric reflux is often not possible, as the ureters may well already be delineated by excreted contrast media. Inadequate detail of the lower urinary tract, due to dilution of the contrast medium, necessitates a formal micturating cystogram with bladder catheterization.

Cystography via bladder catheter

(See Paediatric Radiology, p. 333.) Antibiotic cover should be given to the patient because of tract infection occurring after cystography (see 'Complications' below). The patient is requested to empty the bladder prior to the procedure. A full sterile technique is used, the external urethral meatus being cleansed with a mild antiseptic solution. Local anaesthetic, in the form of 2% lignocaine gel, is applied to the meatus, as well as to the catheter where it also acts as a lubricant. A size 16 or 18F flexible catheter is suitable for adults and a size 6 or 8F for infants and small children. As much urine as possible is drained from the bladder through the catheter. Foley catheters should not be used for cystography.

Barium is no longer used as a cystographic contrast medium because retained barium may form bladder stones and inflammatory changes may follow vesico-ureteric reflux. Sodium iodide was once in vogue, but it is irritative to the bladder mucosa. Conventional triodinated contrast agents in a concentration of 20–25% are adequate for cystography.

Contrast medium is infused through the catheter via polythene tubing from a bottle which is 50 cm above the table top. The bladder has to be filled until there is an uncomfortable desire to micturate, 200 ml or more being required in an adult. A well-distended bladder is most likely to be associated with successful micturition. Difficulties may be encountered in micturating to order in a strange environment, in front of several people, and in an undignified situation. Infants and children are investigated in the supine position while adults are required to micturate in the upright position. Spot radiographs in the oblique position, usually suffice in the recording of urethral delineation and of vesico-ureteric reflux (Fig. 15.11). The gonad dose is of the order of 1–10 rems, depending on the number of radiographs and duration of fluoroscopy. Video and cine may also be used as recording techniques.

Suprapubic bladder puncture

This approach is sometimes of use in infancy in the investigation of lower urinary tract obstruction. The difficulties which may be encountered in this age group with bladder catheterization are avoided by this sterile procedure. The technique is described in Paediatric Radiology, p. 334.

Urethrocystography

The introduction of a water-soluble contrast medium up the urethra and into the bladder, following an

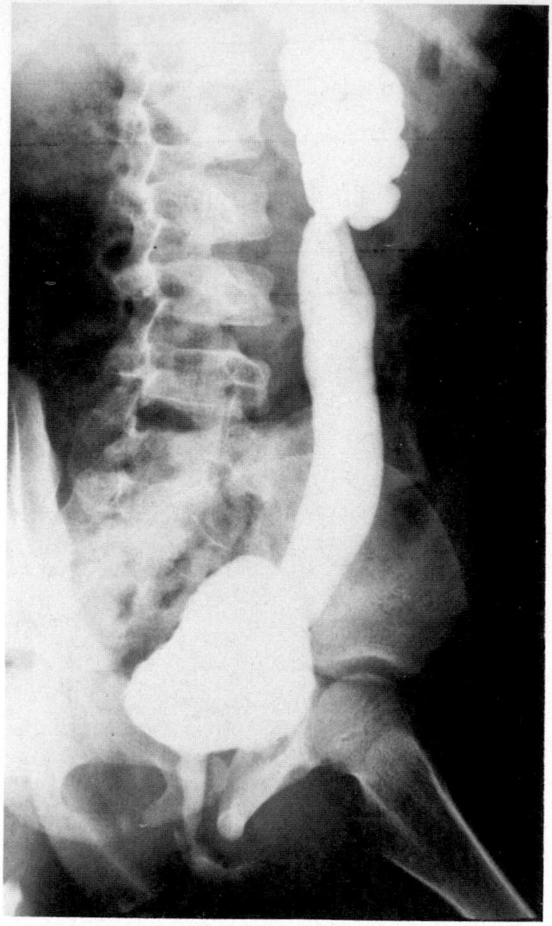

Fig. 15.11 Micturating cystogram in a girl. Gross vesico-ureteric reflux on left side, renal atrophy with dilated pelvi-calyceal system and ureter.

ascending urethrogram via a Knutsson clamp or Foley catheter in the navicular fossa, shows the posterior urethra and bladder in cases where bladder catheterization is not possible. The contrast medium is injected from a syringe under fluoroscopic control.

Variations on basic technique

Double contrast cystography has been used for the diagnosis and assessment of bladder tumours, especially when cystoscopy is not possible. Doyle (1961) injected 150 ml of a sterile suspension of barium sulphate in water (Steripaque) along a bladder catheter. Most of this amount was then aspirated, leaving 20–30 ml in the bladder. Carbon dioxide, 150–200 ml in amount, was then injected through the bladder catheter. The patient was rotated to each side

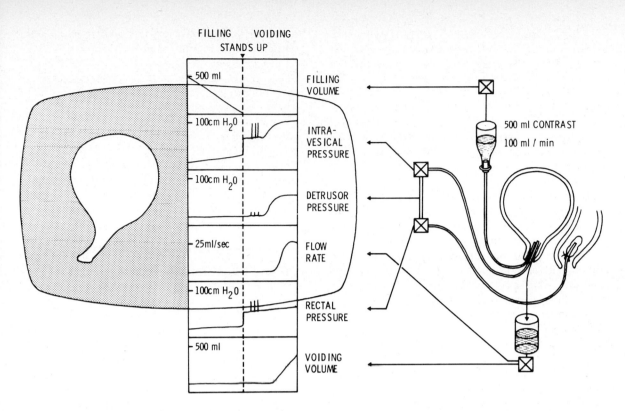

Fig. 15.12 Videocysto-urethrography. Simultaneous recording of bladder and rectal pressure changes during supine cystometry, combined with a display of bladder filling volume, is shown on the left hand side of the polygraph trace. The bladder and rectal pressures during voiding, with the voiding rate and volume, are recorded on the right side of the trace. A television camera selects three parameters (intravesical pressure, detrusor pressure and voiding rate) which are added to the radiographic image of the bladder and recorded with sound commentary on videotape. (Courtesy of S. L. Stanton, and Harper and Row Inc.)

in turn, radiographs being taken with a horizontal beam. Lang (1969) has used this technique to demonstrate bladder diverticula, using multiple radiographic projections. Barium as a cystographic agent carries some risks, as previously mentioned, but double contrast cystography is still occasionally used to show a carcinoma which lies within a diverticulum. Singh and Raghavaiah (1973) have used water soluble contrast medium in the double contrast technique, but inconsistent coating is likely to be the outcome.

Cysto-urethrography combined with pressure flow studies (Bates *et al.*, 1970; Stanton, 1978). The use of cysto-urethrography, with or without a bladder catheter *in situ*, was used for many years in the assessment of disorders of micturition such as urinary incontinence, voiding difficulties and retention. For instance, in cases of stress incontinence, information may be given on prolapse of the bladder base and urethral distortion, as well as the demonstration of incontinence. However, the assessment of bladder function is an important prerequisite in determining the correct treatment in these cases and cannot be determined by radiography alone. Pressure/flow studies are a mandatory addition to the anatomical delineation provided by cysto-urethrography (Fig. 15.12).

Cystography is performed by a bladder catheter. A fluid-filled catheter is then placed alongside the filling catheter and is connected to a pressure transducer to measure the intravesical pressure. Rectal (abdominal) pressure is measured by means of a catheter inserted into the rectum. The electronic subtraction of the rectal pressure from the intravesical pressure gives the detrusor pressure, which is an exact index of detrusor activity. The filling catheter is removed and the patient placed in the erect position, leakage or descent of the bladder base being noted at rest and on straining. The peak flow rate and volume voided during micturition are recorded, voluntary arrest of micturition determining the ability of the posterior urethra to empty back into the bladder. Detrusor irritability may be differentiated from urethral sphincter dysfunction as a cause of stress incontinence. Obstruction may also be assessed from the data and in relation to the cysto-urethrogram image. Radiographic screening is recorded on videotape.

Complications

McAlister *et al.*, (1974) have enumerated a large number of complications which may arise from cystography in children.

Infection   Maskell *et al.*, (1978) found that urinary infection developed over a wide age range in 30% of patients after micturating cystography, all of whom had sterile urine prior to the procedure. The only significant factor influencing the rate of infection seemed to be whether or not the patient was on antibacterial treatment at the time of the investigation. Difficulty in catheterization, the patient's sex, and the presence of urinary tract pathology were not predispositions to infection.

Septicaemia and death from urinary infection, either *de novo* or exacerbated by cystography, may follow the investigation. These dire consequences, rare as they are, are most likely in patients with vesicoureteric reflux, gross hydronephrosis or urinary retention. Post-cystography urinary infection may cause appreciable shrinkage of renal substance over the succeeding several months.

Catheter complications   Trauma to the urethra and bladder during catheterization may cause transient dysuria, frequency and haematuria. Resultant urethral oedema may convert a pre-existing partial obstruction into a complete obstruction. A rigid catheter should not be used as there is a risk of bladder or urethral rupture. A Foley catheter should not be used as it may not deflate prior to removal, or the balloon may be situated within the urethra or bladder neck whereupon injudicious over-distension of the bladder may cause vesical rupture. Using the suprapubic route, a catheter may inadvertently enter the peritoneal cavity or extravesical space.

Complications of bladder filling There should be a negligible risk of bladder rupture in the absence of a balloon catheter and if the patient is not under anaesthesia or heavy sedation. Static vesicoureteric reflux may cause gross upper urinary tract distension with pain and occasionally intrarenal reflux of contrast medium.

Allergic reactions   Absorption of contrast medium through the urothelium and into the systemic circula-tion may theoretically lead to reactions in patients who are allergic to contrast media.

Misdirected insertion of catheter   The catheter may inadvertently be placed within the vagina or, very rarely, into an ectopic ureteric orifice.

Autonomic dysreflexia   Barbaric (1976) has described a marked increase in systolic and diastolic blood pressure as a result of autonomic dysreflexia in cysto-urethrography. This response is the result of distention of the bladder or urethra in patients with a spinal cord lesion at T7 level.

Relationship to other diagnostic techniques

Children with urinary tract infection should have an IVU. A micturating cysto-urethrogram should be done if the IVU is abnormal or if there is recurrent urinary infection. Obstruction may be excluded as a cause of an initial urinary infection in boys by screening micturation following the IVU.

Intravenous radionuclide cystography is a recently developed method of assessing vesico-ureteric reflux (Merrick *et al.*, 1979). The advantages over radiographic micturating cystography are that bladder catheterization is avoided and the radiation dose to the gonads, about 50 millirem, is much less with the isotope method. As with radiographic cystography, the isotope method is especially useful in the investigation of children with urinary infections. An intravenous bolus of 150 µCi/kg Tc^{99m} DTPA is excreted through the kidneys. A gamma camera with a computer-optimized display is used to give images of the urinary tract and also time/activity curves of the renal areas during the initial function study and during micturition. Vesico-ureteric reflux is diagnosed if there is an increase in activity in the renal area on the images and on time/activity curves. Isotope cystography is considered by Merrick *et al.*, to be slightly more accurate than radiographic cystography in the assessment of vesico-ureteric reflux, but the latter method gives superior anatomical detail.

REFERENCES

Barbaric Z. L. (1976) Autonomic dysreflexia in patients with spinal cord lesions: complication of voiding cysto-urethrography and ileal loopography. *Amer. J. Roentgenol.* **127**, 293–5.
Bates C. P., Whiteside C. G. & Turner-Warwick R. (1970) Synchronous cine/pressure/flow/cysto-urethrography with special reference to stress and urge incontinence. *Brit. J. Urol.*, **42**, 714–23.

Fig. 15.13 The Knuttson penile clamp for retrograde urethrography.

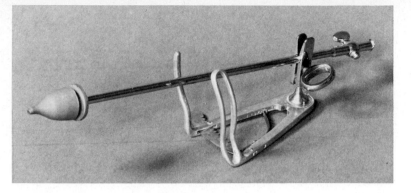

Curriarino G., Weinberg A. & Putnam R. (1977). Resorption of contrast material from the bladder during cysto-urethrography causing an excretory urogram. *Radiology*, **123**, 149–50.

Doyle F. H. (1961) Cystography in bladder tumours. *Brit. J. Radiol.*, **34**, 205–15.

Lang E. K. (1969) Double contrast gas barium cystography in the assessment of diverticula of the bladder. *Amer. J. Roentgenol.*, **107**, 769–775.

Maskell R., Pead L. & Vinnicombe J. (1978) Urinary infection after micturating cystography. *Lancet*, **ii**, 1191–2.

McAlister W. H., Cacciavelli A. & Shackelford G. D. (1974) Complications associated with cystography in children. *Radiology*, **111**, 167–72.

Merrick M. V., Uttley W. S. & Wild R. (1970) A comparison of two techniques of detecting vesico-ureteric reflux. Brit. J. Radiol., **52**, 792–5.

Singh S. M. & Raghavaiah N. V. (1973) Combined double contrast cystography and polycystography in the evaluation of bladder carcinoma. *J. Urol.*, **110**, 70–71.

Stanton S. L. (1978) Preoperative investigation and diagnosis. *Clin. Obstet Gynecol.*, **21**, 705–21.

Turner-Warwick R., Whiteside C. G., Milroy E. J., Pengelly A. W. & Thompson D. T. (1979) The intravenous urodynamogram. *Brit. J. Urol.*, **51**, 15–18.

URETHROGRAPHY

Indications

The object of urethrography is to obtain good anatomical definition of the whole length of the urethra. The urethra is far easier to delineate in the male than in the female. The assessment of urethral stricture and trauma provide the main indications for urethrography in the male. Tumours of the urethra are rare but are well shown by urethrography.

Contra-indications

Urethrography should be delayed for one or two weeks after urethral instrumentation, because of the risk of intravasation of contrast medium from the mucosal damage which is likely to result from the passage of instruments per urethram.

The investigation should not be performed in the presence of active urethritis.

Sensitivity to contrast media is a relative contra-indication as it may provoke an allergic reaction following intravasation.

Technique

Retrograde urethrography is performed either by the application of a Knuttson clamp to the penis, the insertion of a small Foley catheter into the navicular fossa, or by the fixation of a Malstrom-Westerman vacuum cannula.

The patient should empty his bladder prior to urethrography. A sterile technique is employed, the prepuce being retracted and the glans cleansed with a mild antiseptic solution before the insertion of the urethrographic appliance.

The Knuttson clamp (Fig. 15.13) is a time honoured method. The penis is held just behind the glans by the adjustable clamp. The rubber nozzle on the end of the metal cannula is smeared with 2% lignocaine gel before it is inserted into the external meatus and fixed in position. It is not possible to use the clamp in cases of phimosis or hypospadias. Occasionally, the Knuttson clamp may slip off when traction is applied in the uncircumcized patient. Traction is applied to the clamp to delineate the anterior urethra during the injection of contrast medium under fluoroscopic control. Spot radiographs are taken in the appropriate oblique projections to delineate the whole length of the urethra as well as the bladder base. Radiographs to show the posterior urethra have to be taken during the injection of contrast medium. Either a viscous contrast medium, Umbradil, or a conventional water-soluble contrast medium may be used for urethral opacification. Umbradil provides good delineation

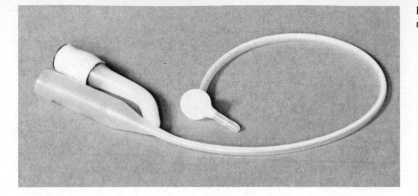

Fig. 15.14 Size 8 Foley catheter for retrograde urethrography.

and distention of the urethra, but should be warmed prior to injection. Standard water-soluble contrast media, such as Conray 280 or Urografin 290, are more likely to leak from the meatus if there has been incorrect application of the clamp. There is more chance of a forceful injection resulting in intravasation, in the presence of a urethral obstruction, with Umbradil than with less viscid contrast media.

A number 8 Foley catheter is often used nowadays in urethrography (Figs 15.14, 15.15). Lignocaine gel is inserted into the external meatus. The catheter is filled with contrast medium to eliminate air bubbles. Following insertion of the catheter tip into the distal portion of the penile urethra, the balloon is filled with about 2 ml of saline in the navicular fossa until it feels a tight fit. This usually provides good anchorage. Occasionally, the catheter may be pulled out during traction, with some risk of traumatizing the external meatus. The Foley catheter technique is applicable in cases of phimosis. The radiologist's hands are more likely to be kept out of the X-ray beam than with the clamp method. Urografin 290 or Conray 280 are the contrast media which are usually used with this technique.

De Lacey and Wignall (1977) have described a method of combining retrograde urethrography with micturating cystography, without catheterizing the bladder, through a Foley catheter which has been inserted into the urethra as described above. The patient lies supine on the X-ray table and is rotated into a 45° right posterior oblique position. Contrast medium is run along the urethral catheter, via polythene tubing, from a bottle containing Urografin 150 or Diodone 25% which is at a height of three feet above the table top. An overcouch 35 × 35 cm radiograph is exposed after approximately 20 ml of contrast medium and shows the urethra as far as the membranous portion. The infusion continues during the processing of this film, a further radiograph being taken after any appropriate adjustment to technique and when the patient feels an urgent desire to micturate. The catheter is then removed and the patient micturates in the supine oblique position. A radiograph during voiding shows the membranous and posterior (prostatic) portion of the urethra. Micturition is arrested by the patient, whereupon a further radiograph is taken to show optimal distention of the posterior urethra following contraction of the external sphincter. Fluoroscopy is not required with this method, thus limiting radiation exposure of the patient and operator. McCallum (1979) uses a similar combination of retrograde and voiding urethrography, stressing their complementary nature and the role of this combined examination in showing the extent of urethral scarring prior to surgery. Normally, the 'milking back' of the internal sphincter prevents good delineation of the posterior urethra. This segment is better distended on micturition and, better still, with the arrest of micturition.

The Malström-Westerman vacuum cannula (see 'Female Genital Tract' p. 246) is an alternative urethrographic appliance, being especially useful in cases of hypospadias (McCallum, 1964). The rubber acorn at the end of the cannula fits into the end of the urethra and a vacuum is applied to the cup as it lies with its rim against the glans. This method has been used in retrograde urethrography on the female (Becker & Gregoine, 1968).

When there is the possibility of urethral rupture following trauma, either the Foley catheter or clamp method can be used with a gentle injection of 20–40 ml of water-soluble contrast medium by hand.

Complications

Intravasation of contrast medium has been recorded in 5.5% of urethrograms (McClennan et al., 1971).

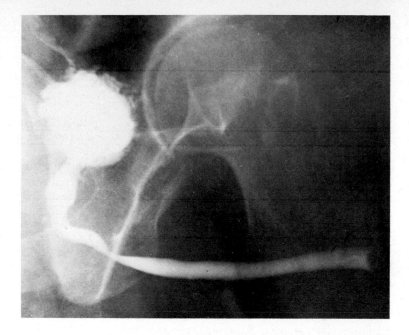

Fig. 15.15 Retrograde urethrogram using Foley catheter. Stricture of the membranous urethra. Filling of the bladder is occurring. There is thickening of the bladder wall.

Bleeding per urethram following intravasation is often minor but is occasionally heavy, although it stops spontaneously within a few minutes. There is the slight potential hazard of a hypersensitivity reaction in the allergic patient. The investigation should be terminated as soon as any intravasation is observed on fluorosocopy. When oil-based contrast media were used for urethrography, intravasation carried the hazard of pulmonary oil embolism. A forceful and clumsy technique, especially in the presence of a tight stricture, recent urethral instrumentation or active urethral inflammation, predisposes to intravasation. Over-filling of the Foley catheter balloon may result in intravasation at the navicular fossa. Antibiotics are often routinely given if there is intravasation. Prophylactic antibiotics should never be mixed with contrast medium, death having been recorded following intravasation when the contrast agent was mixed with Neomycin. As with all procedures involving the lower urinary tract, patients with rheumatic or congenital heart disease are given antibiotic cover to prevent bacterial endocarditis.

Relation to other diagnostic techniques

The urethra may be evaluated on micturition following i.v. urography. It is important that the patient micturates with a full bladder which is achieved by drinking a large amount of water. Fitts *et al.*, (1977) have claimed a successful urethrogram by this method in 87% of cases.

A Zipser penile clamp has been used to increase resistance within the urethra during attempted micturition, the so-called 'choke' urethrogram, with enhanced distention and delineation of the urethra (Boltuch & Lalli, 1975). A satisfactory examination is achieved in many cases, although McCallum (1979) points out that the detail is insufficient for the accurate pre-operative assessment of urethral scarring.

Supplementation of the micturating cysto-urethrogram with pressure/flow studies gives a functional as well as an anatomical appraisal of the urethra.

REFERENCES

Becker J. A. & Gregoire (1968) Retrograde urethrography. *J. Urol.*, **100**, 92–3.
Boltuch R. L. & Lalli A. F. (1975) A new technique for urethrography. *Radiology*, **115**, 736.
Fitts F. B., Herbert S. G. & Mellins H. Z. (1977) Criteria for examination of the urethra during excretory urography. *Radiology*, **125**, 47–52.
De Lacey G. J. & Wignall B. K. (1977) Urography simplified: the drip infusion technique. *Brit. J. Radiol.*, **50**, 138–40.
McCallum A. H. (1964) The MW–VUC cannula modified for male urethrography. *Brit. J. Radiol.*, **37**, 315–16.
McCallum R. W. (1979) The adult male urethra. *Radiol. Clin. N. Amer.*, **17**, 227–44.
McClennan B. L., Becker J. A. & Robinson T. (1971) Venous extravasation at retrograde urethrography: precautions. *J. Urol.*, **106**, 412–13.

HYSTEROSALPINGOGRAPHY

Contrast examination of the uterine cavity was first performed by Rindfleish in 1910, when he injected bismuth emulsion through the cervical canal. A colloidal silver salt was used as a hysterosalpingographic contrast medium by Cary and by Rubin in 1914, but this agent was abandoned because it was not absorbed and caused peritoneal irritation. Lipiodol was used for many years as a contrast medium but was associated with an unacceptable incidence of local and systemic complications. Hysterosalpingography (HSG) with water-soluble contrast media is still a useful and widely employed method of investigating the female genital tract, despite the introduction of direct viewing of the pelvic organs via the peritoneoscope and the development of ultrasonography.

Indications

Infertility   Maldevelopment of the uterus and occlusion of the Fallopian tubes constitute two thirds of all abnormalities demonstrated on HSG in cases of infertility. Congenital abnormalities account for 20% of positive findings in primary infertility cases (Pontifex *et al., 1972),* while evidence of tubal abnormalities are commoner than uterine anomalies in secondary infertility.

Recurrent abortion   The main cause of repeated abortion is cervical and isthmic incompetence. This is suspected when the internal os measures 6 mm or more on hysterography and the cervical canal merges imperceptibly with the uterine cavity. Various balloon catheter devices have been used to assess incompetence.

Abnormal uterine bleeding   Uterine abnormalities such as fibroids, endometrial polyps, adenomyosis and cystic endometrial hyperplasia are sometimes diagnosed on hysterography but are missed on diagnostic curettage. Although not often performed for the investigation of abnormal uterine bleeding, HSG may be regarded as complimentary to curettage. Oligomenorrhoea may be associated with uterine hypoplasia and intrauterine adhesions.

Post-caesarean section   The integrity of the uterine scar following Caesarean section is accurately shown by hysterography, the lateral view being essential. The feasibility of subsequent pregnancies being delivered by the vaginal route or the need for further uterine sections may be assessed from this study.

Before artificial insemination   Structural abnormalities of the genital tract may be excluded by HSG if artificial insemination is under consideration.

After laparoscopic sterilization   Tubal occlusion is confirmed by HSG performed after the sterilization.

Prior to reversal of tubal ligation   The length and gross appearance of the portion of the Fallopian tube proximal to the site of ligation is assessed by HSG.

Following reconstructive tubal surgery   HSG is used to assess the patency of the Fallopian tubes following operations such as salpingolysis, salpingostomy, tubal resection and anastomosis, which have been performed for tubal occlusion.

Evaluation of endometrial carcinoma   HSG is employed in some centres to evaluate post-menopausal bleeding. The technique has been found to be helpful in showing the site and extent of endometrial carcinoma, sometimes when curettage is negative, and as a useful adjunct to radiotherapy planning. There is no convincing evidence that HSG causes dissemination of uterine malignancy.

Following tubal pregnancy   There is a high incidence of adhesions developing in and around the residual Fallopian tube following unilateral salpingotomy for tubal pregnancy. This is presumed to result from fibrosis secondary to bleeding into the pelvic peritoneal cavity, although the original pelvic inflammatory disease may involve both Fallopian tubes. The result is a high recurrence rate of ectopic pregnancy, but assessment of this risk is ascertained by HSG.

Following myomectomy   Extensive resection of intramural and submucosal fibroids may result in gross deformity of the uterine cavity and intrauterine adhesions. HSG shows the shape of the uterine cavity and excludes cornual occlusion.

Ashermann's syndrome Intrauterine adhesions, amenorrhoea and infertility are features of Ashermann's syndrome. The extent of the uterine adhesions is demonstrable on HSG.

Contra-indications

Pregnancy HSG with a pregnant uterus carries a risk of abortion as well as the teratogenic hazards of radiation. Inadvertent HSG during the first two months of pregnancy shows an enlarged, atonic and globular uterine cavity with the gestation sac as a filling defect (Fig. 16.1). Permeation of contrast medium into the thickened endometrium causes a poorly-defined outline to the uterus.

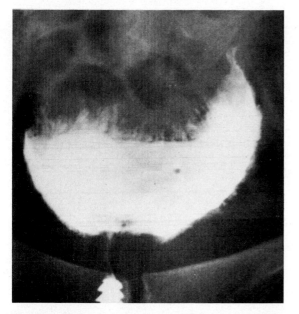

Fig. 16.1 Pregnant uterus. Large globular uterine cavity with the gestation sac seen as a filling defect. Marked endometrial thickening.

Ectopic pregnancy The manipulation and contrast injection associated with HSG carries a risk of dislodging the tubal mole.

Pelvic infection A history of salpingitis in the previous six months precludes HSG until a course of antibiotics has been given and there is clinical assessment of successful treatment. Acute vaginitis and cervicitis carry a risk of ascending infection and should be treated before considering HSG.

*Immediate pre- and post-*menstrual *phases* Spasm of the isthmus and cornua are least likely to occur in

mid-cycle. The thickened and denuded endometriuml which respectively occur before and after the menstrual period, increases the chance of intravasation of contrast medium which will obscure the contours of the uterus and adnexa. There is a risk of performing the investigation in the presence of an early pregnancy in the premenstrual phase.

Sensitivity to contrast medium. Susceptible subjects may have an anaphylactoid response to the contrast medium. The advisability of performing HSG and the need for antihistamine and steroid cover should be assessed in the light of a history of sensitivity to contrast medium or other substances.

Technique

The optimal time to perform HSG is towards the end of the first week after the menstrual period. The isthmus is most easily distended at this time, tubal filling most readily occurs and there is no risk of performing the investigation during an early pregnancy.

Preparation

Premedication is not required in the majority of cases, provided there has been adequate reassurance and explanation of the procedure. The investigation is likely to be uncomfortable and painful in the anxious patient, in whom 5–10 mg of diazepam may be helpful.

Morphia and pethidine should not be given as they stimulate smooth muscle contraction which impedes the filling of the Fallopian tubes with contrast medium. General anaesthesia, or the emotional upset provoked by the thought of it, often precipitates tubal spasm which is unrelieved during anaesthesia.

The patient should empty her bladder immediately prior to the investigation, as a full bladder elevates the Fallopian tubes and causes a spurious radiological appearance of tubal blockage.

Method

The patient is placed in the lithotomy position on the screening table prior to a bimanual pelvic examination. A vaginal speculum is inserted and the external os is swabbed with a non-irritant antiseptic solution such as Hibitane.

The anterior lip of the cervix is grasped by volsellum

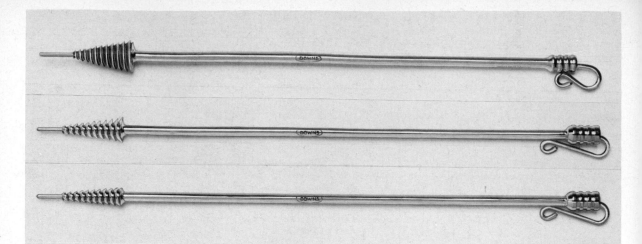

Fig. 16.2 Leech–Wilkinson cannula for hysterosalpingography (Courtesy of Downs Surgical Ltd.)

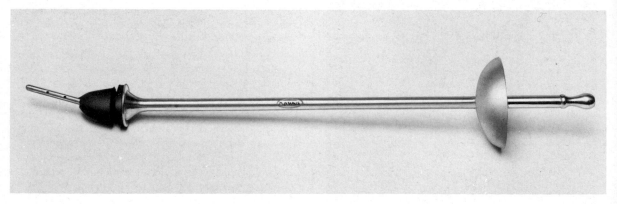

Fig. 16.3 Hayes–Provis cannula with rubber cone (Courtesy of Downs Surgical Ltd.)

forceps. A cannula is then inserted through the external os, followed by removal of the vaginal speculum. Cervical tumours, extensive cervical laceration an an abnormally small cervical canal are causes of failure of cervical cannulation.

The injection cannula The Leech–Wilkinson cannula has a conical, ridged metallic end which is introduced into the cervical canal with a screwing motion (Fig. 16.2). The insertion of this cannula is often painful and there is frequently leakage of contrast medium into the vagina.

The Green–Armytage cannula has a rubber acorn which is variable in position along the length of the straight metal cannula and provides a fairly watertight junction with the cervix. A plunger in the form of a screw allows controlled contrast medium injection.

Other varieties of straight or curved metal cannulae with rubber acorns are available (Fig. 16.3).

The suction type of cannula has become popular in recent years. Although originally described by Kjellman in 1953, the modern modification is the Malström–Westerman vacuum uterine cannula (Wright, 1961) (Fig. 16.4). The special Malström speculum accommodates the Malström–Westerman cannula and is easily removed following insertion of the cannula. Plastic caps, which are in three different sizes, fit over the external part of the cervix. A silicone rubber acorn in the centre of the cup is inserted into the cervical canal. The lumen of the cup is connected by a tube to a unit which produces a vacuum and consists of a pump, a pressure meter and a vacuum bottle. The cervix is drawn into the cup when the tip of the acorn is applied to the external os and a negative

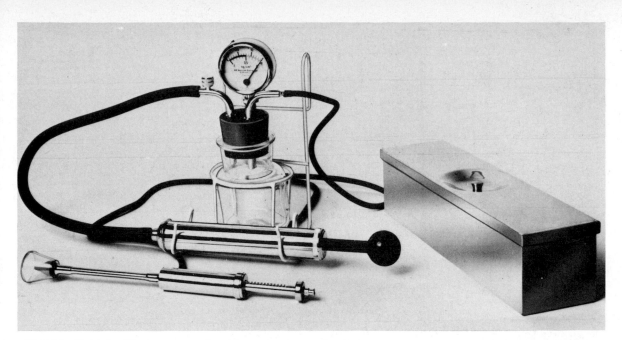

Fig. 16.4 Malström–Westerman cannula, with vacuum pump and syringe.

pressure of 0.2–0.3 kg/cm² is established by the vacuum pump. The acorn is adjustable on the cannula, a distance of 1–2 cm from the distal end usually being a suitable position. The negative pressure is increased to 0.6 kg/cm², which apposes the cannula to the cervix. The injection cannula is connected via a stopcock to a syringe containing contrast medium, care being taken to avoid the introduction of air bubbles. The stopcock is then opened to allow the injection of contrast medium. The advantages of the vacuum method are that the painful application of volsellum forceps is avoided; a watertight junction established between the cannula and cervix; traction is easily applied to the cervix; the patient may be easily rotated without dislodging the cannula; the cervical canal is well demonstrated; and traumatic bleeding is a rare occurrence. Severe cervical laceration or effacement prevent the application of the vacuum cannula. The plastic cups may be sterilized but last for only a few examinations, although aluminium cups have been found suitable.

A further method of cannulation involves the introduction of a Number 8 or 10 Foley catheter into the uterine cavity (Ansari & Nagamani, 1977) (Fig. 16.5). The balloon is then distended with 1–1.5 ml of water. The catheter tip is invariably beyond the internal os. Inevitably, the cervical canal is not visualized, a distended balloon in the mid-portion of the cervical canal causing discomfort and expulsion of the catheter. The isthmus and cervical canal may, however, be demonstrated by injecting contrast medium during the deflation and simultaneous gentle downward traction on the catheter. The timing of this manoeuvre is critical. The advantages of the method are that volsellum forceps are not required, the technique is generally atraumatic and the patient may be easily rotated after catheter insertion.

A preliminary radiograph of the pelvic cavity is only required if some dense opacity is visible on screening. The contrast medium is warmed to body temperature and is gently injected under fluoroscopic control, usually 8–12 ml being required. A lead shield protects the injector's hands. An undercouch radiograph is taken during uterine filling before the contrast opacification becomes too dense, in order to demonstrate small uterine filling defects and deformities (Fig. 16.6). Another radiograph is exposed when the uterus and Fallopian tubes are delineated and peritoneal spill is just occurring from the fimbrial ends of the tubes. A further radiograph is routinely taken 15–20 minutes later to show the pattern of peritoneal spill. While the delayed radiograph is usually taken with the patient supine, an additional radiograph in the prone position is sometimes helpful in the assessment of peritoneal spillage. All the contrast medium should have disappeared by one hour after injection, but usually remains longer in the presence of tubal obstruction. The mean radiation dose to the ovaries

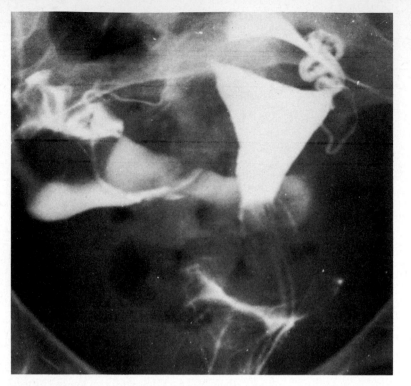

Fig. 16.5 Hysterosalpingogram with Foley catheter. Inflated balloon lies in lower uterine segment.

during HSG is of the order of 1.94 mGy (Sheikh & Yussman, 1976). The radiographic field should be restricted as much as possible. Videotape recording of the screening is a useful adjunct. Oblique and lateral radiographs are sometimes required to demonstrate uterine abnormalities, which increases radiation dose. A lateral view of the contrast filled uterus in mandatory to show the defect caused by previous Caesarean section. The assessment of uterine retroversion and anteversion is made from the pattern of movement of the uterus with traction. Traction on the cannula, and volsellum forceps when present, usually allows good filling of a malpositioned uterus and of the Fallopian tubes. Alternate relaxation and tension on the instruments, the 'butterfly manoeuvre', will also aid tubal filling and may overcome spasm.

Cornual spasm is often prevented by reassurance and a gentle technique. Glucagon is an effective agent for removing uterine and tubal spasm, being more reliable in this effect than atropine, trinitin or amyl nitrite.

The examination is concluded with demonstration of the patency or blockage of the Fallopian tubes.

Contrast media Lipiodol was first used as a contrast medium for HSG in the 1920s. Unfortunately, this oily medium carried a risk of provoking acute tubal blockage. Intravasation of Lipiodol causes pulmonary oil embolism. The high viscosity of Lipiodol necessitated a radiograph 24 hours after the procedure to determine peritoneal spill.

Water-soluble contrast media were also introduced in the 1920s but early agents tended to cause peritoneal irritation. Hysterosalpingographic contrast media must have sufficient viscosity to be retained in the uterus and Fallopian tubes, long enough for their delineation, and yet be able to give a controlled spill from the ampullae without flooding the peritoneal cavity. One group of contrast agents utilizes a large molecular size, or high concentration, to give sufficient viscosity while additives are used for this purpose in the other group.

Urografin 370 (10% sodium diatrizoate and 66% methylglucamine diatrizoate) is a popular contrast medium for HSG which depends on molecular size and concentration for its viscosity. Salpix (53% sodium acetrizoate and polyvinyl pyrolidone), which is no longer available in the UK, and Diaginol Viscous (40% sodium acetrizoate and dextran) are examples of water-soluble contrast media with viscogenic additives.

Metrizamide, a non-ionic contrast medium, has had limited use in HSG but has been found to cause no significant difference in the incidence of discomfort and pain when compared to conventional contrast media of equivalent iodine concentration (Stiris & Andrew, 1979)

Variations on basic technique

Double contrast hysterography, using a water-soluble contrast medium followed by air insufflation, has been a disappointment. There is uneven adherence of contrast medium to the endometrium, with a failure to demonstrate small defects.

Complications

Pain Insertion of the injection cannula may result in transient lower abdominal discomfort. A brief episode of sharp pain occurs when the anterior lip of the cervix is grasped by the volsellum forceps.

Distention of the uterus and Fallopian tubes by contrast medium may cause lower abdominal pain, especially in those who are apprehensive or who have a low pain threshold. A rapid injection of contrast medium also provokes this pain. Usually, this pain subsides within ten minutes.

Tubal spasm or organic tubal obstruction is also associated with pain which is sometimes severe and is maximal lateral to the midline in the lower abdomen.

Some pain often occurs on peritoneal spillage of contrast media, usually lasting for about one hour and relieved by mild analgesics. This pain is thought to result from peritoneal irritation due to the hyperosmolality of the contrast medium.

Pain occasionally commences within an hour or two of the procedure, usually disappearing within 24 hours but occasionally persisting for several days. Pelvic irritation may be the cause of this delayed pain, which must be differentiated from the pain caused by either an exacerbation of pelvic inflammation or by uterine perforation.

Pelvic infection There is a 0.25–2% incidence of pelvic infection after HSG usually an acute exacerbation of a pre-existing infection but sometimes occuring *de novo*.

Haemorrhage Application of the volsellum forceps resulting in slight spotting of blood is a common occurrence. Bleeding from the uterine cavity after HSG suggests the presence of an endometrial polyp or carcinoma. Vigorous uterine sounding or the use of a cannula whose tip extends well beyond the acorn may cause endometrial bleeding.

Uterine perforation Sounding prior to HSG is a potential cause of uterine perforation. Rough application of the cannula may cause severe cervical laceration.

Allergic phenomena Urticaria, asthma and laryngeal oedema may occur as hypersensitivity reactions in susceptible subjects.

Vasovagal attacks sometimes associated with syncope occur in a small proportion of cases.

Venous intravasation (Fig. 16.7) A fine, interlacing network of veins is seen adjacent to the borders of the opacified uterine cavity when there is intravasation of contrast medium into the venous system of the uterus. Large superficial uterine veins and veins which run along the broad ligament into the iliac veins and pampiniform plexi are also seen. The incidence of venous intravasation is 0.6–3.7%.

There are several recognized predisposing causes of venous intravasation, but often none is found. The causes include direct trauma to the endometrium from the tip of the injection cannula; various uterine abnormalities including tuberculosis, carcinoma, hypoplasia and fibroids; and tubal occlusion which leads to a high pressure of contrast medium in the uterine cavity.

Relation to other techniques

Comparative studies of laparoscopy and HSG in sterility have found concordance between both modalities in the assessment of tubal patency in 70–76% of cases (Ladipo, 1976; Kasby, 1980). Horwitz *et al.* (1979) found agreement between HSG and laparoscopic findings in 97% of cases of peritubal adhesions and in 91% of hydrosalpinges.

The unicornuate and bicornuate uterus may be demonstrated on ultrasonography. Fibroids shown or suspected on HSG may be further evaluated by ultrasonography and there is a specific ultrasonic pattern in adenomyosis.

HSG has no place in the localization of intrauterine contraceptive devices (IUCD). Ultrasonography is the preliminary investigation in the assessment of the presence and situation of an IUCD. When the device has been shown not to be within the uterine cavity, a plain radiograph of the pelvis and lower abdomen will confirm its extrauterine site.

Hydrosalpinx is shown by ultrasonography and in some cases distinction may be made between inflammatory disease and endometriosis, both of which are causes of tubal obstruction.

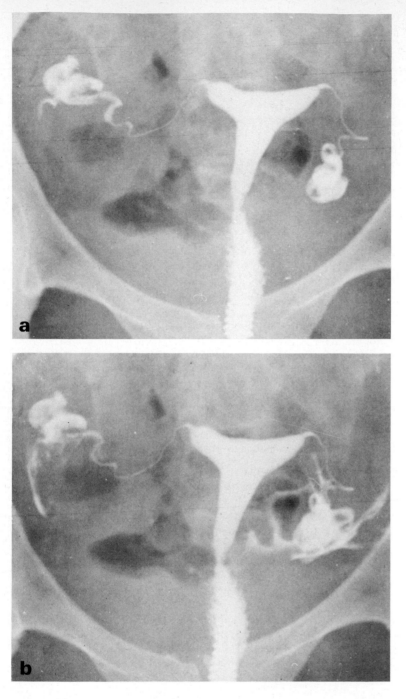

Fig. 16.6 Normal hysterosalpingogram
(a) The uterus is opacified by contrast medium and the Fallopian tubes are delineated to the ampullae.

(b) Slightly later, there is fuller delineation of both Fallopian tubes with early peritoneal spill of contrast medium.

(c) Fifteen minutes after withdrawal of cannula. Contrast medium delineates the pelvic peritoneum with no evidence of loculation.

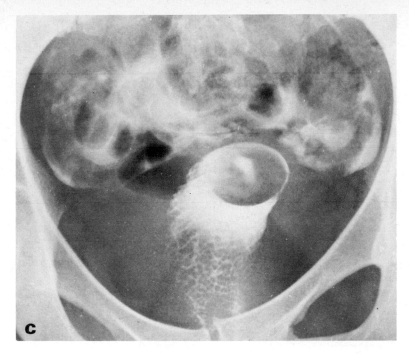

c

PELVIC PNEUMOGRAPHY

Pelvic pneumography (PPG) consists of the induction of a pneumoperitoneum followed by radiography to demonstrate the gas-delineated female pelvic organs (Fig. 16.8). The technique and applications of PPG have mainly been developed by Stein in the 1930s. Laparoscopy and ultrasonography have largely replaced PPG as a means of visualizing the female genital tract.

Indications

PPG has largely been superseded by laparoscopy and ultrasonography. When this is not available, PPG may be of use in the following situations:

1. To delineate the internal genitalia when hystero-salpingography cannot be performed, for instance in vaginal or cervical atresia and stenosis, as well as in children;
2. When adnexal pathology is suspected or cannot be excluded on pelvic examination, for instance in the obese;
3. In intersex states, the presence or absence of a uterus may be ascertained by PPG. The presence or absence of ovaries of abdominal testes may be elicited, although differentiation of ovaries from atypically situated testes or ovotestes is not possible (Lunderquist, 1968). Laparotomy is required to determine the exact gonadal status in many intersex cases, coupled with the removal of abdominal testicular structures which are prone to malignant change.
4. The presence and configuration of the ovaries may be shown in cases of amenorrhoea. The ovaries are totally absent, small or streaked in cases of primary amenorrhoea, for instance in Turner's syndrome. The polycystic ovaries of the Stein–Leventhal syndrome are also demonstrable, although the PPG diagnosis is often indefinite.
5. In infertility cases, congenital abnormalities such as hypoplasia and aplasia of the uterus and ovaries are seen, and differentiation of a bicornuate from a septate uterus may be made. Pelvic inflammatory disease and endometriosis are other causes of infertility which are shown on PPG. Stevens (1967) found a reasonable explanation for infertility in a third of patients subjected to a PPG, which contributory or confirmatory information was given in a further third, and no explanation in the remaining third of cases.

Contra-indications

1. Pelvic infection or peritonitis
2. Ascites, which results in poor visualization of the pelvic organs
3. Large mass lesions which completely fill the pelvic cavity or extend into the abdomen

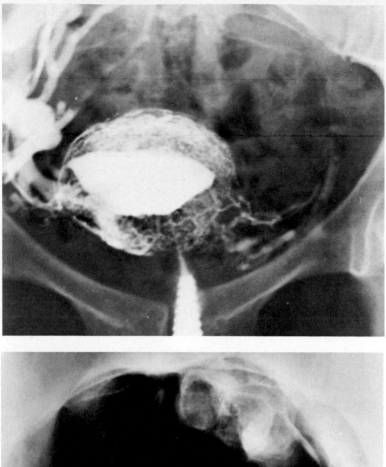

Fig. 16.7 Gross venous intravasation of contrast medium. Opacification of the veins of the uterine wall and pelvic cavity.

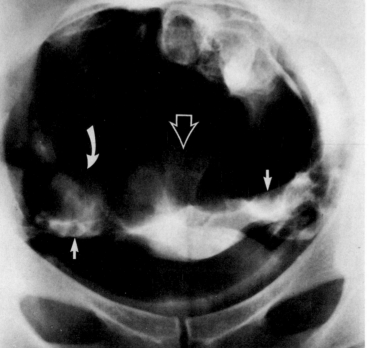

Fig. 16.8 Pelvic pneumogram. Uterus lies in centre of pelvic cavity (open arrow). The broad ligaments (small arrows) run towards the lateral pelvic walls. There is a small cyst of the right ovary (curved arrow).

4. Severe cardiac or respiratory disease, because of reduction in the patient's vital capacity when the peritoneal cavity is distended with gas and by the head down position. Carbon dioxide excretion is impaired in patients with emphysema.

Method

The patient has nothing by mouth for 12 hours, a cathartic agent and a cleansing enema preceding the examination. The bladder is emptied immediately before the establishment of the pneumoperitoneum. Usually no premedication is given to the patient. A control radiograph is taken with the patient lying prone in the head down position on the X-ray table, which is tilted 45° to the floor.

The X-ray beam is perpendicular to the floor, centred on the coccyx, with a focus film distance of 100 cm to limit magnification. Appropriate alterations are made in radiographic factors and patient positioning following the control radiograph.

The X-ray table is restored to the horizontal position and the patient lies supine. The abdomen is daubed with an antiseptic solution. A puncture site is selected immediately lateral to the rectus muscle where it intersects a line between the umbilicus and the anterior superior iliac spine, ensuring that this point is free of scars and an underlying abdominal mass. Infiltrations of the skin and abdominal wall down to the peritoneum is made with 1% lignocaine at the proposed puncture site. A short bevelled 10 cm long No. 18 or 20 spinal needle is introduced through the anaesthetized puncture point. A sudden lack of resistence is felt by the operator when the needle tip enters the peritoneal cavity.

Insertion of the needle is facilitated by the patient flexing her neck, thus increasing the tension in the abdominal musculature. The trochar is removed and the needle is connected by rubber tubing to an apparatus, such as the Maxwell pneumothorax machine, which is suitable for the introduction of gas. Air and oxygen are not used because of the risk of air embolism on accidental intravascular injection. Carbon dioxide avoids this potential hazard and, although it is rapidly absorbed from the peritoneal cavity there is usually sufficient time to obtain a sastisfactory examination. Nitrous oxide is a suitable alternative. When carbon dioxide is used, 1200 ml of gas from a Sparklet cylinder is allowed to enter the peritoneal cavity over 10 minutes. A total of 600 ml is used in infants and 800 ml in children. The inadvertent introduction of gas into the abdominal wall results in palpable crepitus and the lack of a free rise in gas pressure. Injection of gas into the bowel is a rare complication but will be harmless, with colic as an outcome. Shoulder tip pain following the establishment of the pneumoperitoneum is relieved by tilting the patient into a head down position. The needle is removed, a plaster is placed on the puncture site, and the patient is then turned prone. Three radiographs are taken, one as described for the control radiograph and others with the tube angled 10° in caudad and cephalad directions. A lateral radiograph using a horizontal beam is sometimes useful.

Modifications of basic technique

The gas may be introduced into the pelvic cavity by uterotubal insufflation, using a vacuum cannula or a Foley catheter within the cervical canal. This method is unsuccessful in cases of tubal occlusion, where cervical intubation is impossible, and in children.

Complications

1. Shoulder pain, secondary to subphrenic irritation (see Method)
2. Colon perforation (see Method)
3. A pneumothorax will occur in cases where there is a congenital defect in the diaphragm and overlying parietal pleura.

Relationship to other procedures

Laparoscopy, which gives a direct view of the pelvic organs and enables biopsy to be made, and ultrasonography has replaced PPG in most centres. While one of the prime uses of PPG was assessment of the ovaries in the Stein–Leventhal syndrome, it is now recognized that ovarian size is often normal in this condition (Weigen & Stevens, 1967).

VAGINOGRAPHY

Indications

Vaginography is used to demonstrate:
1. Fistulae from the vagina to the ureter, bladder or rectum (Wolfson, 1968)
2. Congenital or acquired abnormalities of the vagina, such as diverticula (Coe, 1963)
3. Reflux of contrast medium up a vaginal ectopic ureter (Katzen & Trachtman, 1954).

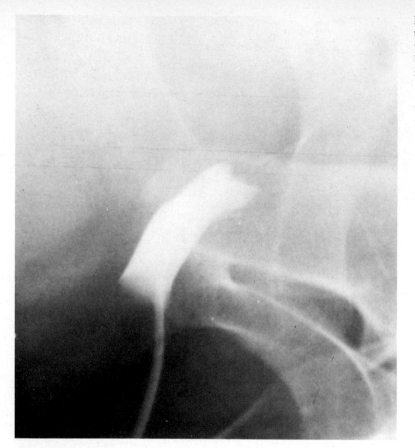

Fig. 16.9 Normal vaginogram. Contrast medium has been injected into the vagina via a balloon catheter. The balloon provided a water-tight junction in the lower part of the vagina.

Contra-indications

1. Acute vaginitis
2. Imperforate hymen or vaginal atresia.

Technique

A Foley catheter is inserted into the vagina and its 30 ml balloon is distended with air. It is imperative that the inflated balloon fits snugly into the lower part of the vagina. Gentle traction is then applied to the catheter to ensure that the inflated balloon fits securely above the introitus. Water-soluble contrast medium, for instance Conray 280 or Urografin 290, is injected through the catheter after a water-tight junction has been established between the balloon and the vagina. Usually 20–30 ml of contrast medium is required and spot radiographs are then taken in the antero-lateral, lateral, and sometimes oblique positions (Fig. 16.9). Steady traction is maintained on the catheter during the injection of contrast medium.

FETOGRAPHY

The injection of water-soluble contrast medium into the amniotic sac has been used in the past to determine fetal abnormalities and viability as well as placental localization. Ultrasonography now provides this information without the disadvantages of amniocentesis and irradiation. There is still, however, a limited use for coating the fetus with a lipid-soluble contrast medium to show soft tissue detail. Fetography has been described by Lennon (1967).

Indications

Soft tissue abnormalities, such as cystic hygromas of the neck and meningocele, are shown by fetography. Intrauterine transfusion may be facilitated when the fetal contour is delineated by contrast medium, particularly as the fetal outline remains visible for about two weeks, when ultrasonography is not available.

Fig. 16.10 Fetography. Normal fetus with its surface delineated by Myodil.

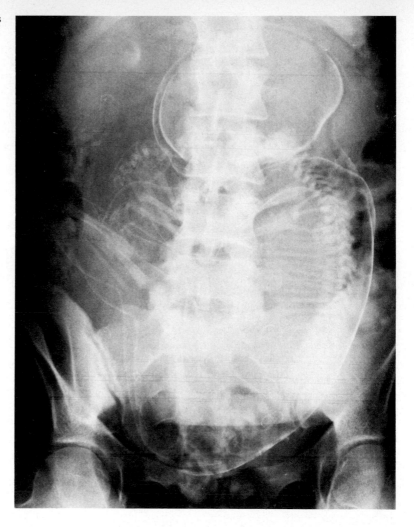

Contra-indications

Fetography should only be performed in the last two months of pregnancy. The technique depends on a lipid-soluble contrast medium combining with the vernix caseosa, which itself contains a large element of fat. Fetography is contra-indicated during labour.

Method

The skin and underlying soft tissues of the maternal abdomen are infiltrated with 1% lignocaine at a point below and lateral to the umbilucus, avoiding the side on which the fetal spine lies. The amniotic cavity is entered from this point by an 18 gauge needle and stylette with a teflon sheath. A small amount of amniotic fluid is aspirated and 6 ml of Myodil (iophendylate) are injected through the Teflon can-

nula. The injection should stop if there is any increase in resistance to the flow of contrast medium or any sudden movement of the fetus. The correct position of the needle is then confirmed by fluoroscopy of the needle before recommencing the injection. The maternal abdomen is then radiographed in the appropriate prone oblique projection 24 hours after the introduction of contrast medium. The fetal soft tissue should be well-delineated by this time (Fig. 16.10).

Complications

The complications of fetography include those of amniocentesis namely premature labour, accidental haemorrhage, infection, fetal exsanguination from laceration of the placenta or umbilical cord, and contamination of maternal circulation by fetal blood cells. Fortunately, all these complications are very uncommon. The inadvertent injection of contrast medium into the soft tissues of the fetus causes skin necrosis (Grech & Spitz, 1977). Careful use of the teflon coated cannula should prevent this complication. Following delivery, there is good healing of the skin necrosis with conservative treatment and the frequent application of 1% mercurochrome.

Relationship to other diagnostic techniques

Centres with good ultrasonographic services would have little or no call upon fetography. However, fetography is useful where ultrasound cannot provide the required information.

REFERENCES

Hysterosalpingography

Ansari A. H. & Nagamani M. (1977) Foley catheter for salpingography, pneumography, tubal insufflation and hydrotubation. *Obstet. Gynec.*, **50**, 108–12.

Horwitz R. C., Morton P. C. G. & Hugo P. (1979) A radiological approach to infertility—hysterosalpingography. *Brit. J. Radiol.*, **52**, 225–62,

Keirse M. J. & Vandervellen R. (1972) A comparison of hysterosalpingography and laparoscopy in the investigation of infertility. *Obstet. Gynec.*, **41**, 685–8.

Ladipo O. A. (1976) Tests of tubal patency. Comparison of laparoscopy and hysterosalpingography. *Brit. med. J.*, **ii**, 1297–8.

Pontifex G., Trichopoulos D. & Karpathios S. (1972) Hysterosalpingography in the diagnosis of infertility (statistical analysis of 3437 cases) *Fertil. Steril.*, **23**, 829–33.

Sheikh G. & Yussman M. A. (1976) Radiation exposure of ovaries during hysterosalpingography. *Amer. J. Obstet. Gynec.*, **124**, 307–10.

Stiris G. Andrew E. (1979) Hysterosalpingography with Amipaque. *Radiology*, **130**, 795–6.

Whitehouse G. H. (1981) *Gynaecological Radiology*. Blackwell Scientific Publications, Oxford.

Wright J. T. (1961) A new method for hysterosalpingography. *Brit. J. Radiol.*, **34**, 465–7.

Pelvic Pneumography

Lunderquist A. (1968) Pneumopelvigraphy in the early diagnosis of intersexuality. *Amer. J. Roentgenol.*, **103**, 202–9.

Stevens G. M. (1967) Pelvic pneumography in the assessment of infertility. *Radiol. Clin. N. Amer.*, **5**, 87–103.

Weigen J. F. & Stevens G. M. (1967) Pelvic pneumography in the diagnosis of polycystic disease of the ovary, including Stein–Leventhal syndrome. *Amer. J. Roentgenol.*, **100**, 680–7.

Vaginography

Coe F. O. (1963) Vaginography. *Amer. J. Roentgenol.*, **90**, 721–7.

Katzen P & Trachtman B. (1954) Diagnosis of vaginal ectopic ureter by vaginogram. *J. Urol.*, **72**, 808–11.

Wolfson J. J. (1964) Vaginography for detection of ureterovaginal, vesicovaginal and rectovaginal fistules, with case reports. *Radiology*, **83**, 438–44.

Fetography

Grech P. & Spitz L. (1977) Fetal complications of amniography. *Brit. J. Radiol.*, **50**, 110–12.

Lennon G. G. (1967) Intrauterine foetal visualization. *J. Obstet. Gynaec. Brit. Cwlth.*, **74**, 227–9.

G. H. WHITEHOUSE

CAVERNOSOGRAPHY

Cavernosography is the delineation by contrast medium of the erectile tissue of the penis.

Indications

Cavernosography is sometimes performed to demonstrate the extent of Peyronie's disease, a condition where fibrous plaques develop within the corpora cavernosa, and in the investigation of priapism (Fitzpatrick, 1973), male erectile dysfunction (Pryor, 1982) and penile trauma (Grossman et al., 1982).

Contra-indications

A history of allergic reaction to contrast medium.

Method

Thomas and Rose (1972), Ney et al. (1976) and Velcek and Evans (1982) have described the techniques and use of cavernosography. The penis is first cleaned by antiseptic solution. The skin, fascia and corpus cavernosum on one side of the midline, just proximal to the glans, are infiltrated with 1% lignocaine. A 21 gauge butterfly needle with polythene connecting tube is attached to a syringe containing 10 ml of normal saline. The needle is inserted into the shaft of the penis at the site of injection with the local anaesthetic agent. A small amount of saline is carefully injected to ensure that the tip of needle is correctly positioned within the corpus cavernosum. A rubber catheter is gently tightened around the base of the penis to prevent the contrast medium from flowing rapidly into the pudendal veins, but a tourniquet may not be used when the venous outflow from the penis is of particular interest.

Urografin 290 or Conray 280 are suitable contrast media, approximately 20 ml being injected through the butterfly needle. The corpora cavernosa on both sides are opacified from a unilateral contrast injection. The penis becomes temporarily erect at this stage. Radiographs are taken in the A–P, lateral and oblique projections (Fig. 17.1). The tourniquet is then released and the butterfly needle flushed through with saline before its removal at the end of the examination.

Complications

Priapism with impotence is a rare complication of cavernosography and is due to venous thrombosis. Haematoma and abscess formation at the puncture site are rare complications (Velcek & Evans, 1982).

REFERENCES

Fitzpatrick T. J. (1973) Spongiosograms and cavernosograms: a study of their value in priapism. *J. Urol.*, **109**, 843–6.
Grossman H., Gray R. R., St. Louis E. L., Casey R., Keresteci A. G. & Elliott D. S. (1982) The role of corpus cavernosography in acute 'fracture' of the penis. *Radiology*, **144**, 787–8.
Ney C., Miller H. L. & Friedenberg R. M. (1976) Various applications of corpus cavernosography. *Radiology*, **119**, 69–73.
Prior J. P. (1982) Cavernosography. *Brit. med. J.*, **285**, 1443.
Thomas M. L. & Rose D. H. (1972) Peyronie's disease demonstrated by cavernosography. *Acta Radiol. Diag.*, **12**, 221–4.
Velcek D. & Evans J. (1982) Cavernosography. *Radiology*, **144**, 781–5.

VESICULOGRAPHY

Opacification of the seminal vesicles by radiographic contrast medium was first performed by Belford some 70 years ago. Vesiculography is not a commonly performed investigation.

Indications

Perineal pain has often been an indication for vesiculography in the past, but is a dubious reason for performing this invasive procedure. Vesiculography has also been performed in cases of infertility. Differentiation between hyperplasia and carcinoma of the prostate has been claimed by vesiculography but is unreliable.

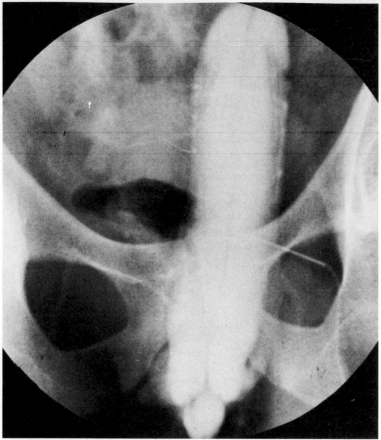

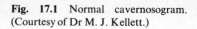
Fig. 17.1 Normal cavernosogram. (Courtesy of Dr M. J. Kellett.)

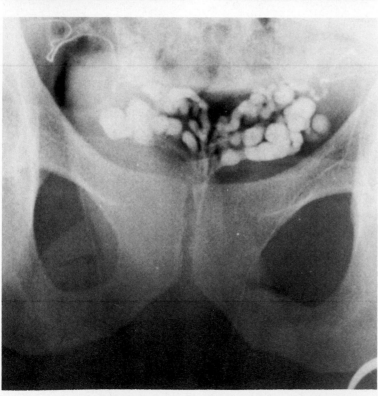

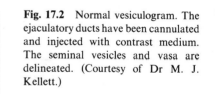
Fig. 17.2 Normal vesiculogram. The ejaculatory ducts have been cannulated and injected with contrast medium. The seminal vesicles and vasa are delineated. (Courtesy of Dr M. J. Kellett.)

Contra-indications

Active prostatitis and epidydimo-orchitis are contra-indications to vesiculography.

Technique

Direct injection of vas deferens (Abeshouse et al., 1954)

The genital region is shaved, daubed with antiseptic solution, and is draped with sterile towels. The vas is palpated in the upper part of the scrotum and is isolated and held in a fixed position under the skin. An injection of 1% lignocaine is made into the skin, subcutaneous tissues and around the vas. The skin is incised for 2 cm in line with, and overlying, the vas. The short segment of the vas is then isolated and cleared of overlying connective tissue. Gentle traction is applied to this segment by means of a loose suture encircling the vas. A 20 gauge, short bevelled needle is inserted into the vas and pointed towards the seminal vesicle. The same procedure is performed on the other side. A small amount of water-soluble contrast medium, 1.5–2 ml of Urografin 290 or Conray 280, is slowly injected into each vas in turn. The vasa, seminal vesicles and ejaculatory ducts are delineated by this method. A single radiograph is taken in the A–P projection with the X-ray beam centred over the symphysis pubis (Fig. 17.2). Suturing of the skin incision completes the investigation. Seminal vesiculography may be incorporated with a surgical exploration of the genitalia under general anaesthesia.

Transurethral route (Herbst et al., 1939)

The orifices of the ejaculatory ducts on the verumontanum may be directly catheterized during urethroscopy. It is a difficult technique and perforation of the ejaculatory duct wall by the catheter is a hazard. A 3 or 4 French gauge ureteric catheter is inserted for 1–3 cm along each ejaculatory duct. The urethroscope has a specially angled guide to assist catheterization. A slow injection of 2 ml Urografin 290 is followed by an A–P radiograph of the pelvic cavity and symphysis pubis.

REFERENCES

Abeshouse B. S., Heller E. & Salik J. O. (1954) Vasoepididymography and vasoseminal vesiculography. *J. Urol.*, **72**, 983–91.

Herbst R. H. & Merricks J. W. (1939) Visualization and treatment of seminal vesiculitis by catheterization and dilatation of ejaculatory ducts. *J. Urol.*, **41**, 733–50.

SECTION 5
THE CENTRAL NERVOUS SYSTEM

The Spinal Canal

R. G. GRAINGER

Myelography is the radiological visualization of the spinal cord, cauda equina and the surrounding subarachnoid space. Contrast medium must be added to the cerebro-spinal fluid (CSF) in the subarachnoid space in order to produce the differential radiological contrast necessary for visualization of the cord and its surroundings.

There are three types of contrast medium which may be so injected, each with distinctive physical and radiographic properties and requiring different radiological techniques. The three types of contrast medium are:

1. Radio-opaque iodinated oil, e.g. iophendylate (Myodil, Pantopaque)
2. Water-soluble iodinated contrast media, e.g. metrizamide (Amipaque), iopamidol (Niopam) and iohexol (Omnipaque).
3. Gas, e.g. air, carbon dioxide or oxygen.

The last ten years have seen a dramatic change in the contrast media and techniques for myelography and a critical reappraisal of the optimal methods to be used for different clinical situations.

Until 1970, practically all myelographic examinations in English-speaking countries were performed with iophendylate oil (Myodil, Pantopaque) because there was no other reasonably safe and convenient myelographic contrast agent. Methiodal was considered to be far too toxic (Shapiro, 1968).

In Scandinavia, and some other European countries, iophendylate oil was regarded as unsuitable for myelography as it causes adhesive arachnoiditis. Instead, gas was used for the radiological demonstration of the spinal cord, and methiodal (Abrodil)—a water-soluble iodinated medium introduced by Lidström and Arnell in 1931—was used for lumbo-sacral radiculography. Methiodal, however, has major radiographic, technical, diagnostic and neurotoxic limitations (Grainger et al., 1971).

Since 1970, first meglumine iothalamate (Conray 280), then meglumine iocarmate (Dimer X) and more recently metrizamide (Amipaque), iopamidol (Niopam) and iohexol (Omnipaque) were introduced as progressively safer and more effective water-soluble myelographic contrast media. Metrizamide has been available since 1977 and has completely displaced methiodal, meglumine iothalamate and meglumine iocarmate (Grainger et al., 1976).

Metrizamide and the newer water-soluble agents, e.g. iopamidol and iohexol have almost completely replaced iophendylate oil for all cauda equina, lumbo-sacral radiculography and lumbar myelography. Water-soluble media are the contrast media of choice for most dorsal myelography and for an increasing number of cervical myelograms. The advantages and disadvantages of metrizamide, iopamidol and iohexol as compared to iophendylate oil and gas myelography are set out in Table 18.1.

Myelography is essentially an in-patient procedure and, except in exceptional circumstances, the patient should be retained in hospital at least 20–24 hours after the procedure.

As water-soluble myelography and oil myelography are completely different radiological examinations, they will be discussed separately. Gas myelography is now rarely utilized as it has been effectively replaced by water-soluble contrast agents. Myelography in infants is described in the section on Paediatric Radiology, p. 331.

Indications for myelography

There must be firm clinical indications for myelography, which is always uncomfortable for the patient and is frequently followed by considerable headache. The essential consideration is that there is the definite prospect that the result of the examination will affect the subsequent management of the patient. Myelography is virtually a procedure for pre-operative assessment and will rarely be indicated if there is no possibility of surgical intervention.

The most frequent indication is the lumbago-sciatica syndrome with suspected compression of a lumbo-sacral nerve root by prolapse of a degenerated intervertebral disc, but only in those patients who have not responded to conservative treatment. The most frequent indication for cervical myelography is degenerative cervical spondylosis with suspected compression of the nerve roots or spinal cord.

Any suspected space-occupying or other operable lesion of the spinal cord, its meninges or the adjacent spinal canal, usually merits myelography. It is very important to localize and to distinguish these poten-

Table 18.1 The advantages and disadvantages of the different contrast media.

Contrast medium	Advantages	Disadvantages
Aqueous: metrizamide, iopamidol iohexol	Optimal visualization of spinal cord, cauda equina, nerve roots, subarachnoid space. Preferred method.	Metrizamide is expensive. Acute neurotoxicity. Cervical myelography rather difficult.
Oil: iophendylate	Sometimes easier technique. Repeatable after single injection. No acute toxicity. Total myelography possible.	Poor visualization of nerve roots. Suboptimal visualization of spinal cord and subarachnoid space. Delayed arachnoiditis.
Gas: air, CO_2, oxygen	Cheap. Non-toxic. Good visualization of varying cord size—'collapsing' cord.	Nerve roots not seen. Very difficult time-consuming technique. Poor radiographic contrast. Now rarely used.

tially operable lesions from non-surgical disease, such as demyelinating or degenerative disease of the spinal cord.

Contra-indications to myelography

Skin sepsis over the spinal puncture site and infection of the subarachnoid space or meninges are absolute contra-indications. Sensitivity to iophendylate or water-soluble agents, e.g. metrizamide or iopamidol, is very unusual, especially with the latter products. The oil examination is best avoided if there is any question of iodine sensitivity. A previous reaction to an injection of intravascular contrast medium is a relative contra-indication to water-soluble contrast myelography. All aqueous contrast agents are potentially epileptogenic and water-soluble myelography, particularly of the cervical spine, is probably best avoided in an epileptic patient. If aqueous myelography is utilized in such a patient, anti-epileptic drugs such as diazepam 5 mg or phenobarbitone 120 mg, should be given both before and after the procedure, and repeated as necessary.

Myelography should be deferred if there has been a lumbar puncture in the preceding 7 days, as the contrast medium may well be injected into a pool of CSF which frequently leaks into the epidural and subdural spaces after a simple lumbar puncture.

WATER-SOLUBLE MYELOGRAPHY

Lumbar myelography and lumbo-sacral radiculography

Contrast medium

Metrizamide (Amipaque) is a substituted amide formulated from a tri-iodinated substituted benzoic acid. Being an amide and not a salt, it does not dissociate in solution. Metrizamide is the first non-ionic iodinated radiological contrast medium and has an osmolality of about one-third of that of solutions of conventional contrast media of the same iodine concentration (*Acta Radiologica* Suppl. Nos. 335 (1973) and 335 (1977); Grainger, 1981).

As metrizamide cannot be autoclaved, it is supplied as freeze-dried lyophilized powder in vials containing 6.75 g (3250 mg iodine) and 3.75 (1807 mg iodine) of the dried powder, together with ampoules of sterile very dilute sodium bicarbonate (5 mg per 100 ml) as solvent.

The volume of solvent required to produce solutions of pre-selected concentrations, is shown in Table 18.2.

The 6.75 g vial is recommended for all lumbar and lumbo-sacral myelography, radiculography and dorsal myelography in the adult. The 6.75 g metrizamide bottle is necessary for cervical myelography performed by the lumbar puncture technique, but 3.75 g may suffice if the examination is being performed by direct cervical puncture. For small children the 3.75 g vial is usually adequate for all myelographic examinations.

A concentration of 170 mg iodine/ml, which is isotonic with CSF, is recommended for lumbar myelography in the small adult. For heavy adults, a solution of 220 or 240 mg iodine/ml is usually preferred.

Almost the entire contents of the 6.75 g bottle, utilizing about 10–16 ml of a solution to give an iodine concentration of 170–240 mg/ml, is used for lumbar myelography and radiculography in the adult. A total dose of more than 3000 mg of iodine, as metrizamide, should not be injected into the subarachnoid space on a single examination.

After the radiologist has 'surgically scrubbed' and

Table 18.2 Dissolution for vial containing Amipaque (metrizamide).

Concentration mg I/ml	3.75 g Amipaque Volume of solvent ml	6.75 g Amipaque Volume of solvent ml
100*	16.4	29.5
110*	14.7	26.5
120*	13.5	24.0
130*	12.2	22.0
140*	11.2	20.2
150*	10.2	18.6
160*	9.6	17.3
170	*8.9*	*16.1*
180	8.3	15.0
190	7.8	14.0
200	7.3	13.2
210	6.9	12.4
220	6.5	11.7
230	6.1	11.1
240	5.8	10.5
250	5.5	10.0
260	5.2	9.4
270	5.0	9.0
280	4.7	8.5
290	4.5	8.1
300	4.3	7.8
	The volume of the final solution will equal the volume of the solvent + 1.7 ml	The volume of the final solution will equal the volume of the solvent + 3.1 ml

* In order to avoid hypotonicity when preparing solutions of lower concentrations than 170 mg I/ml, dilute with solvent to about 170 ml I/ml and then dilute further with cerebrospinal fluid or physiological saline solution.

donned sterile gloves, the solution of metrizamide is prepared by injecting the required volume of solvent into the vial. Complete solution of the powder is essential before injection. Some radiologists prefer to filter the solution through a filter needle or a Millipore filter in an attempt to remove any particulate matter. Palmers (1981) claims a 30% reduction in patient headache following the use of a 22 micron Millipore filter.

Iopamidol (Niopam) synthesized by Bracco Industria Chimica S.p.a. of Milan, Italy, became available for myelography in the UK in autumn 1982, and is still being evaluated.

Iopamidol is the first of the second generation of non-ionic water-soluble contrast agents which, like metrizamide, are substituted amide derivatives of tri-iodinated substituted benzoic acids. The advantages of iopamidol are that it is about one-third the cost of metrizamide, and is stable and autoclavable in solution. It is available in sterile ampoules in concentrations of 200, 300 and 370 mg I/ml.

The amount of iopamidol used for lumbar myelography is the same as for metrizamide, i.e. 2000–3000 mg Iodine. This can be injected either as 10–15 ml of the 200 strength or 7–10 ml of the 300 concentration of iopamidol.

For cervical myelography, 6–10 ml either of the 200 or 300 strength is advised depending on the size of the patient, the clinical circumstances and whether the upper dorsal region is to be visualized. Concentrations of intermediate strength can be readily obtained by diluting iopamidol 300 with CSF or sterile water.

The myelographic technique using iopamidol is identical with that for metrizamide. Iopamidol tends to move and dilute more readily than does metrizamide and care must be exercised to tilt the patient very slowly. It is probable that post-myelographic headache occurs less frequently and less severely after iopamidol than after metrizamide.

Iohexol (Omnipaque) another non-ionic amide, synthesized by Nyegaard & Co., A/S of Oslo, Norway, will be available for myelography in the UK in 1983. Iohexol is similar to iopamidol, but may be even less neurotoxic.

Premedication

No sedative premedication is necessary unless the patient is unusually nervous, when 5 mg diazepam is given by mouth or intramuscular injection. The procedure is explained to the patient and his confidence gained. A Consent Form must be signed by the patient and doctor. An alert, cooperative and relaxed patient is a great asset. The patient should be well-hydrated, but no food or drink is allowed for the previous three hours in order to reduce the possibility of vomiting.

Incompatible drugs

All water-soluble contrast media, are epileptogenic when in contact with central nervous tissue. Drugs which reduce the epileptogenic threshold, such as the phenothiazines (Hindmarsh *et al.*, 1975), should be excluded for the preceding two days and the two days following the procedure. There is, however, some doubt as to how important is this drug incompatibility.

Needle

A pre-sterilized, disposable, thin-walled, short bevel, small gauge needle, 22 SWG, 9 cm long, is recommended. A larger diameter needle makes a larger hole in the theca, permits more CSF to escape after the examination when the patient lies head up, and therefore causes more post-lumbar puncture headache. A long pointed bevel increases the chance of an extra-arachnoid injection.

Puncture site

Conventional frontal and lateral radiographs of the lumbo-sacral spine must always be examined by the radiologist before attempting lumbar puncture for myelography. Congenital or acquired lesions, rotations and scoliosis are noted and the puncture approach is modified accordingly.

Lumbar puncture is recommended at L3/4 interspace, the iliac crest usually being at the level of L4 vertebra.

Local anaesthetic

Local anaesthetic is not recommended as its introduction is probably more painful than the skilful insertion of the 22 SWG lumbar puncture needle. Should the patient be nervous or should a larger needle be used, then 1% lignocaine can be used to infiltrate the skin, subcutaneous tissues and distal portion of the chosen interspinous ligament.

Lumbar puncture

The procedure must be performed with strict asepsis. The radiologist must surgically scrub his hands, wear sterile disposable 'rubber' gloves and use a non-touch technique. Surgical gown and masks are not usually worn but are an added precaution.

The skin over the mid-line lumbar region is shaved if necessary and sterilized with a suitable skin antiseptic, for instance 0.05% Chlorhexide in alcohol. All excess sterilizing agent must be removed by swab and great care is taken to ensure that none has contaminated the needle or the contrast medium.

The patient sits upright on the horizontal X-ray table, with the spine erect and no rotation or lateral tilt, the shoulders being level and horizontal. The patient's legs hang over the side of the table. Just before the lumbar puncture, the patient is asked to lean forwards slightly to reduce the normal lumbar lordosis and to open the lumbar inter-spinous spaces.

An alternative position for lumbar puncture is for the patient to lie in the lateral decubitus position with the spine parallel to the long axis of the horizontal X-ray table. The patient must then lie with the coronal plane perpendicular to the table-top, the knees being flexed towards the chest to induce a lumbar kyphosis. The X-ray table must be tilted 15° foot-down during the injection of contrast medium in order to collect the latter in the lumbo-sacral cul-de-sac.

The erect posture is preferred for lumbar puncture because it is often more comfortable for the patient, as well as distending the lumbar subarachnoid sac and reducing the likelihood of extra-arachnoid injection. The lateral decubitus position is preferred if the patient cannot comfortably sit upright, or if it is desired to fluoroscope during the injection or to take horizontal ray radiographs. In the latter circumstances, the patient lies with the suspected lesion on the dependent side and the first radiographic exposures are made in this position.

The lumbar puncture is made in the conventional way. CSF must flow freely, even when the needle has been rotated to vary the direction of the bevel. Five millilitres of CSF are collected and sent to the laboratory. If the needle does not enter the subarachnoid space at the first attempt, it is withdrawn a little and reinserted in the mid-line with the hub depressed a few degrees and the needle angled upwards. The next cephalad or caudal interspace may be used if the approach through the first attempt at L3/L4 interspinous space is unsuccessful. It is very important to achieve a clean lumbar puncture before the injection of contrast medium. If there is any doubt, then the patient should be assisted to lie down in the lateral decubitus position, the X-ray table tilted 15° foot down and fluoroscopy utilized to confirm that the needle tip is correctly sited. A few drops of contrast medium are injected via a short connecting tube and the contrast medium is seen to drop through the CSF into its most dependent part if the needle has been correctly placed into the subarachnoid space.

Injection of contrast medium

Fluoroscopy is not routine during the injection of contrast agent unless there is uncertainty of the adequacy of the lumbar puncture. If necessary, fluoroscopy during the injection is easily performed, using the undercouch X-ray tube with the patient in the lateral decubitus position.

The contrast medium solution contained in a 20 ml sterile disposable syringe is connected to the inserted lumbar puncture needle, either directly or by a short length of sterile plastic connecting tube. The metrizamide or iopamidol solution is injected smoothly over a period of 30–60 s, rapid squirts of contrast agent cause turbulence in the CSF with unnecessary and undesirable dilution of the contrast medium. Having

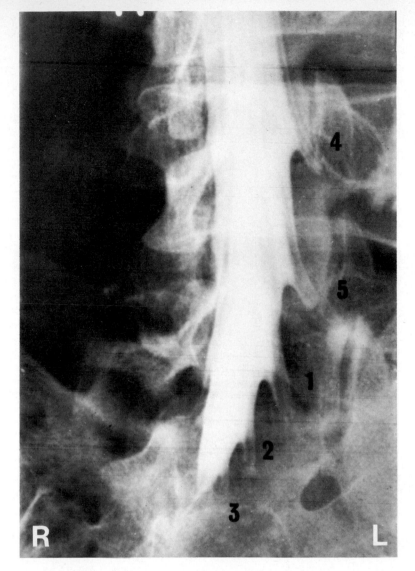

Fig. 18.1 Normal prone-oblique lumbo-sacral water-soluble myelogram.

Patient prone and rotated 20° with left side elevated. Overcouch X-ray tube. Table tilted 45° foot end down. The nerve roots are enumerated.

completed the injection of contrast agent, the lumbar puncture needle is withdrawn and the skin puncture sealed with a sterile dressing.

Patient movement

Jerky, rapid patient movements must be avoided at all costs in order not to disperse and dilute the injected aqueous contrast medium with CSF.

Before the patient is moved from the sitting position, the X-ray table is tilted 20° foot end down. The patient is then gently and slowly assisted to change posture from the sitting position into the prone position. It is essential always to maintain the patient's sacrum *below* the level of the upper lumbar spine.

X-ray table tilt

Table movement must be smooth, jerky movement being avoided in order to retain the bolus of contrast medium. For water-soluble myelography of any region, a table head-down tilt of more than 25–30° is rarely required.

The first radiographs to show the sacral cul-de-sac of the subarachnoid space are taken with the patient prone and the X-ray table tilted 45° foot end down (Fig. 18.1 and 18.2a). The table is then brought into the horizontal position and radiographs are taken of the upper and mid-lumbar region (Fig. 18.2b). A slight adverse tilt, 10° head down is often necessary to move the bolus of contrast medium into the dorsi-lumbar junction region.

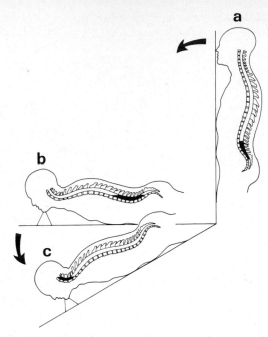

Fig. 18.2 (a) Patient erect. Contrast medium occupies lumbo-sacral subarachnoid cul-de-sac.
(b) Patient tilted horizontal. Head and neck extended. Contrast medium in upper- and mid-lumbar region prevented from entering dorsal region by lumbar lordosis and dorsal kyphosis.
(c) Patient tilted 20–30° head end down. Head and neck well extended exaggerating cervical lordosis in which contrast medium collects.

Fluoroscopy

Fluoroscopy with an image intensifier, on the undercouch or overcouch tube, is necessary to control the movement of the contrast medium, to obtain radiographs which cover the entire lumbo-sacral region and to select optimal oblique projections. Lateral fluoroscopy with a horizontal tube is not necessary for lumbar or dorsal water-soluble myelography but it facilitates oil myelography of the lumbar dorsal or cervical region.

Radiography

As the radio-opacity of metrizamide or iopamidol is much less than iophendylate and as it becomes progressively less dense due to dilution, dispersion and absorption during the procedure, radiography is commenced within a few minutes of the injection and maximal radiographic contrast is provided by a low kV (60–75) for the frontal and oblique projections and high Ma with a fast film-screen combination. A short

exposure time is advisable to reduce movement blur. All exposures must be taken with an absorption grid and with a well collimated X-ray beam.

Radiographic projections

The first radiographs are taken with the foot end of the table tilted at 45° down. The frontal films are taken with the patient prone (Fig. 18.2). The prone oblique films are taken with the patient rotating in his own long axis, the entire right side and then the entire left side of the patient being rotated in turn off the table about 15–25° in order to align parallel to the table top the lumbo-sacral nerve roots as they emerge through the exit foramina. The nerve roots on the elevated side, with the patient prone, are projected on the radiograph (Fig. 18.1 and 18.3b). All these radiographs are taken on the explorator under fluoroscopic control using the frontal (undercouch) X-ray tube. Several radiographs with different degrees of obliquity may well be necessary to see optimal detail of all of the lumbo-sacral nerve roots.

A lateral view of the lower lumbar spine and lumbo-sacral junction is then taken in either of two ways:

1. The patient turns slowly into lateral decubitus: the X-ray table is still tilted 45° foot down. A true lateral radiograph is then taken on the explorator using the undercouch (frontal) tube (Fig. 18.4b), or
2. The table is still tilted 45° foot down. A shoot through lateral view may be obtained, without moving the prone patient, by using a second (lateral) X-ray tube shooting horizontally across the table (Fig. 18.4a).

Method 1 is simpler, quicker and does not require a second X-ray tube. There is little practical advantage in method 2 for water-soluble myelography, but that technique is essential for oil lumbar myelography (Fig. 18.4a).

Having checked the radiographs of the lumbo-sacral region, the X-ray table is then tilted into the horizontal with the patient prone. This moves the bolus of contrast medium into the upper and mid-lumbar spine; frontal, oblique and lateral radiographs of this region are obtained as previously described (Fig. 18.2b).

Accessory radiographic projections

Lateral decubitus projections are taken with a horizontal ray from a second (lateral) X-ray tube. The contrast medium, being heavier than CSF, layers on the dependent side of the subarachnoid space. This view is therefore most appropriate when the contrast

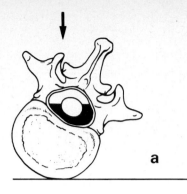

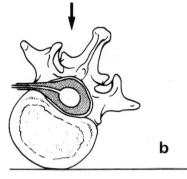

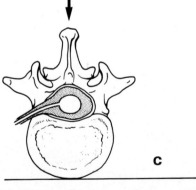

Fig. 18.3 Oblique projections to show emerging spinal nerve roots and their subarachnoid sleeves.
(a) Patient rotated 20–30°. Using oily medium, the nerve root sleeve parallel to the table top (the upper most nerve root) *may not* be exposed to the contrast medium.
(b) Patient rotated 20–30°. Using a water-soluble medium, the nerve root parallel to the table top *is* well exposed to the contrast medium and, being parallel to the films, is ideally projected.
(c) With patient prone, a vertical X-ray beam will foreshorten the projection of the nerve roots and their sleeves.

medium has been injected with the patient in the lateral decubitus position with the suspected disease side dependent. With the patient's back towards the lateral X-ray tube and the patient's abdomen adjacent to the cassette, rotation of the (lateral decubitus) patient 15° upper side towards the cassette and away from the tube will project the dependent nerve roots parallel to the film (Fig. 18.5). The dependent nerve roots are particularly well-demonstrated on this oblique lateral decubitus projection but only occasionally does it reveal lesions which are not adequately seen on good quality prone oblique radiographs taken on the explorator with the undercouch (frontal) tube. Having checked the diagnostic quality of the first lateral decubitus radiograph, the patient may be gently rotated through 150° about his long axis into the opposite oblique lateral decubitus and a further film taken of the lumbo-sacral nerve roots which were previously uppermost but are now dependent.

As the lower lumbo-sacral nerve roots are usually under suspicion in the lumbago-sciatica syndrome, the X-ray table should be tilted 15–30° foot down for the above lateral decubitus views.

Erect lateral radiographs   The table is gently brought into the vertical position. The patient is turned so that his coronal plane is perpendicular to the table top and lateral exposures are made on the explorator with the patient stooping in flexion and then in full extension. Some disc protrusions are only seen with extension of the spine.

Tomography   is a useful accessory technique as it may demonstrate lesions which may be hidden in the conventional views. Tomography during myelography (patient prone, oblique or in lateral decubitus) is most readily performed on a remote control table with an overcouch fluoroscopic tube and tomographic facilities, such as Televix and Futuralix.

Dorsal myelography

Dorsal water-soluble myelography is a simple extension of lumbo-sacral myelography. The same quantity and concentration of metrizamide or iopamidol is used and the lumbo-sacral region is usually examined first if there are any symptoms referable to that area.

Having checked all the radiographs of the lumbo-sacral subarachnoid space for technical quality and diagnostic content, the contrast medium is then run up into the dorsal (thoracic) region.

For dorsal water-soluble myelography, the patient is turned into the lateral decubitus position and the X-ray table tilted head down whilst the radiologist observes the movement of the bolus of the contrast medium on the TV monitor. The table tilt is stopped

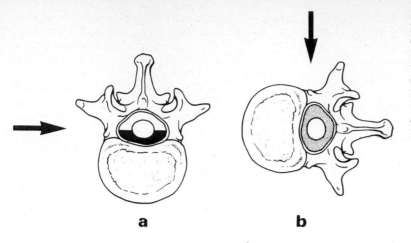

Fig. 18.4 Lateral projections during lumbar myelography.
(a) Using oily medium, the patient *must* be prone, using the lateral X-ray tube with horizontal ray.
(b) Using a water-soluble medium, the lateral radiograph may be taken with a vertical ray with patient in lateral decubitus, or position 18.4a may also be used.

a

b

after the first 10° tilt, and then subsequently after each additional 5° tilt, as the bolus of contrast medium may take several seconds to begin to move. Once it has started to move, it may move very quickly and be lost into the cervical region and skull. In order to prevent the contrast medium entering the skull, the neck of the patient should be flexed laterally on a high pillow towards the uppermost shoulder, raising the head from the table (Fig. 18.6).

Usually a head down tilt of 10–15° is sufficient to move the contrast medium bolus into the mid- and lower-dorsal region. A deep inspiration lowers the diaphragm as the contrast medium moves cephalad, and gives a much improved view. A lateral radiograph is exposed from the undercouch tube on the explorator with the patient in lateral decubitus. A low kV radiographic exposure is required for this radiograph.

Having checked the lateral film, the patient is slowly turned on to his back, the table still being tilted 10–15° head down. The head and neck are raised off the table top on a high pillow. This manoeuvre pools the bolus of contrast medium in the dorsal kyphosis and a frontal radiograph is taken on the explorator from the undercouch tube with the patient supine.

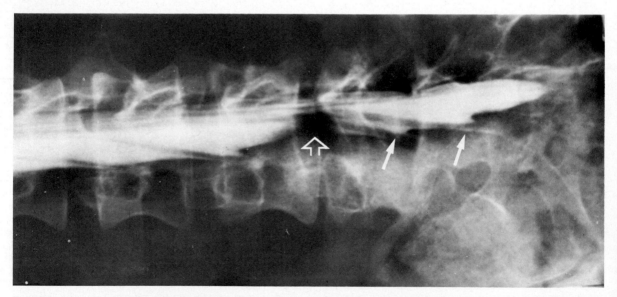

Fig. 18.5 Lateral oblique decubitus position to show the lumbar nerve roots. Patient's back to the X-ray tube, abdomen adjacent to the cassette, patient's upper side rotated 15° towards the cassette and away from the tube. Table tilted 30° foot down. Horizontal ray lateral X-ray beam. Water-soluble myelogram.

Large lateral disc prolapse at L4/5 ⇗ causing marked medial displacement, compression and oedema of the right L5 and S1 nerve roots

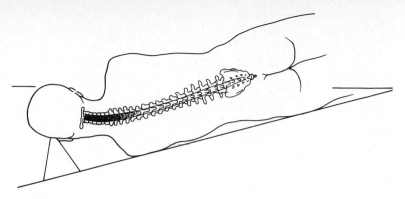

Fig. 18.6 Lateral decubitus position, head well raised on pad to create lateral curvature of the cervical spine region in which the contrast medium collects.

The film 'Right' and 'Left' markers on the explorator need to be reversed, as the original frontal films of the lumbar spine were taken with the patient prone but the frontal views of the dorsal spine are taken with the patient supine.

The above films demonstrate the dorsal subarachnoid space from D5–D12 (Fig. 18.7).

Having checked the films of the lower- and mid-dorsal region, the tilt of the table is increased in 5° increments head end down until the contrast medium reaches the upper dorsal region when a frontal (supine) radiograph is taken on the explorator. The head of the patient must be elevated from the table by a high pillow to prevent the contrast medium entering the head. The patient is then turned slowly into an oblique lateral position, and an off-lateral view is obtained of the upper dorsal spine.

Cervical myelography

Water-soluble cervical myelography is a more difficult technical procedure than oil cervical myelography, and should only be attempted after the radiologist has become confident in his ability to control the bolus of contrast medium during lumbo-sacral and dorsal water-soluble myelography.

There are two completely different methods of performing water-soluble cervical myelography, depending on the route of injection of the contrast medium.

Both lumbar injection and direct cervical injection have their advantages and disadvantages. As each technique offers advantages in certain clinical situations, expertise should be developed in both methods.

Both techniques are much facilitated by a second X-ray tube with a horizontal beam shooting across the X-ray table top, this being essential basic equipment for cervical myelographic radiography. The addition of lateral tube fluoroscopy is strongly recommended.

Lumbar injection of contrast medium

Much of the advice given in the preceding sections on 'Examination of the Lumbar and Dorsal Spinal Cord' is applicable. Only the differences are considered here.

Contrast medium As the aqueous contrast medium becomes progressively more dilute and dispersed as it is transported from the lumbar to the cervical region, it is important to inject contrast medium at high concentration when the cervical region is being examined following lumbar administration. Ten millilitres of metrizamide or iopamidol of 250–300 mg I/ml concentration is used.

Premedication No water-soluble contrast agent is well tolerated by the cerebral cortex. It may induce an epileptic attack even in a person with no history of fits. As some spill or contrast agent into the skull may well occur during cervical myelography with any technique, some radiologists prefer to give an anti-epileptic drug such as phenobarbitone sodium (120 mg) or diazepam (5 mg) either by mouth or by intramuscular injection 30 minutes before the myelogram.

Incompatible drugs It is important in cervical myelography that the patient is not given phenothiazine or other incompatible drugs for the previous 48 hours and for the following two days.

Patient movement and table tilt Unlike oil myelography, it is always difficult and sometimes impossible to produce diagnostic lumbar, dorsal and cervical myelographic radiographs from one injection of aqueous contrast medium. If the cervical region is the only one of clinical interest, the contrast medium should be taken up to the cervical spine immediately after its injection.

There are two methods of moving the bolus of

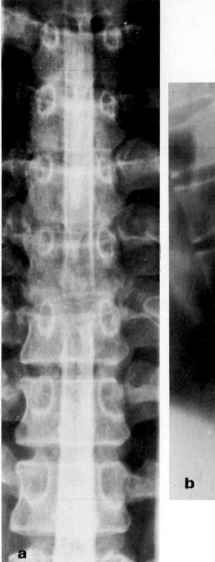

Fig. 18.7 Dorsal water-soluble mye-logram. Patient horizontal.
(a) Antero–posterior view.
(b) Lateral view (tomogram). Patient in lateral decubitus. Vertical X-ray beam.

Demonstrating recent fracture of dorsal vertebra with swollen damaged spinal cord. Paraplegia.

contrast medium from the lumbar region, where it was injected, into the cervical region which is being investigated. Both methods are satisfactory but the lateral decubitus technique is preferred, particularly if there is a prominent dorsal kyphosis.

LATERAL DECUBITUS TECHNIQUE

The patient is placed in lateral decubitus in order to avoid running the contrast medium through the full curvature of the lumbar lordosis and dorsal kyphosis.

The lumbar puncture has been performed and the metrizamide or iopamidol injected with the patient sat upright on the horizontal X-ray table. The foot end

of the table is tilted 20–30° down in order to keep the contrast bolus in the lumbo-sacral region. The patient is assisted to turn slowly into lateral decubitus and a thick pillow is placed under his head and neck in order to flex the head towards the uppermost side and to produce a curvature, convexity downwards, in the cervical spine where the bolus of contrast medium will be eventually trapped (Fig. 18.6).

The X-ray table is then tilted horizontal. A 10° head-down tilt of the table is made with the patient in the lateral decubitus position. The radiologist fluoro-scopes, preferably with the horizontal ray tube, the upper margin of the bolus of contrast medium which will be in the upper lumbar spine. If the bolus does

Fig. 18.8 (a) Patient returned from position 2c into horizontal position. Head and neck still well extended maintaining contrast medium in the exaggerated cervical lordosis. Radiographs of the mid- and lower-cervical spine can be taken in this position or with controlled reduction of cervical lordosis.

(b) Pad removed from patient's chin. Head and neck gradually flexed under fluoroscopic control until contrast medium flows through foramen magnum to flow on to the clivus. This position is used for the frontal open mouth occipito-atlanto-axial projection and for the lateral cervical spine projection in flexion.

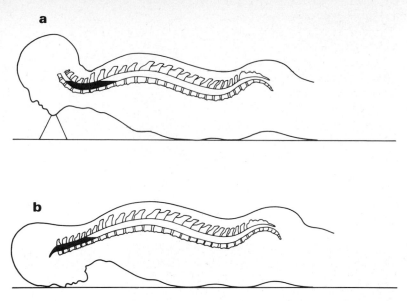

not move within one minute, a further 5° head-down tilt of the table is made and the bolus will almost certainly begin to move into the lower dorsal region. As soon as this occurs, the radiologist should move the explorator, preferably a horizontal ray tube, over the cervical area and watch the contrast medium slowly arriving and accumulating in the concavity produced by the head pillow. The patient is of course still in lateral decubitus with the head and neck laterally flexed and raised off the table (Fig. 18.6).

If the bolus has not arrived in the cervical region within 2 minutes, a further 5° head-down tilt of the table is made. This will almost certainly produce enough gravitational influence to shift almost all the contrast medium into the concavity of the cervical area where it is allowed to accumulate. This movement may take a further one or two minutes. The patient must remain in the lateral decubitus position with their head well-flexed towards the uppermost shoulder throughout this manoeuvre. If the patient begins to slide down the table he should be supported either by a previously applied harness or by a nurse steadying his shoulders. Once the bolus of metrizamide or iopamidol has been collected in the cervical region, the table is gently returned to the horizontal plane, the patient still in the lateral decubitus position with the neck laterally flexed to the uppermost shoulder.

The next manoeuvre is very important for, if it is clumsily performed, the bolus of contrast medium will be dispersed and some may enter the head or run down the spine. The radiologist leaves the explorator and holds the patient's head in both hands. The patient is then assisted to rotate head and body, slowly and gently into the prone position. The patient's neck is maintained in extension throughout the procedure and a triangular radiolucent pad is placed under the chin when the prone position has been gained (Fig. 18.8a). The contrast medium bolus is now in the extended cervical spine and is prevented from running either into the head or down the spine by the cervical lordosis. During the entire manoeuvre of turning the patient from lateral decubitus into the prone position, the head and shoulders must not be allowed to rise above the patient's trunk and the head must not be allowed to become lower than the neck.

Radiographic projections   Having collected the bolus of contrast medium in the concavity of the extended cervical spine, with the patient prone and the X-ray table horizontal, a frontal A–P film is taken from the undercouch tube on the explorator. The radiologist then slowly turns the patient's head and neck and shoulder into a 20–25° prone oblique position, the patient following the rotation with his body. The nerve roots on the side elevated are now parallel to the explorator (Figs. 18.3b and 18.9) and a vertical ray exposure is made (Fig. 18.9).

Having checked these films, the radiologist holds the patient's head and rotates it into the opposite 20–25° prone oblique and a further radiograph is taken to see the nerve roots of the now uppermost side. Having checked the film, the patient is then returned slowly into the prone position.

It is essential that all of these movements are smoothly and gently executed as jerky movements disperse the water-soluble contrast medium. The

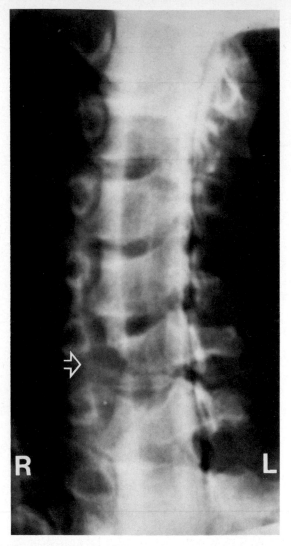

Fig. 18.9 Frontal oblique cervical water-soluble myelogram. Patient prone, right side raised 20°. Vertical X-ray beam. Demonstrates right cervical nerve roots. Large disc lesion C5/6 right side ⇨ .

movements must be performed without raising or lowering the head, whilst the cervical spine is maintained in a moderate degree of extension.

The lateral cervical film is then taken, with the patient prone, from a second X-ray tube shooting horizontally across the table. The patient's arms and shoulders are pulled well down in order to visualize the lower cervical spine (Fig. 18.10). Lateral tube fluoroscopy with horizontal beam shooting across the table is most helpful at this stage in order to cone down adequately with the light beam diaphragms and to adjust the degree of neck flexion accurately so that

the contrast medium just reaches the foramen magnum.

Accessory projections

Extension and flexion lateral films of the cervical spine are very helpful as some disc protrusions are only visible in extension. The extension film is taken first, followed by the flexion film, both being made from the lateral tube horizontally across the horizontal table, with the patient prone.

For the flexion film, the chin is tucked well down and some contrast medium will trickle on to the lower part of the clivus (Fig. 18.8b). A minor degree (5°) of head down tilt of the table may be necessary to allow the contrast medium to reach the clivus. After the flexion film has been taken, the neck is immediately extended in order to retain the contrast medium in the concavity of the extended cervical spine.

Tomography If the radiological equipment is equipped with a tomographic attachment on the lateral tube, mid-line lateral tomography with the patient prone is sometimes helpful as mid-line cervical disc lesions may be obscured on the conventional lateral film.

Open-mouth view of occipito-atlantal axis region If the conventional frontal view has not adequately demonstrated this area, a further frontal view may be obtained with the patient prone and the table horizontal with the head gently flexed under frontal fluoroscopic control until the contrast medium just passes through the foramen magnum. When this situation has been gained, the patient opens the mouth wide, dentures having been removed, to provide a window through which to visualize the occipito–atlantal region and a frontal view is obtained on the explorator.

Shoot through lateral swimmer's view can be taken with the patient prone, one arm carefully extended and stretched out parallel to the side of the head, with the other arm pulled down towards the feet. As the objective is to visualize the lower cervical and upper dorsal spine on this view, the X-ray table will probably have to be tilted 10–15° foot down under fluoroscopic control to move the bolus of contrast medium down from the mid-cervical region. The patient is rotated about 10° off lateral to prevent having to radiograph through the full thickness of the shoulders. An off-lateral film is then taken with the horizontal ray lateral tube. A high kV is necessary to penetrate the upper dorsal region and a rice or water bath can be used as a

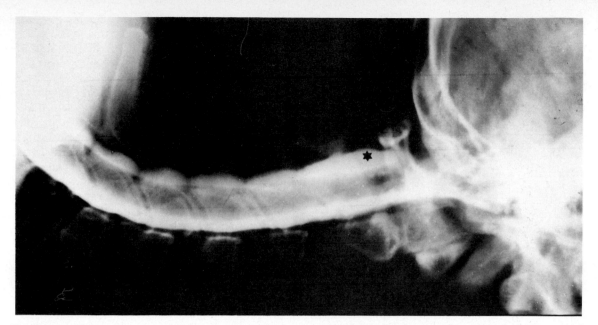

Fig. 18.10 Normal cervical water-soluble myelogram. Lateral projection. Neck in slight extension, table horizontal, arms well pulled down, horizontal ray lateral X-ray beam. Water-soluble contrast medium injected by C1/C2 lateral puncture at ★.

filter adjacent to the neck to prevent over-exposure of the cervical region.

The myelographic examination of the cervical spine is now completed and the patient is assisted to sit upright on the X-ray table, care being taken to prevent lowering of the head. The contrast medium runs down into the lumbar region and he is returned to the ward with head and shoulders well propped up.

Prone position

The bolus of contrast medium may be transported from the lumbar region, where it has been injected, into the cervical region by tilting the patient head end down in the prone position. This technique is less reliable than the lateral decubitus method, particularly if there is a prominent lumbar lordosis or dorsal kyphosis which may even render this method inapplicable. All other features of this technique are exactly the same as for the lateral decubitus technique, except for the transportation of the bolus of contrast medium into the neck.

X-ray table tilt   Immediately after the injection of the contrast medium (10 ml metrizamide or iopamidol 250–300 mg I/ml) into the lumbar region, the table is tilted 30° foot end down and the patient is assisted to lie prone on the table top. As more head down tilt of the table is required for the prone technique than for

the lateral decubitus method, a restraining harness will almost certainly be needed to prevent the patient slipping head-first down the table and it should be fitted before the patient lies prone. The patient's neck is fully extended and supported in this position by a radiolucent triangular pad under the chin throughout the tilt procedure. Unless good cervical extension is achieved, the contrast medium will run into the head and this will compromise the procedure.

The X-ray table is then brought into the horizontal plane and the radiologist fluoroscopes the upper limit of the contrast medium bolus in the lumbar spinal canal. If available, horizontal ray lateral fluoroscopy is preferred to frontal fluoroscopy.

The table top is tilted 10° head end down, and further head down tilts of 5° increments are added until the bolus begins to move down towards the head. The radiologist should wait 30–60 s after each increment of tilt as the bolus movement may begin slowly. Once the bolus begins to move, it usually moves quite quickly cephalad. Once the bolus begins to flow cephalad, the explorator, which is preferably on lateral fluoroscopy, is moved to the neck region and the arrival and collection of the contrast medium bolus in the concavity of the extended cervical spine is awaited (Fig. 18.2c). This transportation of contrast medium may take two minutes and should not be hastened by unnecessarily applying further head down tilt to the table. Usually 20–30° is adequate but more may be required if there is a prominent dorsal kyphosis. Once the complete bolus of contrast medium has been collected in the cervical region, the table is returned to the horizontal plane, the extension pad is carefully removed from under the patient's chin and a lesser degree of cervical extension is maintained.

Radiographs are now taken exactly as described for the lateral decubitus technique. After completing the radiography and checking the films, the radiologist holds the patient's head and keeps it well elevated whilst the patient sits up on the table to allow the contrast medium to run down into the lumbar region. The patient is then returned to the ward with the head and shoulders well propped up.

CERVICAL WATER-SOLUBLE MYELOGRAPHY BY LATERAL
CI-2 PUNCTURE

This technique is not difficult to learn but must only be practised after the radiologist has observed an experienced operator. Lateral fluoroscopy is essential. The technique is best described by Lamb (1981).

The objective is to insert a spinal needle at C1–C2 level, behind the spinal cord, and to inject water-soluble contrast medium into the cervical subarachnoid space (Fig. 18.10). The contrast medium is injected *in situ* and is not transported within the spinal cord as with the techniques previously described.

Contrast medium As little dilution will occur in the absence of transportation of the bolus, 8–12 ml metrizamide or iopamidol 200/250 mg I/ml is recommended.

Needle A larger gauge (SWG20) is preferred for water-soluble cervical myelography because CSF may not drip through the narrower gauge needle, even after a satisfactory cervical spinal puncture.

Cervical spinal puncture The patient lies prone on a thick (10 cm) radiolucent mattress on the horizontal X-ray table. The hair is shaved over and caudal to the mastoid process and any loose strands of hair are restrained by adhesive tape or a hair net.

The patient's neck is gently extended with a triangular polyfoam pad or perspex angled support under the chin. The patient must be comfortable in this position and be able to breath easily. A lateral shoot-through radiograph is taken from the lateral tube with horizontal beam and it is examined to assess anatomy and pathology in order to avoid inappropriate puncture.

The puncture site is determined by positioning a metal pointer just caudal to the tip of the mastoid process, so that on lateral fluoroscopy it is projected over the interspace between the C1 and C2 posterior neural arches and just anterior to the posterior boundary of the cervical subarachnoid space (Fig. 18.10). The usual optimal site for puncture is 5–10 mm caudal to the mastoid tip and 5 mm anterior or posterior to the tip. This point for the puncture is marked with indelible ink. The area about the entry point is surgically cleaned and local anaesthetic (1% lignocaine) is infiltrated into the skin, subcutaneous and ligamentous tissues. The 20 gauge spinal needle is then inserted, precisely directed parallel, to the horizontal table top, in the coronal plane of the patient, perpendicular to the long axis of the patient, pointing neither cephalad nor caudal. Intermittent lateral fluoroscopy is a great help in maintaining this line of approach and any necessary adjustments to the needle direction are made if the needle is not exactly in the desired line. It is a great comfort for the patient, and a help for the operator, if a nurse placed at the head of the table steadies the patient's head.

The dura is punctured at a depth of about 5 cm from the skin, but this varies considerably with the thickness of the neck. If the operator is concerned that the needle tip has passed beyond the mid-sagittal plane, a few seconds A–P fluoroscopy will be very helpful. The patient may feel a little discomfort as the dura is punctured and the radiologist also appreciates the penetration. The needle tip is advanced 2 mm further to clear the arachnoid, the stilette of the needle is removed and CSF should drip slowly from the hub. The first few millilitres are collected for the laboratory and the syringe, previously loaded with metrizamide or iopamidol at 200–250 mg I/ml concentration, is connected by flexible tubing to the needle. The first few drops of contrast medium are then injected under lateral fluoroscopic control, and should descend through the CSF to lie against the posterior aspects of the mid-cervical vertebral bodies. Having confirmed the free entry of the contrast medium into the subarachnoid space, a further 3–4 ml of contrast medium is injected under intermittent lateral fluoroscopy. Any obstructing lesion in the cervical subarachnoid space will now become evident and if there is such an obstruction no further contrast medium should be injected as it will probably spill into the skull.

In the absence of an obstructing lesion, a further 3–4 ml contrast agent is injected, again under intermittent lateral fluoroscopic control. The entire cervical subarachnoid space should now be demonstrated on the fluoroscope; if not, a further 2–3 ml contrast medium may be added, but the total should not exceed 12 ml. The table top may need to be tilted 5° or even 10° either head or foot end down, and the degree of the patient's neck extension may need adjustment to ensure that the contrast medium reaches from the foramen to C_7 without spilling into the head. The needle is left *in situ*, still connected by the plastic tubing to the syringe. Radiography can now commence.

Radiographic projections   With the patient prone and neck slightly extended, frontal, 20–30° right and left prone oblique and lateral projections are made as previously described (Figs. 18.9 and 18.10). The lateral films are taken with the lateral tube firing horizontally. As the contrast medium is moderately concentrated, two lateral exposures at conventional and higher penetration (kV) are taken in order to visualize both the spinal cord and the subarachnoid space to best advantage. Having checked these radiographs, the needle is removed and the puncture wound covered by plastic skin or sterile adhesive.

Accessory projections   Lateral radiographs of the cervical spine in flexion and extension taken with horizontal ray from the lateral tube are almost always advisable with this technique.

An open mouth view of the occipito-atlanto-axial region is also usually advisable to supplement the conventional frontal projection. If a lesion of the lower cervical or upper dorsal spine is suspected, then a shoot through swimmer's view taken from the lateral tube is usually necessary. These accessory views are described previously. When all the films have been checked, the radiologist holds the patient's head to prevent it becoming dependent as the patient sits up on the horizontal X-ray table.

Post myelographic posture and care

Whether the water-soluble contrast medium is introduced by lumbar or cervical puncture, the patient is sat up immediately after the procedure in order to run the medium into the lumbo-sacral region. The patient is returned to the ward by chair or trolley with head and shoulders propped up on pillows. He is encouraged to remain in bed in this position for six hours and must be told not to lower his head during this period. He should be encouraged to drink fluid. Headache should be treated by reassurance and aspirin or paracetamol. Nausea and vomiting are best treated by metaclopramide (Maxalon). Phenothiazines such as Stemetil, Largactil must be avoided for at least two days. The nursing staff must be specifically informed about this restriction, for phenothiazine drugs may otherwise well be given for vomiting.

OIL MYELOGRAPHY

This method of myelography, particularly the movement of the bolus of contrast medium and the technique of lateral radiography, is quite different from the water-soluble method described above. Iophendylate oil droplets remain undiluted and can be collected as a bolus at any time of the procedure by appropriate tilting of the table. The entire spinal subarachnoid space can be examined at the first procedure and repeated later if necessary. Despite these advantages, the crudity of the diagnostic images and the danger of delayed adhesive arachnoiditis make oil myelography a much less sophisticated, less precise and generally a less desirable technique.

Contrast medium

The only oil-based myelographic contrast medium approved in the UK and USA is Iophendylate (also known by the registered name of Myodil, Pantopaque, Ethiodan, Neurotrast).

Iophendylate is ethyl 10-p iodophenylundecylate, having a single iodine atom firmly attached to a benzene ring. It has a molecule weight of 416 and an iodine content of 30.48%. Iophendylate is a colourless, viscous, oily liquid, considerably heavier than CSF with a specific gravity of 1.26. Iophendylate is not miscible with CSF and tends to globulate into discrete, intensely radio-opaque droplets reducing its radiographic potential. It is therefore important during myelography to prevent droplet formation by tilting the patient smoothly.

Iophendylate must not be injected in a polystyrene syringe as this plastic is seriously affected by the oil. Polypropylene or glass syringes are not so affected. The oil is supplied in ampoules containing 3 ml. As the iodine tends to be liberated in sunlight, the ampoules should not be exposed to daylight.

The volume of iophendylate required for adult myelography is usually 6 ml for the lumbar and dorsal regions, and 9 ml for cervical myelography, but up to 20 ml have been used, although this is not advisable.

Needle   A larger (20SWG) gauge short bevel needle is preferred for oil myelography as the oil is quite viscous. Escape of CSF through the lumbar puncture hole is less of a problem than following water-soluble myelography because the patient is nursed flat after oil myelography.

Lumbar puncture position   The lateral decubitus position is recommended as it is much more important to monitor the injection with fluoroscopy in order to prevent epidural or subdural injection of iophendylate which will remain for weeks or months.

Fluoroscopy during the introduction of the contrast medium is much easier with the patient in the lateral decubitus position, using the undercouch tube, than when the lumbar puncture is performed with the patient sitting upright. The patient is made comfortable in the lateral decubitus position, knees well-flexed into the abdomen, shoulders rolled forwards, the coronal plane perpendicular to the table and the spine parallel to the long edge of the table top. The X-ray table is tilted 20° foot down to allow the heavy iophendylate oil to pool in the lumbo-sacral subarachnoid cul-de-sac.

The skin, subcutaneous tissues and superficial portion of the interspinous ligament should be infiltrated with local anaesthetic (1% lignocaine) when the 20 SWG needle is used. The lumbar puncture needle is inserted as previously described in the L3/4 or L4/5 interspace.

Injection of contrast medium A few millilitres of CSF are collected for the laboratory. The syringe pre-loaded with 6–9 ml iophendylate is then injected, followed by removal of the lumbar puncture needle.

Patient movement, table tilt, fluoroscopy and radiography with the table tilted 20–40° foot down, A–P prone, and 20° right and left prone oblique radiographs are taken from the undercouch tube on the explorator.

With oil as contrast medium, the posterior aspects of the vertebral bodies and intervertebral discs are only seen with the patient prone and using a horizontal ray lateral X-ray tube (Fig. 18.4a). With an aqueous contrast medium, there is usually sufficient mixing with CSF to permit satisfactory lateral films with the patient in lateral decubitus using a vertical X-ray as discussed above (Fig. 18.4b). A lateral film of the lower lumbo-sacral spine is therefore taken with the patient prone, table tilted 40° foot down, horizontal X-ray beam from the lateral tube.

Having checked the radiographs of the lower lumbo-sacral region, the table is returned to the horizontal plane and A–P prone, right and left 20° prone oblique films are taken on the frontal explorator, and a lateral film is then exposed from the lateral tube using a horizontal beam. Lateral radiography is greatly facilitated by lateral fluoroscopy. While lateral fluoroscopy is not essential, it becomes increasingly valuable for examination of the dorsal and cervical regions.

With oil contrast medium, usually only two to four lumbar vertebrae are covered by the contrast medium in any one position of the table. Fluoroscopy is necessary to ensure that the whole of the region under suspicion is examined with the iophendylate in the necessary position. The table must be tilted as required to achieve this objective and two or even three different degrees of table tilt may be necessary to move the oil in order to visualize the entire lumbo-sacral subarachnoid space.

The dorsal subarachnoid space is then examined by tilting the prone patient head end down until the oil moves into the dorsal region. The necessary tilt may be 20–45°, depending on the degree of lumbar lordosis and dorsal kyphosis. The tilt needed is considerably more than necessary in water-soluble myelography and the patient needs a restraining harness to prevent him slipping down the table. In order to prevent the contrast medium entering the head, the neck is maintained in a well-extended position on a triangular pad during the head down tilt.

When the iophendylate oil has reached the dorsal spine, prone A–P films of the dorsal spine are taken on the undercouch tube. Two or three radiographs with slightly different degrees of table tilt may be necessary to visualize the whole of the dorsal spine. Horizontal ray, low kV lateral exposures are made of the dorsal spine in full inspiration with the patient prone.

A few minutes is allowed for the oil to move gently through the dorsal region. Excessive head down tilt is uncomfortable for the patient and does not allow optimal radiography. If there is a spinal block, a head down tilt of 60–90° for several minutes may be necessary to confirm the block and to radiograph its features. The patient harness must therefore be secure, safe and inspire patient confidence.

When all the oil has passed through the dorsal subarachnoid space, it will accumulate in the concavity of the extended cervical spine. Cervical extension is maintained throughout the head down tilt. When all the oil has been collected in the cervical spine, the table is returned to the horizontal position and the degree of cervical spine extension is reduced under fluoroscopic control until the oil is spread out along the cervical spine.

Prone frontal, 20–30° prone oblique films of the cervical spine are taken from the undercouch tube on the explorator. One or more horizontal ray lateral radiographs are exposed from the lateral X-ray tube. The appropriate degree of cervical spine flexion and table tilt necessary for these films is more easily assessed by lateral fluoroscopy. Usually the cervical spine needs to be moderately well-flexed to allow the oil to run cephalad to the foramen magnum. The patient's arms should be well pulled down towards the feet for the lateral views.

The iophendylate oil will probably not cover the

entire cervical spine in any one degree of cervical flexion or table tilt. The oil is therefore moved gently while altering the degree of cervical spine flexion and table tilt. When the entire cervical spinal subarachnoid space has been radiographed satisfactorily, accessory views such as 'frontal-prone-open mouth', lateral films in cervical extension, flexion and swimmer's position may be taken as required (p. 274). Lateral fluoroscopy is particularly useful for the lateral projections especially for the flexion film, where the objective is to allow the oil to trickle on to the back of the lower clivus without much spilling into the head (Fig. 18.8b).

Supine oil myelography Should a knowledge of the posterior aspect of the subarachnoid space be needed, the patient is turned supine and horizontal ray lateral radiographs exposed at the spinal level under review. For adequate supine films, the patient must lie on a 10 cm mattress on the table top at the beginning of the procedure, in order to raise the posterior aspects of the spine from the table.

Oil myelography by cervical puncture

Cervical myelography is usually a simple procedure after the oil has been introduced by lumbar puncture. Direct cervical injection is rarely indicated unless there is a complete spinal block or if there is a contra-indication to lumbar puncture.

If necessary, the oil may be introduced by either suboccipital or lateral C1/C2 puncture (p. 276). A volume of 3–6 ml is usually adequate and the upper limit of the spinal block is demonstrated by tilting the patient (lying prone or supine) steeply feet down.

Having checked the above radiographs, the patient is sat up for a few minutes to allow the oil to collect in the lumbo-sacral cul-de-sac and he is returned to the ward, lying horizontal with the head on a single pillow.

Post myelographic posture and care after iophendylate

The patient should lie in bed for at least 6 hours, head flat or raised on one pillow. The oil will not usually flow into the head in this position. Headache may be treated by increasing fluid intake and aspirin or paracetamol. Vomiting is unlikely and may be treated by anti-emetics, including phenothiazines, e.g. Stemetil, as there is very little danger of causing a fit after oil myelography.

Aspiration of iophendylate

As iophendylate is absorbed so slowly from the subarachnoid space (about 1 ml per year) and as it frequently causes adhesive arachnoiditis, most radiologists remove the oil by aspiration following the myelogram. In America, large volumes of iophendylate, up to 20 ml, are sometimes injected into the subarachnoid space—'the full column method', removal of the oil being mandatory with this technique. Even when smaller quantities (6–9 ml) are injected, it is desirable but perhaps not mandatory, to aspirate the oil. Medico-legal considerations favour removal of the contrast medium, but it must be appreciated that there is no evidence that post-myelographic adhesive arachnoiditis is dose-dependent, removal of the oil is time-consuming, may be difficult, painful, and may even damage a nerve root.

Iophendylate oil is removed by the lumbar puncture needle which can be left *in situ* after the original lumbar puncture and throughout the examination, taking due care not to disturb the needle during the procedure. Supine radiography is obviously precluded. An alternative method is to remove the original lumbar puncture needle and reinsert another needle after completion of the myelogram. A minimum needle calibre of 20SWG is necessary, for the oil is quite viscous. There are some specially designed needles, such as the Hinck needle, with elongated slits just proximal to the needle tip to facilitate aspiration of the oil from the subarachnoid space.

With the patient prone, the oil is collected into the lumbo-sacral arachnoid cul-de-sac by tilting the patient into the steep foot down position. The table is then tilted towards the horizontal until the oil is moved to lie under the needle tip.

The hub of the needle is connected by a short connecting tube to a 5 or 10 ml syringe and gentle aspiration is applied under continuous fluoroscopic control to remove as much of the oil and as little CSF as possible. The needle tip may have to be advanced forwards a few millimetres to enter the oil which pools in the anterior part of the subarachnoid space as the patient lies prone throughout the procedure. Several adjustments of table tilt are necessary to bring all of the oil droplets into contact with the hole(s) in the lumbar puncture needle. When no more oil can be aspirated, or if the procedure becomes too uncomfortable, the needle is removed and the skin puncture covered by plastic skin spray or a sterile adhesive dressing. The aspiration should be terminated if the patient becomes distressed or if the lumbo-sacral nerve roots are irritated by the needle.

Following the aspiration, the patient should drink freely and be nursed lying down in bed, preferably with foot end elevated, for 6–12 h in order to reduce leakage of CSF.

Variations on basic technique

The above description refers to the use of conventional radiological equipment which may be found in any well-equipped X-ray department. Lateral X-ray tube horizontal fluoroscopy and radiography is not essential for lumbar and dorsal water-soluble myelography but is virtually essentially for cervical aqueous myelography, especially when the contrast medium is injected by cervical puncture.

Lateral tube horizontal ray radiography is essential for oil myelography of any region of the subarachnoid space, being the only projection which demonstrates the posterior aspects of the vertebral bodies and the intervertebral discs (Fig. 18.4a). Horizontal ray fluoroscopy is very useful for oil myelography, especially for the cervical region. An X-ray table with head down tilt of 90° is necessary for oil myelography in some patients with a compromised subarachnoid space, but a head down tilt of more than 40° is rarely required for water-soluble myelography. Specially designed myelographic equipment reduces to a minimum, rotation movements of the patient which may disperse and dilute the water-soluble medium and thereby making the examination more difficult and less valuable. Equipment is available which enables the X-ray tube to be rotated on a C or U arm around the patient so as to obtain frontal, oblique and lateral radiographs (and fluoroscopy) without requiring the patient to make any movement. Examples of this equipment are the Orbiskop and the Mimer III—the former being particularly suitable—its use for water-soluble myelography being well described by Morris and Cail (1981). While such purpose-built myelographic equipment greatly facilitates the examination, the patient must of course still be tilted in his long axis to move the contrast medium into the desired area of the spine, although the need for patient rotation is eliminated.

Spinal block

Kendall and Valentine (1981) have described a modification of the lateral decubitus injection technique to demonstrate a spinal block and to induce some contrast medium to pass cephalad beyond the obstructing lesion in order to demonstrate its upper margin.

Metrizamide or iopamidol or iohexol are injected with the patient in the lateral decubitus position on the X-ray table. The patient's spine is bowed and positioned so that the suspected site of the obstructing lesion is most dependent, with the spine both cephalad and rostral to the lesion sloping upwards. The contrast medium is slowly injected by lumbar puncture under screen control so that the obstruction is immediately apparent, the table tilt and bowing of the spine being adjusted under fluoroscopy. On completion of the injection, conventional radiographs are taken. With this technique, both the upper and lower margins of the obstructing lesion are almost always demonstrated, and the 'complete' spinal block is found to be a rarity.

Complications

Water-soluble myelography

Headache, nausea, vomiting and dizziness are the most frequent adverse reactions, usually beginning 4–6 hours after the investigation and lasting another 4–6 hours. Some 20–30% of patients develop post-myelographic headache, and about 10% will have more severe and more prolonged headache.

Female patients develop more frequent post-myelographic symptoms than males, but the headache is usually mild and transient, requiring only reassurance and simple analgesics. Approximately 10% of patients develop more severe headache, worse on sitting up, lasting for one to two days or even longer. In the author's experience, prolonged and severe headaches are less frequent with iopamidol than with metrizamide myelography.

Controversy exists as to the cause of these symptoms. Escape of CSF through the puncture hole in the arachnoid is the usual explanation, for the patient is propped head up after the procedure. An analysis of the international literature by Nyegaard (1981) suggests that headache following metrizamide myelography is no more frequent or serious than following iophendylate. The author's distinct impression however, is that metrizamide myelography is more frequently followed by headache than iopamidol or iophendylate.

Headache is probably aggravated by dehydration and reduced by over-hydration. It is advised that the patient drinks freely before the examination, but not in the immediately preceding 3 hours, and also after the procedure. Eldevick *et al.* (1978) found considerable reduction in headache after 2 litres fluid had been given intravenously before the metrizamide myelography. Aggravation of the pre-myelographic lumbago and sciatica may occur after the myelogram, probably related more to the loss of CSF and disturbance of the nerve roots than to the contrast agent.

Epileptic fits are the most serious complications of water-soluble myelography but are very rare, mild and usually single after lumbar or dorsal myelography. In the cervical examination, the incidence of an epileptic fit is increased to about 0.5 to 1% of examinations, occurring particularly when an excess of undiluted contrast medium is allowed to enter the skull and reach the cerebral cortex. With increasing experience of the operator, the incidence of an epileptic fit after cervical myelography is considerably reduced to about 0.1% as a smaller quantity of contrast medium tends to be used and less enters the intracranial cavity.

Seizures tend to be short-lasting and are usually abolished by intravenous diazepam 10 mg repeated if necessary. Many radiologists advise pre-operative diazepam or phenobarbitone (120 mg) in an attempt to reduce the frequency of fits following cervical aqueous myelography.

Meglumine iocarmate (Dimer X) myelography was more frequently followed by fits and by spasm of the spinal muscles, which was sometimes severe enough to cause fractures. The earliest sign of muscle irritability is a very important warning and must always be treated by intravenous diazepam, repeated as necessary. Fortunately, spasm of spinal muscles is extremely rare and usually mild after metrizamide or iopamidol myelography.

Mental reactions Confusion, time-space disorientation, hallucinations, aggression and depression may occasionally follow metrizamide and possibly iopamidol myelography, especially of the cervical region. These mental reactions are uncommon, usually mild, but not always, and transient, rarely lasting more than two days. Computed tomography may show considerable brain penetrance and cerebral oedema in these patients.

Adhesive arachnoiditis is discussed more fully under 'oil myelography'. It probably does not occur following clinical myelography with metrizamide or iopamidol but has been induced by injecting high doses of metrizamide into the subarachnoid space in monkeys (Haughton *et al.*, 1977).

Earlier water-soluble myelographic contrast media such as methiodal, meglumine iothalamate and meglumine iocarmate all caused arachnoiditis in up to 50% of patients, but the arachnoiditis is usually not as severe as that following iophendylate injection and rarely causes symptoms.

Fortunately, myelography with metrizamide or iopamidol in the doses and concentrations advised above appears to be free of this complication.

Oil myelography

Iophendylate is not an acute neurotoxin and rarely, if ever, is responsible for precipitating an epileptic attack, muscle spasm or paralysis.

Headache, nausea, and vomiting are the most frequent acute complications following iophendylate myelography. The subject is discussed under 'water-soluble myelographic complications', p. 280.

Pain in buttocks and thighs following myelography tends to be more frequent and more severe following iophendylate than after metrizamide myelography.

Arachnoiditis Although iophendylate is not an acute neurotoxin, its prolonged retention in the arachnoid space is a definite irritant and causes an inflammatory reaction—an adhesive arachnoiditis—in the majority of patients.

The radiological signs of this arachnoiditis are narrowing of the subarachnoid space because of thickening of the meninges, stenosis of the lower end of the subarachnoid sac which terminates more cephalad than it did before the myelogram, obliteration of the lumbo-sacral nerve root sleeves by adhesions, and irregularity and distortion of the contours of the subarachnoid sac. The nerve roots descending in the cauda equina tend to move peripherally toward the meninges, to which they become adherent. This results in a homogeneous column of contrast medium within the narrowed and shortened subarachnoid sac, without the normal longitudinal striations due to the nerve roots. All of these changes are most marked at the lower end of the sac and there is usually a fairly abrupt change between the normal subarachnoid space above and the arachnoid change below. Drops of iophendylate are almost always permanently present in the abnormal area, often immobilized by adhesions, and sometimes seem fixed in the nerve root sleeves.

Arachnoiditis is best recognized by a second myelogram, preferably with water-soluble media. Post myelographic arachnoiditis is primarily a radiological entity and in most patients its major significance is that it prevents complete visualization of the lumbo-sacral nerve roots at a second myelographic examination.

Post-myelographic arachnoiditis is usually asymptomatic but it may cause pain in the lower back and legs. In a very few patients, the adhesions and thickening of the arachnoid may severely compress the nerve roots and spinal cord, causing neurological damage of varying severity, including dense paraplegia.

Aspiration of the oil is recommended after the myelogram, to prevent these delayed irritant reactions to iophendylate, but there is no proof that the arachnoiditis is dose dependent.

Subdural and epidural injection · Injection of iophendylate into the epidural (extradural) or subdural space may occur during the myelographic injection, particularly if there has been difficulty during the lumbar puncture or if a long bevel needle has been used. When the oil is injected into the *epidural space*, it tends to spread outside the spinal canal along the lumbo-sacral nerve roots and surrounds the subarachnoid space. The oil does not move freely when the patient is tipped and does not fall to the dependent aspect of the subarachnoid space as best seen on horizontal ray radiographs.

Subdural injection of iophendylate can usually be readily recognized by the slow movement of the oil, the unusual contour of the 'space' which it outlines, and the fact that it does not drop to the dependent part of the subarachnoid space. Subdural oil may, however, move fairly quickly under the influence of gravity and it may not be immediately apparent that the oil lies outside the subarachnoid space.

Injections outside the subarachnoid space are more likely to involve both subdural and epidural space than either space alone, and usually some oil is also injected into the subarachnoid space. It is very important to recognize when oil has been injected into an inappropriate space. Epidural injections can be readily recognized, but subdural oil may produce confusing appearances during fluoroscopy and be difficult to differentiate from subarachnoid injection until horizontal ray radiographs have been critically examined.

Subdural and/or epidural injections of water-soluble contrast agents may of course also occur, but they are quickly absorbed within hours, rather than days or months or years which follow iophendylate extra-arachnoid injection.

Choice of oil or water-soluble contrast medium

Ten years ago, virtually all myelograms in English-speaking countries were performed with oily iophendylate. The situation is nowadays quite different, as metrizamide and more recently iopamidol and iohexol, are becoming universally acceptable as safe and reliable water-soluble myelographic agents.

The author recommends that all lumbar myelograms and all mid- and lower-dorsal myelograms should be performed with metrizamide, iopamidol, or iohexol or other safe aqueous contrast media which may become available, unless the patient is epileptic or has previously demonstrated sensitivity to aqueous contrast media. Even these adverse circumstances are not absolute contra-indications but they indicate that exceptional care should be taken. If a prolapsed

lumbar or dorsal intervertebral disc is suspected, then water-soluble myelography is very strongly indicated because it provides greatly improved detail of the nerve root sheaths than does an oil medium.

Cervical and upper-dorsal myelography pose a different problem because there is no doubt that these examinations are easier to perform with oil than with aqueous contrast agents. When the contrast medium is introduced by lumbar puncture, it is more difficult to manipulate and to maintain the bolus of the aqueous product as compared with the oil medium. This difficulty is greatly reduced when the radiologist has had considerable practice with the technique.

Direct cervical puncture, whether lateral C1/C2 or suboccipital, is a rather intimidating technique until the radiologist has gained confidence by learning the method from an expert.

The considerable advantage of cervical water-soluble myelography is that much greater detail of the subarachnoid space, cervical cord and nerve roots is obtained. Few experienced myelographers would choose oil for the examination.

If the suspected lesion is at the cervico-dorsal junction, and if the patient has broad shoulders, it may be very difficult to obtain good lateral radiographs with aqueous media which are much less radio-opaque than iophendylate. The oil medium may be preferred if it is important to perform total myelography on a single examination, or if it is anticipated that rescreening will be required within the next few days. With these exceptions, metrizamide, iopamidol or iohexol are recommended for virtually all myelographic examinations.

Relationship to other imaging modalities

There is no technique other than myelography which provides comparable radiological detail of the spinal cord and subarachnoid space.

Some pathological conditions investigated by myelography are lesions in the epidural space which compress the spinal cord and nerve roots. The most frequent of these conditions is degenerative spondylosis with intervertebral disc prolapse, and some radiologists examine the epidural space of these patients by alternative techniques such as *epidurography* and *spinal venography*. These latter techniques avoid puncture of the subarachnoid space and avoid escape of CSF, with a considerable reduction of post-puncture headache and debility, but they do not demonstrate the lumbo-sacral nerve roots as well as does myelography.

Direct puncture *discography* is a technique less frequently utilized in the investigation of suspected prolapse of an intervertebral disc, usually lumbar but occasionally cervical, but it involves traumatic puncture of the disc with possible complications.

At the present time, myelography is used as the prime method of investigation of the spinal cord and its coverings; with epidurography, spinal venography and discography reserved as back up investigations for suspected but unproven epidural lesions.

Computerized tomography (CT) on modern general purpose scanners provides excellent quality transverse sections of the spinal canal at all levels, and is therefore the optimal investigation for suspected spinal bony stenosis or metastases. However, unenhanced CT does not usually produce good visualization of the individual nerve roots as they descend in and leave the cauda equina. High quality CT scanning, even without injection of water-soluble contrast medium, can demonstrate (lumbar) disc prolapse with increasing accuracy.

If a small quantity of water-soluble contrast agent is injected, the spinal cord, subarachnoid space and their lesions are very well visualized by CT scanning and disc protrusions are even better demonstrated.

Ultrasonography is used by a few enthusiasts (Porter, 1981) in an attempt to measure the oblique diameter of the spinal canal and to identify those patients with a small diameter canal who are therefore more liable to compression of nerve roots. Many investigators, however, have been unable to reproduce Porter's findings and further assessment is necessary. CT provides much more accurate information of the shape and size of the bony spinal canal, but ultrasonography is very much cheaper and avoids X-radiation. It is hoped that improved ultrasonography will eventually provide adequate and reliable information to support Porter's original observations.

Recently developed *Nuclear Magnetic Resonance* (NMR) permits excellent visualization of the spinal cord and subarachnoid space, in transverse or longitudinal tomographic sections. No contrast medium is required as the necessary detail is provided by the differing concentrations of protons in the different tissues. The nerve roots are not adequately shown by NMR, but when the technique is fully developed it could well be a procedure of choice for the demonstration of the spinal cord and subarachnoid space.

REFERENCES

Amundsen P. & Skalpe I. O. (1975) Cervical myelography with metrizamide. Technical aspects. *Neuroradiology*, **8**, 209–12.

Bonati F. & Felder E. (1977) Iopamidol: a new non-ionic contrast medium. Preliminary clinical studies. XLV International Congress on Radiology (Rio de Janeiro).

Drayer B., Suslavich F., Luther J., Rommel A., Allen S., Dubois P., Heinz R. & Bates M. (1982) Clinical trial of iopamidol for lumbosacral myelography. *Amer. J. Neuroradiol.*, Jan–Feb **3** (1), 59–64.

Grainger R. G. (1975) Water-soluble radiculography. In *Recent Advances in Radiology* (Eds. Lodge T. & Steiner R. E.), Vol. 5, pp. 37–50. Churchill Livingstone, Edinburgh.

Grainger R. G. (1979) Further developments in water-soluble myelography 1974–1977. In *Recent Advances in Radiology and Medical Imaging.* (Eds. Lodge T. & Steiner R. E.) Vol. 6, pp. 177–94. Churchill Livingstone, Edinburgh.

Grainger R. G., Kendall B. E. & Wylie I. G. (1976) Lumbar myelography with metrizamide. *Brit. J. Radiol.*, **49**, 996–1003.

Grainger R. G. (1981) Contrast media for myelography. In *Myelographic Techniques with Metrizamide.* (Eds. Grainger R. G. & Lamb J. T.) Chapter 1, pp. 11–18. Nyegaard (UK) Ltd., Mylen House, 11, Wagon Lane, Sheldon, Birmingham BS26 3DU.

Grainger R. G. (1981) The technique of lumbar myelography with metrizamide. In *Myelographic Techniques with Metrizamide.* (Eds. Grainger R. G. & Lamb J. T.) Chapter 3, pp. 31–36. Nyegaard (UK) Ltd., Birmingham.

Haughton V. M., Ho K. C., Unger G. F., Larson S. J. & Correa-Paz F. (1977) Experimental production of arachnoiditis with water-soluble myelographic media. *Radiology*, **123**, 681–5.

Hindmarsh T., Grepe A. & Widen L. (1975) Metrizamide-Phenothiazine inter-action. *Acta Radiol. Diagn.*, **15**, 497–507.

Johnson A. J. (1981) Thecal scarring due to myelography. In *Myelographic Techniques with Metrizamide.* (Eds. Grainger R. G. & Lamb J. T.) Chapter 20, pp. 167–78. Nyegaard (UK) Ltd., Birmingham.

Kendall B. E. & Valentine A. R. (1981) Myelographic study of the obstructed spinal theca with water-soluble contrast medium. *British Journal of Radiology*, **54**, 408–412.

Lamb J. T. (1981) Cervical myelography by C1–C2 puncture. In *Myelographic Techniques with Metrizamide.* (Eds. Grainger R. G. & Lamb J. T.) Chapter 6, pp. 59–74. Nyegaard (UK) Ltd., Birmingham.

Morris J. L. (1974). Personal Communication.

Morris J. L. & Cail W. S. (1981). C-arm X-ray Unit for use in water-soluble myelography in Grainger R. G. and Lamb J. T. *See* Further Reading No. 3, Chapter 8, 79–94.

Nyegaard & Co. A/S (1981) Headache after myelography. An analysis of Published papers, in Grainger R. G. and Lamb J. T. *See* Further Reading No. 3, Chapter 21, 179–204.

Occleshaw J. V. (1981) Metrizamide myelography in the lumbar region. In *Myelographic Techniques with*

Metrizamide. (Eds. Grainger R. G. & Lamb J. T.) Chapter 4, pp. 37–52. Nyegaard (UK) Ltd., Birmingham.

Palmers (1981) Personal communication.

Porter R. W. (1981) The value of myelography and ultrasound measurement of the spinal canal to the orthopaedic surgeon. In *Myelographic Techniques with Metrizamide*. (Eds. Grainger R. G. & Lamb J. T.) Chapter 22, pp. 205–12. Nyegaard (UK) Ltd., Birmingham.

FURTHER READING

The following texts deal comprehensively with water-soluble myelography with particular reference to metrizamide. Grainger and Lamb (1981) particularly reflects this author's views.

Acta Radiologica (1973) Metrizamide—a non-ionic water-soluble contrast medium. Supplementum No. 335.

Acta Radiologica (1977) Metrizamide—Amipaque. Further clinical experience in neuroradiology. Supplementum No. 355.

Grainger R. G. & Lamb J. T. (Eds) (1981) Myelographic techniques with metrizamide. Nyegaard (UK) Ltd., Mylen House, 11, Wagon Lane, Sheldon, Birmingham BS26 3DU, UK.

Sackett J. F. & Strother C. M. (Eds) (1979) *New Techniques in Myelography*. Harper and Row, Maryland, USA.

Shapiro R. (1975) *Myelography*. Year Book Publishers, Chicago, USA (Oil Media).

Skalpe I. O. & Sortland O. (1978) *Myelography—Textbook and Atlas*. Tanum-Notli, Oslo, Norway.

ACKNOWLEDGEMENTS

Figs. 18.1, 5 and 10 are reproduced with kind permission of the Editors and Publishers of Recent Advances in Radiology No. 5 (1975) and No. 6 (1979). Churchill Livingstone, Edinburgh and London, from chapters written by the present author.

B. S. WORTHINGTON

The advent and subsequent refinement of computed tomography (CT) has transformed the practice of neuroradiology. This non-invasive and safe method of investigation reveals a wealth of information about intracranial and intraorbital structures. It is the only procedure required for patient management in many cases of congenital malformations, degenerative disorders, intracranial suppuration and cranio-cerebral trauma. Computed tomography is the initial procedure of choice in the evaluation of patients suspected of harbouring an intracranial tumour. Angiography, however, still has a role in demonstrating the anatomy of intrinsic vascular disorders and in the differential diagnosis of lesions which give similar CT appearances. Furthermore, the development of interventional procedures following on superselective angiography has now extended its applications. The intrathecal injection of contrast medium or air as adjuncts to CT allows the diagnosis of small tumours which encroach on the basal cisterns. In addition, direct coronal scans and reformatted sagittal and coronal images from multiple contiguous transverse scans now provide a much needed multiplanar facility in CT. These developments have led to the almost total abandonment of pneumoencephalography and ventriculography in centres where a modern CT scanner is available. The occasional need for such studies, however, requires that a few specialists retain the necessary expertise to carry them out.

CEREBRAL ANGIOGRAPHY

Indications

The introduction of CT in 1972 by Hounsfield has led to a reappraisal of the indications for cerebral angiography. While CT can provide useful information in intrinsic disease of the blood vessels, including aneurysm, arterio-venous malformation and venous thrombosis, particularly about their sequelae, angiography is usually necessary to define the precise morphology of the underlying lesion and its connection to cerebral vessels. In the management of patients with cerebro-vascular disease, angiography is required to demonstrate related extra-cranial and intra-cranial vascular occlusions, stenoses and ulcerated atheromatous plaques. The examination also shows patterns of collateral blood supply when main vessels have been compromised. While CT alone may provide sufficient information in tumour cases to determine further management, there are many instances where angiography assists the differential diagnosis and provides information about vascular anatomy useful to the surgeon. Computed tomography has replaced angiography in the management of cranio-cerebral trauma, except where associated vascular damage such as carotid dissection is suspected.

Contra-indications

1. Where there is a contra-indication to arterial puncture itself. This includes patients with bleeding disorders or severe hypertension.
2. Although the age of the patient is no bar to cerebral angiography, due regard must be taken of the increasing prevalence of atherosclerotic changes with advancing age which will render the procedure potentially more hazardous.
3. In patients with known sensitivity to contrast media, it is clearly preferable to avoid angiography if possible. Appropriate precautions must be taken when it is deemed necessary to carry out the procedure (see Urography, p. 223).

Technical aspects

The introduction of arteriography took place in 1927 when Egan Moniz reported the radiographic visualization of cerebral vessels by the injection of 25% sodium iodide solution into the surgically exposed carotid artery. The original name of 'arterial encephalography' applied to the technique has been replaced by 'cerebral angiography'. Continuous improvements in contrast media and X-ray equipment have increased the diagnostic quality of the examination whilst reducing the risk to the patient.

Contrast media

Thorotrast, a 25% colloidal suspension of thorium dioxide, was adopted in 1931 as a contrast medium which was well-tolerated and gave excellent radiographic contrast. It was a far from ideal medium, however, since any leakage into the tissues was associated with a dense fibrotic reaction. Since it is radioactive and retained in the reticulo-endothelial system, it has the late complication of tumour induction—particularly in the liver. The evolution of the preparations of iodine-based contrast media, associated with a progressive reduction in their toxicity, is described in Chapter 25. All conventionally used contrast media for cerebral angiography until very recently were ionic salts of tri-iodinated substituted benzoic acid, with the meglumine salts having a lower toxicity than sodium salts. A suitable contrast medium is Conray 280 (60% w/v meglumine iothalamate) with an iodine concentration of 280 mg/ml. The introduction of the non-ionic contrast media, such as metrizamide and iopamidol, represents a significant advance; for they cause far less pain on intra-arterial injection, with considerably less endothelial damage and increase in permeability of the blood–brain barrier than previous contrast media, and a consequent reduction in neurotoxicity.

X-ray equipment

In order to make a precise analysis of intra-cranial vascular anatomy and to obtain information about regional contrast flow rates, bi-plane serial angiography is a basic necessity. This requirement was foreseen by Moniz himself, but it was not until 1952 that Fredzell introduced a rapid cut-film changer suitable for cerebral angiography and which could expose as many as 30 films at rates of up to 3/s. Fluoroscopy and a high quality image intensifier are required for catheter studies, coupled with a table which has a movable top capable of a wide range of excursions to follow catheter manipulations. For magnification studies, an X-ray tube with a small focal spot (0.1–0.3 mm) and a 3 phase generator are essential.

Techniques

Whilst cerebral angiography can be carried out by direct puncture or by retrograde filling from injection of a remote vessel, the majority of studies are now carried out by catheterization of individual vessels.

Catheter techniques

Direct catheterization of the four major vessels is usually carried out by the femoral route although, when this is precluded, the axillary route is an alternative. The percutaneous introduction of a catheter into the femoral artery and the general conduct of a catheterization procedure is described in Chapter 8.

Most studies in adults can be carried out under local anaesthetic with basal sedation. A variety of suitable end hole catheters is commercially available for cerebral angiography, personal preference and experience dictating which is selected. Some radiologists prefer to make their own catheters from soft, thin-walled 5F polythene tubing. A simple hook configuration is sufficient in the majority of cases. Preformed 'headhunter' catheters of more complex shape, especially when formed of stiffer material to provide better torque control, are suitable where tortuous ectatic main vessels are encountered.

Under fluoroscopic control, the catheter is advanced into the ascending arch of the aorta and is then rotated until the tip is pointing cranially. The orifices of the main vessel can then be engaged by advancing and withdrawing the catheter. Further catheter advancement, for example in superselective studies, can be achieved with the use of a guide wire. After confirming a correct catheter position by a small test injection of contrast medium, definitive injections are made. Conray 280 (10 ml) is suitable for common carotid angiography with a smaller volume (6–8 ml) being adequate for vertebral angiography, the amount being tailored to the size of the vessel. The catheter is removed after completing the study and sufficient pressure is maintained·on the puncture site for 10–20 minutes to prevent haematoma formation.

Carotid arteriography by the direct puncture technique

Although percutaneous puncture of the carotid artery can be carried out under local anaesthesia, general anaesthesia is required for children and patients unable to provide the necessary degree of cooperation because of anxiety or neurological disturbance. A puncture site is chosen in the lower part of the neck, where the common carotid artery can be palpated medial to the sternomastoid muscle. If the vessel lies very medial, it may be necessary to dislocate it laterally before attempting puncture. A variety of needles and cannulae have been used. The author prefers a simple 18 gauge needle, with a short bevel, mounted in a plastic hub which is continuous with a short length of plastic tubing. The skin and superficial fascia are perforated with a skin needle. A 10 ml glass syringe and a simple two-way tap are connected to the needle assembly and the whole is filled with saline. The index and middle finger palpate the artery with the head slightly extended, the needle then being advanced down to the artery at an angle of approximately 60°. An assistant now disconnects the saline-filled tubing from the tap and the artery is transfixed with a quick thrust. The needle is then slowly withdrawn, applying pressure on its undersurface so that a definite click is

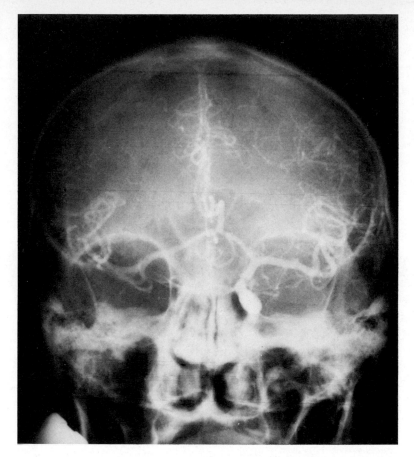

Fig. 19.1 Cross-circulation arteriographic study. The left common carotid artery has been injected with simultaneous compression of the right carotid. The arterior cerebral arteries are elevated by a suprasellar mass.

felt as it passes through the posterior arterial wall. When blood is seen to flow freely into the tubing, it is connected to the tap. The hub of the needle is depressed and the latter stabilized by draping several moistened swabs over it. The needle is intermittently flushed with saline during the procedure. The tap should be turned off whilst saline is still flowing to ensure that there is no backflow of blood into the needle. Serial injections of 10 ml of contrast medium are then made by hand, calling for the exposure to be made close to the end of the injection. As with catheter angiography, intermittent pressure must be maintained over the puncture site for 10 minutes to avoid haematoma formation. Instructions are given to the ward to observe the patient for further bleeding or swelling of the neck which, if bilateral, can cause tracheal compression.

Variations on the basic technique

Compression studies

By compressing the opposite carotid artery during the injection of contrast medium, filling of the contralateral intra-cranial vessels can be achieved to a degree which depends on the patency of the anterior communicating artery (Fig. 19.1). This manoeuvre is valuable when main vessel ligation is being considered as an option in aneurysm surgery. By compressing the vessel above the needle during injection of the right carotid artery, there is reflux of contrast medium into the brachio-cephalic trunk with subsequent filling of the right vertebral artery.

'Trickle' arteriography

Elegant studies of pathology involving the post wall of the carotid artery can be achieved by taking films after the slow injection of 5 ml of contrast medium at 2 s intervals for 8 s. This contrast medium enters the slowly moving sleeve of fluid on the dependent wall of the artery, permitting the identification of small thrombi and pathological stasis associated with atheromatous plaques (Hugh, 1970) (Fig. 19.2).

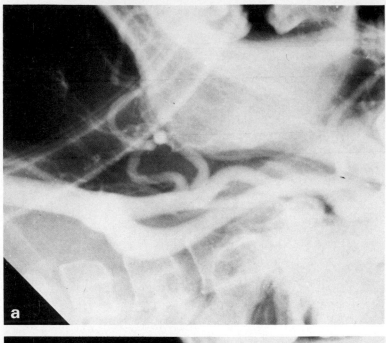

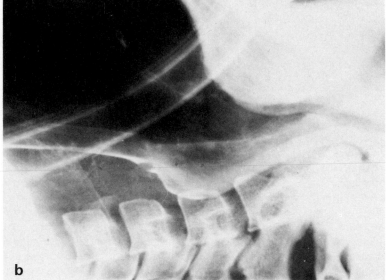

(b) Trickle arteriogram in the same patient. The contrast layer on the posterior wall outlines thrombus at the carotid bifurcation.

Vertebral arteriography

Because of the small lumen of the vertebral artery, needles such as that introduced by Sheldon in 1956 with a blocked tip and a small proximal side hole, are preferred to those with an open bevel. With the head slightly extended and the carotid dislocated laterally, the needle is directed upwards and laterally between the lateral border of the vertebral bodies and medial to the palpable anterior tubercle of the transverse processes. The object is to puncture the vessel in the mid-cervical region as it passes between adjacent transverse foramina. Hypoplasia of the vertebral artery, which is more frequent on the right, precludes successful puncture. Five to 6 ml of contrast medium are injected slowly by hand. An alternative method of direct puncture, described by Maslowski, involves entering the artery above the arch of the atlas from a lateral approach below the mastoid process. Injection of one vertebral artery normally results in sufficient filling of the distal segment of the opposite vertebral artery to outline the posterior inferior cerebellar artery.

Retrograde injection techniques

In 1933 Moniz described the first radiographic demonstration of the vertebral artery by exposing the subclavian artery and making a retrograde injection of Thorotrast. Adopting the same principle, Barbieri and Verdecchia in 1957 described vertebral angiography by percutaneous puncture of the subclavian artery from a supraclavicular approach as this vessel crosses the first rib. The retrograde flow of contrast medium is facilitated by a sphygmomanometer cuff on the upper arm inflated above the systolic pressure. Care must be taken not to allow the needle to pass medial to the first rib, because of the danger of penetrating the lung apex and causing a pneumothorax. When puncture is achieved, the needle is stabilized by lying it flat and taping down the hub. Serial films are exposed at the end of the injection of 20 ml of Conray 280. Although the quality of films may fall short of that achieved by direct injection of the vertebral artery, there is no risk of damaging the wall of the vessel or of dislodging artheromatous plaques from its orifice. Puncture of the right subclavian artery allows the simultaneous display of the right carotid artery as well as the vertebrobasilar system. Similar retrograde studies can also be carried out from cannulation of the brachial artery, although this vessel is more liable to spasm and there is the risk of median nerve damage.

Radiographic procedure

Routine views of the intra-cranial circulation are obtained in at least two projections: the lateral and the antero–posterior. For the latter, the central ray is inclined 15° to the orbito-meatal line to superimpose the superior rim of the orbit and the petrous ridges in carotid studies. The angulation should be increased to 25° in vertebral angiography so that the principal vessels are not superimposed on the skull base. A variety of oblique projections are used principally to clarify the relationship of aneurysms to their parent and adjacent arteries. Delayed films (4–10 s) in the half-axial oblique position after carotid injection are valuable for demonstrating the anatomy of the principal venous sinuses. Evaluation of the extra-cranial carotid vessels requires coned views in the lateral and A–P projections. Magnification angiography using an X-ray tube with a fine focal spot gives an improved demonstration of pathological vessel changes, as in tumours or small arterio-venous malformations. If the plane of the vessels to be studied is 4.5 cm from the tube, with a 0.3 mm focal spot and a focus film distance of 100 cm, a magnification factor of 2.25 then allows vessels as small as 120 μm to be shown.

Photographic subtraction was introduced by Ziedes de Plantes in 1934 and is a valuable adjunct to angiography, particularly in areas where contrast-delineated vessels are superimposed over dense portions of the skull. A standard sequence of films, which allows visualization of the intra-cranial vessels from the arterial phase through to late venous phase, is 2 films/s for 3 s followed by 1 film/s for 4–6 s. Where there is rapid regional blood flow, as in arterio-venous malformations, a more rapid sequence may be required; whereas delayed films are necessary for studying the venous anatomy in sinus thrombosis. Only single films are required for the oblique projections when studying aneurysms. Stereoscopic angiography has few advocates but is regarded by the author as being of value in defining the mutual topographical relationships of the vascular components in arterio-venous malformations and to clarify the relationship of aneurysms to parent and adjacent vessels.

Complications

Cerebral angiography is not without risk, but the most experienced angiographer will have a serious complication rate of less than 0.5% (Mani & Eisenberg, 1978). These authors stress the importance of an experienced operator, finding that a neuroradiologist is twice as safe as a general radiologist and nine times safer than a trainee. The level of experience can be translated into a shorter procedure time and the use of a smaller amount of contrast medium to complete a study, both factors contributing to a reduced morbidity. The local complications associated with femoral catheterization are discussed in the chapter on Arteriography and only specific complications are discussed here.

Damage to the arterial wall Improper placement of the needle tip in direct puncture procedures may lead to the injection of contrast medium beneath a flap of intima, which can lead to partial or even complete arterial occlusion. This may be followed by permanent neurological deficit when the intra-cranial collateral pathways are poor. The use of glass syringes allows the operator to feel the transmitted arterial pulsation in addition to seeing a free back flow of blood into the tubing, both criteria being necessary to ensure correct needle placement. Intimal damage can also follow the forcible advancement of a catheter, particularly if this is made of a rigid material.

Embolization Both the puncturing needle and intra-vascular catheter can dislodge fragments of atheroma, which is particularly likely to happen after prolonged catheter manipulations in the aortic arch of elderly subjects. Both intra-vascular needles and catheters form a nidus for thrombus formation, particularly in prolonged examinations. The catheter and needle system should be irrigated at frequent intervals with heparinized saline.

Contrast medium toxicity Complications due to contrast medium are thought to be due to alteration in the permeability of the blood–brain barrier. This can cause an increase in cerebral oedema in patients with a cerebral tumour, leading to subsequent clinical deterioration. Sodium salts are more toxic in this regard than meglumine salts. Transient cortical blindness, which has been described following vertebral angiography, is thought to be due to a direct toxic effect of contrast medium on the occipital cortex. Care must be taken to avoid complete occlusion of small vertebral vessels by the catheter, which would prevent adequate wash-out of contrast medium.

Current developments in angiography

Supraselective angiographic examination of smaller branches of the extra-cranial and intra-cranial vessels has allowed the development of a variety of occlusion procedures. These have been used to close anterio-venous fistulae, to obliterate vascular malformations, and to reduce the blood supply to vascular lesions prior to surgery. Digital vascular imaging is a recent innovation which is based on real time electronic subtraction of a mask from image intensifier images following injections of contrast medium. The computer enhancement of the digital intensifier image gives a great increase in low contrast detectability. This permits excellent visualization of extra-cranial vessels following an i.v. injection of contrast medium. Excellent images are also produced in cerebral arteriography with small amounts of contrast medium of much lower concentration than is required in conventional techniques.

AIR ENCEPHALOGRAPHY AND VENTRICULOGRAPHY

The ventricular system was first studied by contrast radiography in 1918 when Dandy introduced air into the lateral ventricles by either a fontanelle puncture or a burr hole. It was quickly appreciated that the method was of value in studying cases of hydrocephalus and in the localization of tumours. In the following year, Dandy outlined the cerebrospinal fluid pathways by introducing air through a lumbar puncture. This approach allows the basal cisterns and ventricular system to be studied and is referred to as 'air encephalography'.

Indications

Whereas air studies were used extensively in former times to evaluate cases of suspected intrinsic and extrinsic space-occupying lesions and in the assessment of hydrocephalus and atropic conditions, these examinations have been rendered virtually obsolete by computed tomography. Limited encephalograms are occasionally used to study the brain stem, because of the excellent display in the sagittal plane, and to evaluate lesions within the suprasellar cisterns, particularly if it is required to show their relationship to the optic chiasma prior to surgery.

Contra-indications

Air encephalography is contra-indicated in the presence of raised intra-cranial pressure, when lumbar puncture may be followed by the development of a pressure cone.

Technique

Air encephalography is potentially a very unpleasant examination which may provoke severe and persistent headache and vomiting. The incidence of these symptoms has, however, been greatly reduced by the introduction of neuroleptanalgesia with droperidol and phenoperidine combined with atropine premedication. Hydrocortisone cover is essential in patients with hypopituitarism. During the initial part of the study, the patient sits in a chair facing the skull table top which is inclined at approximately 70° to the horizontal. Following lumbar puncture, a slow injection of 10 ml of air is made, the head being flexed so that the orbito-meatal line is inclined 15° below the horizontal to optimally fill the ventricular system. The cisterna magna, fourth ventricle, aqueduct and posterior half of the third ventricle are outlined in this position. Films are taken in the lateral and reverse Towne's projection (Fig. 19.3a). Delineation of the midline ventricular system may be improved if the patient's head is slowly rotated from side to side to produce an autotomogram (Fig. 19.3b). Filling of the basal cisterns is achieved by extending the head and rapidly injecting 10 ml of air. The needle is removed when adequate ventricular filling has been achieved after the injection of 20–30 ml of air. The patient is then laid down and serial films are taken to show the different parts of the ventricular system. In the supine or brow up position, air outlines the anterior horns and body of each lateral ventricle and the anterior end of the third ventricle (Fig. 19.3c). The patient is next turned prone into the brow-down position to show the posterior part of the lateral ventricles. The temporal horns are filled by somersaulting the patient forwards from the prone position back to the brow up position. Study of the front end of the third ventricle and suprasellar cisterns is carried out by extending the head and is facilitated by dropping the skull table below the level of the patient table.

Ventriculography differs from pneumoencephalography in that air is injected directly into a lateral ventricle via a ventricular cannula, which is then manoeuvred through the ventricular system by a series of positions similar to those described for encephalography. In ventriculography, however, the supratentorial structures are studied first and filling of the ventricular stem within the posterior fossa is achieved by a backward somersault from the brow up position into the brow-down position.

Complications of air encephalography

1. Headache, pallor, sweating and vomiting may occur when air is introduced into the basal cisterns.
2. Mild pyrexia, which is unrelated to the volume of injected air.
3. The production of a pressure cone in a patient with raised intra-cranial pressure. This potential complication requires that the procedure is only carried out where immediate neurosurgical assistance is available.

Positive contrast ventriculography

Outlining the mid-line ventricular system with a small quantity of positive contrast medium allows impinging

lesions to be shown with greater ease and less upset to the patient than occurs with air ventriculography. With the patient sitting and head flexed, 2 ml of Myodil are injected through a catheter whose tip is positioned in one anterior horn. Under screen control, the head is canted slightly and slowly extended so as to run the oil along the medial wall of the ventricle and through the foramen of Monro into the front end of the third ventricle. Further passage of contrast medium can be followed by fluoroscopy. The patient is laid down and films are taken as the Myodil outlines the posterior part of the third ventricle, aqueduct and fourth ventricle (Fig. 19.4).

Cisternography

Cisternography refers to the study of the basal cisterns with contrast medium in order to demonstrate small tumours in the cerebello–pontine angle and suprasellar cisterns.

The cerebello–pontine angle cistern

It is widely accepted that CT with contrast enhancement becomes unreliable when tumours, such as acoustic neuromas, project less than 1 cm into the cerebello–pontine angle. Introduction of contrast medium into the cerebello–pontine angle cistern affords a method of detecting or excluding a very small tumour in the angle and internal auditory meatus. Myodil was the first contrast medium to be used for this purpose. 2–3 ml of Myodil are injected by lumbar puncture and then screened into the cervical region with the patient prone. The patient's head is now rotated through 45° and, with the affected side down, the table is slowly tilted while the contrast medium is screened as it runs through the foramen magnum and then outlines the cerebello–pontine angle cistern. Care must be taken to ensure that no contrast medium escapes through the tentorial hiatus, because it cannot be subsequently retrieved. A–P and a horizontal beam lateral radiographs are then taken. After returning the oil to the cervical region, the procedure can be repeated to obtain comparative views of the other side. CT following the intra-thecal injection of metrizamine to outline the basal cisterns is an alternative procedure. Both methods, however, have been rendered obsolete by the introduction of CT assisted gas cisternography (Sortland, 1978). For this, the patient lies on his side on the scanner table with the affected side uppermost and the shoulders elevated. In order to outline the angle cistern, 5–6 ml of air are injected by lumbar puncture. The patient

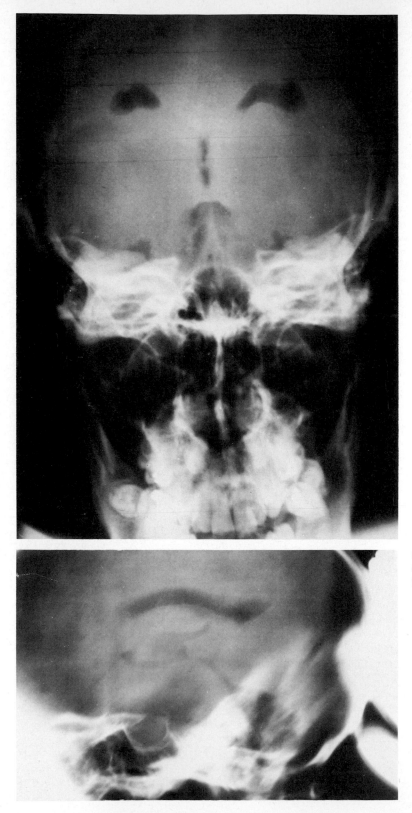

Fig. 19.3 Air encephalogram
(a) Reverse Towne's projection with the patient erect. Air is seen in the lateral ventricles, the third and fourth ventricle and in the cerebello–pontine angle cisterns.

(b) Autotomogram with the patient erect showing excellent visualization of the midline ventricular system.

(c) Brow up lateral film showing a suprasellar extension of a pituitary tumour outlined by air.

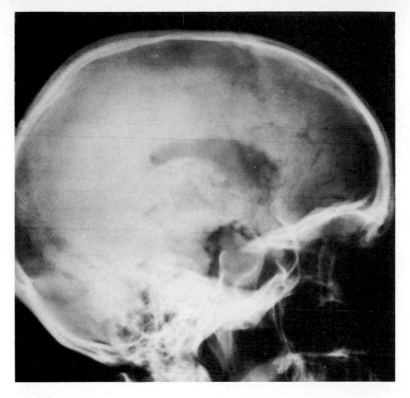

Fig. 19.4 Myodil ventriculogram. Brow up lateral film showing the contrast outlining the midline ventricular system.

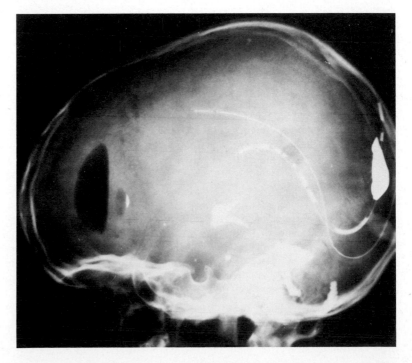

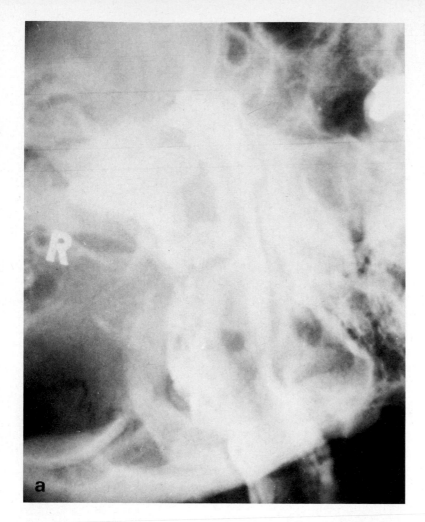

Fig. 19.5 (a) A–P film in a normal myodil cisternogram. There has been excellent filling of the cerebello–pontine angle cistern and adjacent internal auditory canal.

may report a transient discomfort in the ear, which indicates successful filling. The patient is then moved into the scanner and sections are obtained at the level of the internal auditory meatus. The opposite angle cistern can be studied by turning the patient prone and then on to his other side (Fig. 19.5).

The supra sellar cisterns

Investigation of pituitary and para-pituitary lesions can be exacting because their clinical manifestations, including visual failure and endocrinological disturbances, may occur early when the lesion is small. Precise localization and a distinction between the different pathologies is required, to that the appropriate operative route or field size for irradiation can be chosen. It is also valuable to have follow-up studies to assess the results of treatment by radiotherapy or drugs on tumour size. After plain skull X-rays, CT in

the transverse axial plane is usually the next diagnostic method. Despite the high quality of CT images now available, difficulty can sometimes be experienced in assessing the precise extent of the extra-sellar extension of a pituitary tumour and in diagnosing microadenomas. Air encephalography may be required to confirm a suspected diagnosis of the empty sella syndrome and to determine the relationship of any mass to the optic chiasm.

An alternative technique is to opacify the suprasellar cisterns with metrizamide and carry out CT in the transverse, axial and coronal plane. Several authors have pointed out the advantages of screening the contrast medium into the basal cisterns and taking plain radiographs supplemented by tomography to show the anatomy in the sagittal plane. The contrast medium (12 ml of metrizamide, 250 mg I/ml) is injected by lumbar puncture and screened into the suprasellar cisterns using a lateral image intensifier.

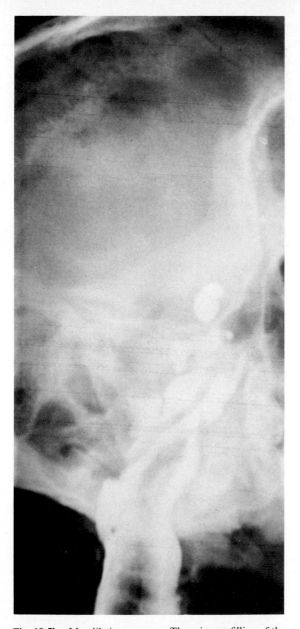

Fig. 19.5b Myodil cisternogram. There is non-filling of the cerebello–pontine angle system and the medial margin of an acoustic neuroma has been outlined.

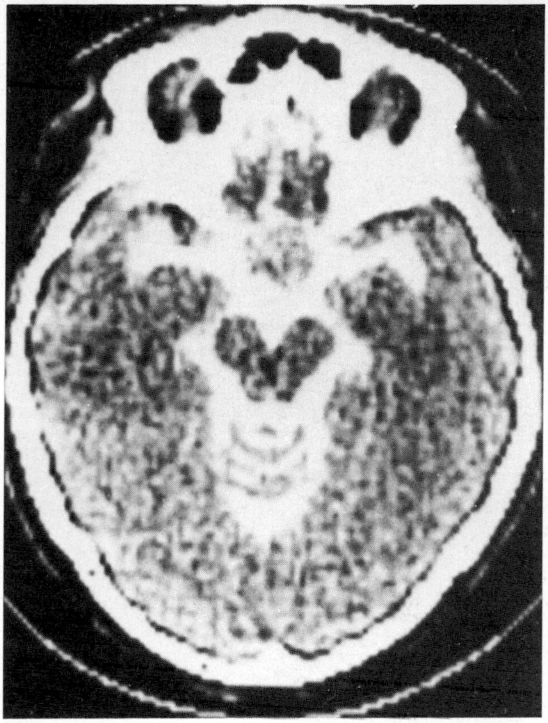

A smaller volume can be used if lateral cervical puncture is adopted. The contra-indications and side effects of the procedure parallel those outlined in the chapter on myelography; a greater frequency and severity of side effects being associated with higher concentrations of metrizamide (Fig. 19.6).

Fig. 19.6 Computer tomographic assisted metrizamide cisternogram. The suprasellar cisterns have been outlined and a rounded filling defect is seen anteriorly which represents an upward extension of tumour from a pituitary adenoma.

REFERENCES

Barbieri P. L. & Verdeccia G. C. (1957) Vertebral arteriography by percutaneous puncture of the subclavian artery. *Acta Radiol.*, **48**, 444.

Dandy W. E. (1918) Ventriculography following the injection of air into the cerebral ventricles. *Ann. Surg.*, **68**, 5.

Dandy W. E. (1919) Röntgenography of the brain after the injection of air into the spinal canal. *Ann. Surg.*, **70**, 397.

Hugh A. E. (1970) Trickle arteriography: demonstration of thrombi in the origin of the internal carotid artery. *Brit. med. J.*, 574.

Mani R. L. & Eisenberg R. L. (1978) Complications of catheter cerebral angiography. *Amer. J. Roentgenol.*, **131**, 867.

Maslowski, A. A. (1955) Vertebral angiography: percutaneous lateral atlanto-occipital method. *Brit. J. Surg.*, **43**, 1.

Moniz E. (1927) Arterial encephalography: its importance in the location of cerebral tumours. *Rev. Neurol.*, **48**, 72.

Moniz E. (1940) Die cerebral Arteriographie und Phlebographie in Monographien aus dem Gesamtgebiet der Neurologie und Psychiatrie. Springer, Berlin.

Sheldon P. (1956) A special needle for percutaneous vertebral angiography. *Brit. J. Radiol.*, **29**, 231.

Sortland O. (1978) X-ray diagnosis of expanding lesions in the cerebellopontine angle. Meeting of the Nordic Society of Radiology.

Ziedes de Plantes B. G. (1961) *Subtraktion*. Thieme, Stuttgart.

FURTHER READING

Burrows E. H. (1975) Positive contrast examination (cerebello-pontine cisternography) in extra-meatal acoustic neurofibromas. *Brit. J. Radiol.*, **42**, 902.

Hall K. & McAllister V. L. (1980) Metrizamide cisternography in pituitary and juxta-pituitary lesions. *Radiology*, **134**, 101.

Newton R. H. & Potts D. G. (Eds) (1977) *Radiology of the Skull and Brain*. Vol. 2. Book 1. Angiography Technical Aspects. Vol. 4. Ventricles and Cisterns. Mosby, St Louis.

Sortland O. (1979) Computer tomography combined with gas cisternography for the diagnosis of expanding lesions in the cerebello–pontine angle. *Neuroradiology*, **18**, 19.

G. A. S. LLOYD

Plain radiography

The plain X-ray examination of the orbit consists, in the first instance, of standard skull projections; that is, postero–anterior (P–A), lateral and Towne's projections.

In the presence of a unilateral proptosis, the standard projections are augmented by views of the optic foramina. The radiographic position for these is obtained by tilting the orbito–meatal baseline of the skull 30° upwards from the occipito–frontal position and rotating the head 39° away from the affected side, thus projecting the optic canal into the infero-lateral quadrant of the orbit. A useful modification of this optic canal view in cases of suspected enlargement of the superior orbital fissure is obtained by using slightly less angulation of the orbito–meatal line, 25° instead of 30°, and less obliquity of the head than that normally employed for optic canal projections. This gives better visualization of the apex of the orbit and surrounding structures and is the optimum method of demonstrating erosion of the optic strut by plain radiography.

An occipito–oral view should be used routinely in an orbital skull series. The radiographic position is similar to that of the standard occipito–mental view used in the radiography of the paranasal sinuses, but with the orbito–meatal line tilted 35° to the film. A similar projection is obtained by placing the head in the position for a P–A view with 35° of caudal tube angulation. The central ray is then directed along the horizontal axis of the orbit so that the roof is more completely seen than in the standard P–A view, with less foreshortening, and the petrous temporal bases are projected below the inferior orbital margin.

Tomography

Tomography is an essential part of the X-ray investigation of the orbit and the related paranasal sinuses. Abnormalities not readily visualized on plain radiography may be demonstrated on tomography; while changes seen on standard films are often better delineated in terms of size, extent and relationship to adjoining structures by this means.

Complete tomography of the facial skeleton requires radiography in three planes: namely coronal, lateral and axial.

Coronal plane

The patient is placed prone. An under-tilted occipito–mental position is preferred for demonstrating the orbits, the orbito–meatal line being angled 30–35° cephalad. In this view, the central ray is projected roughly along the central axis of the orbit. The same projection is used to demonstrate the maxillary antra. However, the posterior ethmoids and sphenoid sinuses are better demonstrated by adjusting this position to correspond to a P–A projection, the nose and forehead being placed in contact with the table top, and the orbito–meatal line at right angles to it.

The most important application of tomography in the coronal plane is the demonstration of expanding processes and bone destruction, either inflammatory or neoplastic, in paranasal sinus disease and for the delineation of fractures involving the orbit and sinuses.

Lateral plane

The patient is placed in the prone oblique position with the uppermost leg raised and the knee bent. This helps to maintain a true lateral position when the head is turned in a lateral direction. Lateral tomography is used to demonstrate 'blow out' fractures of the orbital floor, including a pre-operative estimation of the posterior extent of the fracture. In cases of mucocele of the frontal sinus invading the orbital roof, it is sometimes possible to demonstrate a thin rim of expanded bone forming the inferior border of the mucocele on lateral tomography. In addition, lateral tomography is also important in the assessment of the naso-pharynx, sphenoid sinus and basisphenoid.

Axial tomography

Pluridirectional tomography is mandatory for this technique. Hypocycloidal tube movement gives the best results, but other rotational tomographic movements yield adequate results in most instances. The position of the patient is illustrated in Fig. 20.1. A light wooden platform is placed on the table top so that the submento-vertical (SMV) position of the skull is obtained with the patient lying horizontal. While a standard SMV projection with the orbito–meatal line placed parallel to the film, is adequate for axial

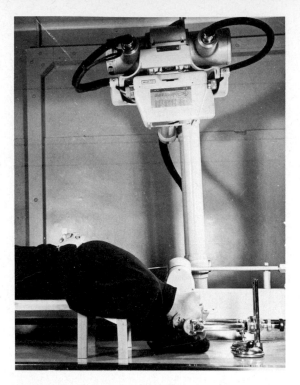

Fig. 20.1 Position of the patient for axial tomography. The wooden platform has an angled end to help the patient maintain the extended position of the head and neck.

tomography of the orbits and paranasal sinuses, a more hyperextended position is required to show the optic canal in the axial plane. Since this is physically impossible for most patients, it becomes necessary to angle the radiograph in the cassette holder. The attachment for macrotomography on the Polytome apparatus allows angles of inclination of 45° or more. The film has to be inclined 25–30° for the tomographic cut to lie in the plane of the optic canal with the patient in the SMV position. The inclined plane method is also very useful in patients who have difficulty in maintaining a full SMV position, for instance the elderly or patients with a dorsal kyphosis, the inclination of the film compensating for any under-tilt of the head.

Axial tomography is an essential part of the investigation of the ENT causes of proptosis. The majority of lesions which cause exophthalmos and originate in the paranasal sinuses are demonstrated by plain radiography, but early expansion or erosion of the medial orbital wall from lesions arising in the ethmoid cells may be very difficult to appreciate without either conventional or computed tomography. Axial tomography provides a plan view of the whole of the ethmoid labyrinth on a single radiograph so that the exact extent of a tumour can be demonstrated, showing any encroachment across the mid-line or into the sphenoid sinuses or a breach of the medial-orbital wall with orbital involvement. The presence and degree of orbital involvement is particularly important in malignant disease of the sinuses since it influences the decision to exenterate the orbit at surgery.

Computed tomography (CT) of the orbit

CT scanning has revolutionized the radiological investigation of orbital disease in the past decade. The presence of fat in the orbit acts as a natural contrast medium. Following plain radiographic examination of the skull, CT scanning is now the principal method of investigating patients with uni-lateral exophthalmos and suspected intra-orbital mass lesions. Other modalities, namely orbital venography, carotid angiography and ultrasonography are ancillary to this method.

An all-purpose scanner is preferred for orbital CT rather than a dedicated head scanner, since the design of the latter makes coronal scanning difficult or impractical as a routine procedure. In addition to axial scans, coronal, oblique and even sagittal sections are feasible in body scanners because of their larger scanning apertures. For axial scans of the orbit, the prone position is preferred when there is an overcouch gantry and tube mounting. In this way the incident beam of X-rays is directed for the most part through the back of the skull, reducing the radiation dose received by the lens and cornea to less than one-sixth of that received when the patient is supine. It is important that the attitude of the patient's head allows the optimum scanning plane to be obtained through the orbits. Satisfactory scans should include the globes, showing the lens, optic nerve, lateral and medial rectus muscles on the same cut. To do this, the position of the head should be adjusted so that the scanning plane forms an angle of 16° caudally from the orbito–meatal line, which is marked on the skin prior to scanning. Optimum orbital scans are obtained if the posterior clinoids are shown on scans which also include the optic nerves and clearly show the globes on both sides.

For coronal scans the patient lies prone (Fig. 20.2) with the chin elevated, so that the radiation port is principally through the skull vault for scanners designed with an overcouch tube mounting. A similar position can be obtained by placing the patient supine with the head hyper-extended, a position which is

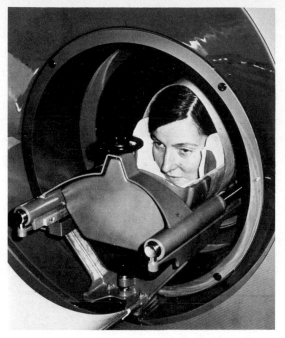

Fig. 20.2 Position of the patient for coronal CT of the head.

preferable in rotate-translate scanners with an under-couch tube.

Contrast medium

The injection of contrast medium for orbital CT scanning is no longer a routine procedure. Post-contrast scans to show tissue enhancement are to be avoided if possible, since the injection of contrast medium converts a totally non-invasive procedure into one which carries a similar morbidity and mortality to i.v. urography. Initial studies (Lloyd & Ambrose, 1976) showed that specific tissue recognition is unlikely from the behaviour of the attenuation values before and after contrast medium injection. In general, therefore, contrast medium should only be used to show up doubtful space-occupying lesions in better detail or when there is suspicion of intra-cranial spread and involvement of the blood–brain barrier. The administration of contrast medium if a clearly defined lesion is shown on the unenhanced scans is usually unnecessary.

REFERENCE

Lloyd G. A. S. & Ambrose J. A. E. (1976) An evaluation of CAT in the diagnosis of orbital space occupying lesions. In *Computerized Axial Tomography in Clinical Practice*. p. 154. Springer Verlag, Berlin.

ORBITAL VENOGRAPHY

The investigation of orbital space-occupying lesions by filling the superior ophthalmic veins with contrast medium was first described by Dejean and Boudet (1951) and Yasargil (1957). In the original technique, the superior ophthalmic vein was filled from an injection into the angular vein by either a cut-down or a percutaneous puncture. This method has largely been superseded by the method of frontal vein injection, described by Vritsios (1961) (Fig. 20.3). In the majority of patients, the venepuncture into a frontal vein or main tributary is easy to perform and to maintain during radiography.

Before injection, a rubber band is placed around the forehead at the hairline to prevent the escape of contrast medium over the scalp. Compression of the facial veins is also required to prevent loss of contrast medium and is achieved by instructing the patient to compress the veins on either side of the nose with the fingers. In some patients the most prominent forehead vein is the anterior temporal branch, and it can be used successfully to make the injection provided the temporal vein is occluded above the angle of the jaw by finger pressure. A 23-gauge scalp vein needle is used for the injection, unless the veins are large enough to accommodate a 21-gauge needle which results in a more rapid injection and better venous filling. Ten millilitres of Conray 280 or an equivalent contrast medium is used, radiographs being exposed after delivery of 5 ml and immediately prior to the end of the injection. A preliminary control film is also obtained for subtraction studies.

Both orbital venous systems normally fill, provided sufficient contrast medium is used, the frontal vein approach having the advantage of allowing minor degrees of displacement of the veins on the abnormal side to be detected by comparison with the opposite normal side. Routine A–P and undertilted axial film series are taken and, where necessary, lateral views. The latter are generally the least informative because of the overlap of the venous system on the two sides in this projection. Frontal venography is performed without anaesthesia and on an out-patient basis in at least 80% of patients. A general anaesthetic is required in children, and in adults with difficult veins in which venipuncture has failed initially.

Orbital venography causes little pain and has a low morbidity. The only complications in a series of over 700 venograms have been subcutaneous extravasations of contrast medium at the injection site, which have resolved without incident. Hypersensitivity to the contrast medium is the principal risk, so that the

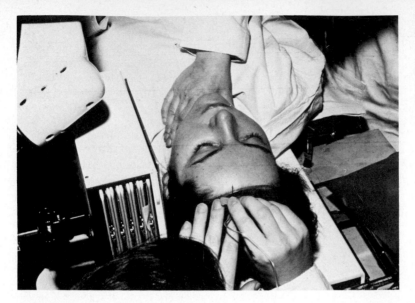

Fig. 20.3 Method of venepuncture for orbital venography. A rubber band is placed at the hairline to prevent reflux of the contrast medium. The neck veins are compressed at the moment of puncture to create venous distension over the forehead.

overall morbidity and mortality of this investigation is similar to that of i.v. urography.

The majority of space-occupying lesions in the orbit are demonstrated by venous displacement. The pattern of displacement indicates the location of the lesion in the orbit; for example whether it has an intra- or extra-conal situation. To a large extent, orbital venography has been superseded by soft tissue imaging techniques, notably computed tomography. Venous obstruction may be caused by tumours, especially those in the apex of the orbit, by venous thrombosis of the superior ophthalmic vein and by retro-orbital masses obstructing the cavernous sinus. A caroticocavernous fistula also causes non-filling of the veins on the affected side.

A pathological circulation gives additional evidence of the presence of a tumour, usually being associated with malignancy but sometimes with benign tumours such as cavernous haemangiomas. The grossest venous abnormalities are, however, seen most often in patients with congenital venous malformations or orbital varices.

REFERENCES

Dejean C. & Boudet C. (1951) *Bull. Soc. Fr. Ophthalmol.* **64**, 374.
Vritsios A. (1961) *Archs. Soc. Ophthalmol. Grece.* **12**, 223.
Yasargil M. G. (1957) *Die Rontgendiagnostik des Exophthalmus unilateralis.* Karger, Basel.

CAROTID ANGIOGRAPHY

The introduction of computed tomography has made carotid angiography less necessary for the routine investigation of unilateral exophthalmos. CT scanning has largely superseded carotid angiography in the exclusion of intracranial lesions causing proptosis. Soft tissue imaging has also made pre-operative intra-orbital diagnosis far more exact and surgery may be undertaken without the morbidity associated with carotid puncture or catheterization. Carotid arteriography should therefore only be carried out on selected patients; principally those with suspected vascular anomalies in either the orbit or middle fossa; for example, an arterio-venous malformation or infraclinoid aneurysm. Arteriography may also be required pre-operatively to identify the feeding vessels of a highly vascular tumour or for the purposes of embolization.

In a patient with proptosis, an elaboration of normal carotid arteriographic technique is required to combine an adequate study of the intra-cranial vessels with a detailed investigation of the orbit. Straight needle puncture is to be avoided, selective catheterization of the carotid vessels via the femoral artery being the method of choice.

Three projections are used for the angiogram series. These are all magnified geometrically using a high energy X-ray tube with a focus of 0.3 mm or less.

1. A standard lateral arteriogram series of the skull and a series of lateral macro-angiograms coned to the orbit.

2. An A–P series. The latter projection is modified from that normally used in carotid angiography. The orbito–meatal line is angled cranially 10°, with the central ray at right angles to the film. This projects the ophthalmic artery through the orbit, at the same time giving adequate visualization of the internal carotid and the anterior and middle cerebral vessels. The ophthalmic artery is seen end on in this view, which is therefore an unsatisfactory second plane of visualization of this vessel when used in conjunction with the lateral series. This demonstration is provided by the third projection.
3. Modified axial view. This provides a plan view of the ophthalmic artery and its main branches. It is neither necessary nor desirable to obtain a full axial or SMV view. In the latter the lower jaw is projected through the orbits making good subtraction studies difficult, particularly if the patient has a full set of teeth. In the position recommended, the head and neck are extended and the tube angled cranially to make an angle of 75° to the orbito–meatal line while the central ray is directed through the roof of the mouth. The lower jaw is then projected entirely below the orbit and the ophthalmic vessels are seen through the maxillary antrum. This position could be described as a reversed over-tilted occipito–mental view. Selective internal carotid injection of contrast medium is essential for a good angiogram series in this position, since filling of the external carotid obscures the orbital vessels. Subtraction films should be routine.

DACRYOCYSTOGRAPHY

Dacrocystography was originally described by Ewing (1909) who used bismuth subnitrate as a contrast medium to outline a lacrimal sac abscess cavity. The conventional technique derived from his method consists of cannulation of the inferior or superior canaliculus, the injection of contrast medium into the duct system, followed by P–A and lateral radiographs taken after the removal of the cannula. Campbell (1964), using this method of injection, introduced a radiographic enlargement technique and showed the advantages of the enhanced radiographic detail obtained by macrodacryocystography. Iba and Hanafee (1968) described a method of distension dacryocystography, drawing attention to the advantages of making the radiographic exposure during the injection of the contrast medium. The technique to be described is a combination of these two methods and, when combined with subtraction studies, is the optimum way of radiographically demonstrating the lacrimal

duct system. The greater detail of the canalicular system is of critical importance in deciding the surgical approach to abnormalities of the common canaliculus.

The technique is based on a continuous injection method, described by Jones (1959) particularly to show the common canaliculus, and has been combined with radiographic enlargement. The magnification technique has been modified from that of Campbell (1964), in that the patient is placed supine using a standard skull table or serial changer. Geometrical enlargement of the radiograph is obtained by using an X-ray tube with a 0.3 mm focal spot or less. Normally two macrograms are obtained and a control exposure is made prior to injection for subtraction studies. Subtraction allows bone-free visualization of the ducts, particularly the common canaliculus.

The radiographic exposure is made during the actual injection of contrast medium through the catheter. This is important in obtaining optimal filling of the duct system and in most instances produces an image of the contrast medium which is continuous throughout the duct system. Before catheterization of the inferior canaliculus, a drop of amethocaine is instilled into the conjunctival sac and any mucus in the duct system is expressed by pressure over the inner canthus. A non-viscous contrast medium is used, since the bore of the catheter is too small to allow a brisk injection of Lipiodol which is generally used in dacryocystography. A dose of 2 ml Lipiodol ultrafluid is drawn up into a syringe which is then connected to a 12 in intravenous catheter (outside diameter 0.63 mm) and any air bubbles are expressed. The punctum is dilated with a Nettleship dilator and the tip of the catheter is then introduced into the canaliculus. This manoeuvre is greatly facilitated if the punctum is drawn laterally and the tip of the catheter is rotated between the finger and the thumb during its introduction. In order to obtain the best radiographs, it is essential not to advance the tip of the catheter more than 3–4 mm into the canaliculus. The catheter is held in place by sticking plaster applied to the cheek at the outer canthus. Slight pressure is applied to the loop of the catheter so that it is under tension and thereby held in position during the injection (Fig. 20.4). The lower canaliculus is usually chosen as it is more convenient and functionally more important. The upper canaliculus is normally outlined by reflux of the contrast medium. In special circumstances, the upper canaliculus is catheterized and injected either individually or simultaneously.

The narrow lumen of the catheter and the low viscosity of the contrast medium allow only a small positive pressure to be created, even if considerable

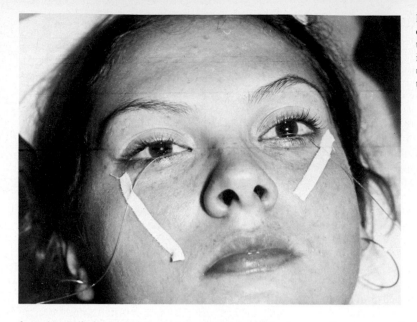

Fig. 20.4 Method of securing the catheters for intubation macrodacryocystography. Both inferior canaliculi are intubated and the catheters are kept under slight tension by fixing them to the cheek with sticking plaster.

force is applied to the syringe. In order that sufficient contrast medium circulates in the system, an interval of 3 s is allowed after starting the injection and before exposing the radiographs. The macrograms are exposed in the A–P plane during injection of the contrast medium and a lead-rubber screen is therefore needed to protect the operator from scattered radiation.

It is the usual practice to perform bilateral intubation macrodacryocystograms simultaneously, because of the high incidence of bilateral abnormalities and the useful information which can be obtained by comparison with the normal macrogram. It is wise to take a subsequent upright lateral film to ensure that the contrast medium has had an opportunity to reach the nasopharynx, thus confirming the patency of the system. If bilateral macrodacryocystograms have been carried out, the same information can be obtained from an oblique film.

In summary, the method employs:

1. Intubation to produce distension of the duct system and better contrast filling, particularly of the common canaliculus.
2. Macroradiography to produce better radiography definition.
3. Subtraction to produce bone-free visualization of the ducts, particularly the common canaliculus.

REFERENCES

Campbell W. (1964) The radiology of the lacrimal system. *Brit. J. Radiol.*, **37**, 1–26.

Ewing A. E. (1909) Roentgen ray demonstration of the lacrymal abscess cavity. *Amer. J. Opthalmol.*, **26**, 1–4.

Iba G. B. & Hanafee W. N. (1968) Distension dacryocystography. *Radiology*, **90**, 1020–2.

Jones B. R. (1950) Personal communication.

SECTION 6
MISCELLANEOUS

Arthrography 21

E. J. ROEBUCK

'The diagnostic value of arthrography of any joint in radiological practice is directly proportional to the interest and experience of the Radiologist using it.' *Editorial Comment Year Book of Radiology*, 1970.

Arthrography is the radiological examination of a joint, following the injection of contrast medium, in order to demonstrate details of congenital or acquired abnormalities which might not otherwise be apparent.

A single contrast technique may be used for small volume joints. Large capacity joints, particularly where detailed visualization of intra-articular structures is required, are examined by a double contrast technique.

While arthrography is mostly performed on synovial joints, other types of articulations such as the intervertebral body joints can also be examined (discography).

While the procedure itself is relatively simple, accurate interpretation of arthrograms usually requires considerable experience. Attention to radiographic detail is essential, with high quality radiography being mandatory. In particular, accurate positioning by fluoroscopy is essential for most joints (Sachs *et al.*, 1950; Butt & McIntyre, 1969; Ricklin *et al.*, 1979; Stoker, 1980).

CHOICE OF CONTRAST MEDIUM

Negative contrast medium

A single contrast technique, using only a gas, is rarely employed nowadays, although it may still have a role in differentiating a popliteal cyst rupture from deep vein thrombosis or in individuals with a history of severe hypersensitivity to contrast media.

Air is now almost universally employed in double contrast techniques, the risk of air embolism being extremely small. When relatively large volumes of gas are required, as in the knee joint, the use of carbon dioxide results in joint distension and consequent discomfort of minimal duration because of the rapid absorption of this gas (Butt & McIntyre, 1969; Stoker, 1980). However, air still results in only slight patient incapacity under the same circumstances (Roebuck, 1977).

Positive contrast media

Positive contrast is obtained by the injection of an iodine—containing water-soluble contrast medium. Several compounds are available, each having disadvantages and advantages.

A contrast medium with a large molecule, such as Hexabrix (May & Baker), has a slower rate of absorption into the cartilagenous surfaces, and facilitates the differentiation between pathological damage and intact surfaces. Moreover, when a procedure is prolonged, due to supplementary projections or tomography, the rapid rate of absorption of monomeric compounds causes unsharpness of normal joint surfaces (Roebuck, 1977). The disadvantage of Hexabrix is the cost, which is higher than that of simple monomeric compounds. Urografin 310 (Schering Chemicals) and Conray 280 (May and Baker) are cheaper and, in common with Hexabrix, give rise to little synovial irritation. The dilution of the contrast medium by synovial fluid, resulting from synovial membrane irritation, is virtually avoided by the use of non-ionic contrast media; namely metrizamide (Amipaque, Nyegaard), iopamidol (Niopam, Merck) and iohexol (Omnipaque Nyegaard). However, these agents are very expensive and their use is scarcely justified for arthrography.

The addition of 0.3 ml of 1 in 1000 adrenalin to the positive contrast reduces synovial secretion by inducing a reduction in blood flow (Hall, 1974), but this also delays the return of the knee to normality (Roebuck, 1977).

BASIC TECHNIQUE

A strict aseptic technique is essential, in order to avoid the risk of septic arthritis. The operator should wear gloves, but a mask and sterile gown are not usually worn.

The patient should have the procedure explained in full prior to the examination, and should be warned as each successive step is undertaken. Sedation is then rarely necessary in adults, but general anaesthesia is often advisable for children since full cooperation and muscle relaxation is not easily achieved in the very young.

It is important that a full plain radiographic examination of the joint is performed prior to arthrography. The injection site is subsequently chosen and should be as remote as possible from any clinically or radiologically suspected abnormality.

The patient is positioned on the radiographic table and the skin over the chosen injection site, identified on fluoroscopy, is marked with an indelible pen. The skin is cleansed with a suitable antiseptic solution and the injection site is infiltrated with local anaesthetic. The needle of choice is then advanced into the joint space. If a syringe partially filled with air or saline is attached to the needle, the correct positioning of the needle point is confirmed by a reduction of resistance to injection and a lack of 'bounce back' of the syringe plunger on release of pressure. Positioning of the needle may be confirmed by fluoroscopy.

Contrast medium is introduced following correct positioning of the needle. When a double contrast technique is employed, the injection of air is followed by a water-soluble positive contrast medium. Commonly, this in turn is followed by a further injection of air or carbon dioxide. Small volume joints, such as the wrist and ankle, are satisfactorily examined by using only a positive contrast medium.

The needle is removed on completion of the injection and the puncture site is sealed with Nobecutane or collodian. Active or passive movements ensure even distribution of the contrast medium within the joint. The patient is then ready for radiography.

RADIOGRAPHY

In order to obtain high quality radiographs, it is essential to pay attention to many points of technique. The focal spot size should be the smallest possible. A 0.3 mm focal spot is ideal but, if a 0.6 mm or 1.2 mm size is necessary for reasons of tube loading, the resultant degradation of image quality may be acceptable.

Accurate and maximum beam collimation is necessary. A purpose designed, small aperture lead diaphragm is often advantageous, particularly for knee arthrography.

Geometrical unsharpness should be minimized by using the largest possible tube–object to object–film ratio. This is difficult when films are taken during fluoroscopic examination with an undercouch tube, but the use of elevating pads on the radiographic table may be helpful. The use of a grid to eliminate scatter should be avoided, if possible, in cases where there is only minimal soft tissue overlying the joint.

The particular film screen combination is of great importance. The speed should be sufficiently fast to avoid movement blur, but high definition is the most important requirement.

Patient positioning is best achieved by fluoroscopic control, although this is not essential or even practicable for some joints. Stress views are commonly required, with the use of restraining bands to reduce the risk of movement blur.

Contra-indications to arthrography

The presence of local sepsis is an absolute contra-indication to arthrography because of the risk of inducing an acute septic arthritis. Arthrography should also be deferred if a patient is suffering from an acute generalized infection.

KNEE ARTHROGRAPHY

Indications

The investigation and elucidation of suspected meniscal or cruciate ligament injury provides the main indications for knee arthrography. Arthrography should be regarded as an adjunct to clinical evaluation, the inter-relationship of arthroscopy and arthrography being clearly defined within each unit (Table 21.1).

Table 21.1 Relative value of arthrography and arthroscopy

	Arthrography	Arthroscopy
Meniscus tears		
Anterior	Good	Good
Posterior	Good	Difficult
Inferior surface	Good	Impossible
Small	Poor	Better
Meniscus degeneration	Poor	Good
Meniscus fragment removal	Impossible	Possible
Chondromalacia patellae	Very poor	Good
Osteochondritis dissecans	Good	Good
Cruciate ligaments	Good	Variable
Popliteal cyst	Excellent	Difficult
Synovitis	Poor	Good

The presence or rupture of a popliteal cyst is readily confirmed by arthrography.

Technique

A lateral injection site is usually the most convenient, although a medial injection is no more difficult. The patient lies supine on the radiographic table. A 19 gauge needle is introduced about 1 cm lateral (or medial) to the mid-point of the patellar border. Manual displacement of the patella towards the injection site creates a larger subjacent joint cavity and considerably facilitates accurate needle positioning and subsequent injection.

It is important to aspirate any synovial effusion as completely as possible, prior to the injection of contrast medium, in order to avoid dilution and to minimize bubble formation.

Following the injection of about 20 ml of air, 3 ml or positive contrast medium are injected, followed by the remainder of the air or carbon dioxide. The total volume required varies with the capacity of the individual joint, 50–80 ml being usual but up to 100 ml may be necessary. A sufficient volume is determined by palpating the tension in the supra-patellar pouch.

Meniscus examination

It is necessary to apply an abduction force, to 'open up' the medial side of the joint space, for the demonstration of the medial meniscus. Similarly, an adduction force is necessary to show the lateral meniscus. These forces are best applied by positioning the patient prone on suitable elevating pads and passing a looped band around the thigh. This band is attached to the side of the table medial to the joint under examination when an abduction force is applied to the knee, and to the lateral side when applying an adduction force. The levering force is obtained by manipulation of the leg, which is held at ankle level by the examiner.

In cases where the prone position is impracticable, adequate films may be obtained with the patient supine (Roebuck, 1977). Radiologists should familiarize themselves with both prone and supine techniques, the examination being occasionally facilitated by reversing the patient's position when there is difficulty in demonstrating a specific region of an individual joint.

Using a suitable spot film device, a series of 8–12 films are taken of each meniscus to give a cross-section view of the whole length of the meniscus. The radiographs are exposed by an assistant, while the examiner applies an abduction (or adduction) force to the leg and ensures by fluoroscopic observation that the section of tibial plateau underlying the portion of meniscus being examined is exactly in line with the central X-ray beam (Fig. 21.1).

Patello–femoral joint examination

Although arthrographic abnormalities are rare in chondromalacia patellae, examination of the patello–femoral joint should be undertaken as a routine in all patients undergoing arthrography in whom there is any clinical suspicion of patello–femoral abnormality.

Both axial and lateral projections of the patello–femoral joint are obtained by using a horizontal X-ray beam and overcouch tube technique. It is important that the knee should be flexed through no more than 40° during this procedure, otherwise there will be no visualization of that portion of the femoral articular surface which is normally in contact with the patella (Fig. 21.2).

Cruciate ligament examination

The anterior cruciate ligament should be examined routinely because, although it may be ruptured as an isolated injury, it is commonly damaged in association with medial meniscus or medial ligament tears.

Although the cruciate ligaments are extra-synovial in situation, they may be visualized in two planes. A modified tunnel view gives a sagittal projection (Roebuck, 1977) but a lateral projection is the preferred view for demonstrating tears, laxity or avulsion. It is important that the knee is flexed through at least 60°, otherwise visualization may be impossible (Liljedahl et al., 1965). Radiographs are taken with a vertical beam, using either a fluoroscopic spot film device or an overcouch tube. A radiograph should routinely be taken under stress, with the tibia pulled anteriorly—the 'drawer sign' manoeuvre.

A very satisfactory technique is that advocated by Freiberger (1979) and by Stoker (1980). The patient sits on the end of the radiographic table with his thigh supported on a pad and the leg hanging vertically. Two radiographs are exposed with a horizontal X-ray beam, one at rest and one with the calf actively pressed against the vertical edge of the table.

Popliteal cyst examination

High intra-articular pressure, due to a traumatic effusion or haemarthrosis, or to an effusion secondary to a synovitis such as rheumatoid arthritis, may cause a rupture of the posterior capsule of the joint with the subsequent formation of a popliteal bursa or cyst.

Occasionally, an acute rupture may give rise to clinical signs similar to those of deep calf vein thrombosis. Similar signs may arise if the high pressure state recurs subsequent to the formation of a popliteal cyst, which may itself then rupture or extensively dissect distally between the calf muscles.

A simple lateral film of the leg following either a

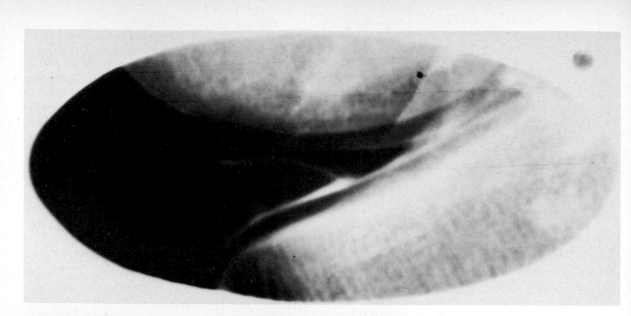

Fig. 21.1 Knee arthrogram. Spot radiograph of meniscus.

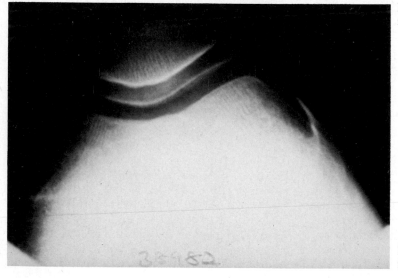

Fig. 21.2 Knee arthrogram. Patello–femoral joint.

single or double contrast injection is sufficient to establish the diagnosis (Fig. 21.3).

HIP ARTHROGRAPHY

Indications

The main indication for hip arthrography is the management of congenital hip dysplasia (CHD) (Grech, 1972). Specifically, arthrography is indicated when there is clinical doubt regarding the diagnosis or when there has been a failure of closed reduction. In some centres it is regarded as being an essential investigation prior to open reduction. Arthrography is also of value in recurrent hip dislocation, or dislocation secondary to muscle paralysis.

In Legg Calvé Perthes disease, arthrography has little to contribute in the early or late stages, but enables a more accurate prognosis to be made in the intermediate stage (Kutz, 1968).

Some assistance in the management of the complications of total hip replacement has been reported (Salvati *et al.*, 1971) and, with the assessment of articular surface damage, provides the main indication for arthrography in adults.

Technique

If the patient is younger than 10 years old, it is usually necessary to perform hip arthrography under general

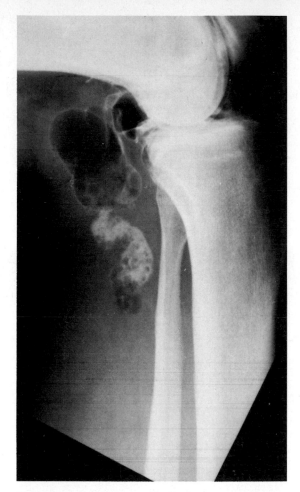

Fig. 21.3 Knee arthrogram. Popliteal cyst.

anaesthesia. Only light sedation is usually required in other cases.

The patient is placed supine on the radiographic table, with the hip in a relaxed neutral position. Following cleansing of the skin, a point directly anterior to the supero-lateral aspect of the femoral head is identified by fluoroscopy. When the capacity of the hip joint is suspected to be increased, or where the femoral head is completely dislocated, the skin marking for injection should be over the infero-medial aspect of the femoral head. A 20 or 22 gauge, short bevelled needle with a stilette is introduced vertically from this point until the tip is felt to impinge on the femoral head. The stilette is then replaced by a syringe containing a few millimetres of saline. When the needle is correctly positioned, it is possible to inject 0.5–1 ml of the saline without difficulty. Pressure on the plunger is then released and the syringe slowly refills due to the intra-articular pressure, thus confirming correct positioning of the needle.

The saline syringe is then replaced by one containing the contrast medium. Between 1 and 4 ml of contrast medium are injected, correct positioning being confirmed after the first 0.5 ml by fluoroscopy. The exact quantity of contrast medium varies according to the age of the patient and the degree of laxity of the joint, the correct volume being judged by the resistance of injection and fluoroscopic appearances.

While the anterior approach as described above is most commonly used, some examiners prefer a lateral approach with the needle being passed just above the greater trochanter and along the femoral neck. An inferior approach has also been employed, the needle being introduced under the adductor tendons while the contralateral leg is in adduction.

Radiographic technique

Radiography is by spot films or continuous video tape recording or, ideally, the simultaneous use of both. The spot films are taken with a fluoroscopic spot film device, or 100 or 105 mm format camera. (Fig. 21.4)

It is important to perform a full range of hip movements and stress studies. A full list of suggested positions is given by Grech (1972). Variations of the full technique may be made when limited information is required from the examination, as in a repeat examination to monitor response to treatment.

There are several key observations which contribute to accurate interpretation, and particular attention should be paid to their demonstration during the investigation. These are: capsular capacity, location of the labrum acetabulare, the parallelism and the smoothness of the joint surfaces, femoral head deformity, and stability of the femoral head in the acetabulum. The advantages of video tape recording and the necessity for stress views are readily appreciated in the assessment of stability.

SHOULDER ARTHROGRAPHY

Indications

Arthrography of the shoulder is of value following acute injury, when it is necessary to estimate the degree of damage to the rotator cuff tendons and the joint capsule before considering operative repair.

The commonest indication is in cases of persistent pain and/or limitation of movement where arthrography may demonstrate surgically remediable lesions or may provide evidence that operative exploration is unnecessary (Preston & Jackson, 1977).

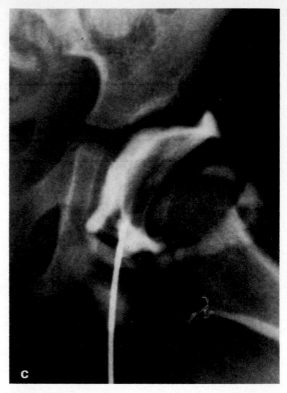

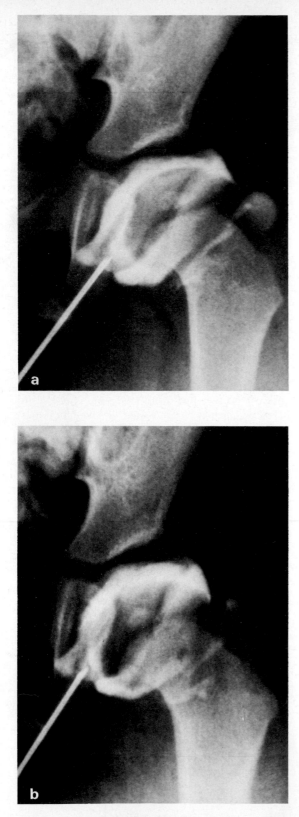

Fig. 21.4 Hip arthrogram.
(a) neutral position
(b) external rotation
(c) frog leg projection

In cases with recurrent dislocation, arthrography may demonstrate damage or defects in the labrum glenoidale and thus influence operative management.

Technique

The patient lies supine on the radiographic table and the injection is made 2 cm inferior and lateral to the tip of the coracoid process, which is identified by fluoroscopy.

A two inch 20 gauge needle with a short bevel is inserted from the skin mark with 5° medial angulation, correct positioning within the joint being confirmed by a small injection of air or positive contrast medium. The injection of 10 ml of positive contrast medium is followed by 10 ml of air under fluoroscopic control. Occasionally, either patient discomfort or a reduction in joint capacity necessitates a smaller injection volume. In addition to confirming correct positioning, fluoroscopy during injection allows assessment of the size of a capsular tear by observation of the rate of leakage from the joint. On completion of the injection, the needle is removed and the joint is put through a passive range of movements to ensure adequate dispersal of contrast medium within the joint cavity and to facilitate the passage of contrast medium through any capsular defect.

Radiographic technique

Axial radiographs of the shoulder with the patient supine and prone are followed by A–P projections with the arm in external rotation and internal rotation. The A–P projections are then repeated with the patient erect. An axial projection of the bicipital groove may also be taken. (Fig. 21.5)

Video-tape recording during a full range of active and passive movements is valuable in cases where instability is either suspected or is present.

ANKLE ARTHROGRAPHY

Indications

It may be impossible to assess clinically the degree of ligamentous damage following trauma to the ankle, arthrography being indicated in such cases. For more detailed evaluation of tears of the calcaneo-fibular ligament, it may be necessary to inject contrast medium directly into the peroneal tendon sheath (Minford et al., 1982).

Technique

The patient is placed on the radiographic table with the ankle in the lateral position. An injection site is chosen on the anterior aspect of the joint, just lateral to the dorsalis pedis artery. Following cleansing of the skin, a 22 gauge needle is introduced horizontally with slight cranial angulation so as to pass between the overhanging anterior tibial margin and the talus. The position is checked by fluoroscopy. The normal capacity of the joint is between 8 and 10 ml, 0.5–1 ml of positive contrast medium being sufficient for double contrast demonstration.

Radiographic technique

Radiographs are taken in A–P, lateral and both oblique projections, together with stress films in cases of ligamentous damage. Tomography is often considerably valuable in demonstrating damage to the cartilageneous joint surfaces and also osteochondritis dissecans.

ELBOW ARTHROGRAPHY

Indications

The majority of cases referred for elbow arthrography have suspected articular surface damage or loose intra-articular bodies.

Technique

The patient's arm is placed on the radiographic table, with the elbow flexed to 90° and the radial aspect uppermost. The patient may either be prone on the table or be seated alongside. The radio–capitellar joint is identified by fluoroscopy and a skin marking is made directly over it. Following infiltration with local anaesthetic, a 22 gauge needle is introduced vertically to the joint until reduced resistance indicates entry into the joint space. About 8 to 10 ml of air, together with 0.5 ml of positive contrast medium, is sufficient to demonstrate the adult elbow joint.

Radiographic technique

Radiographs should be taken in A–P, lateral and both oblique positions. Tomography is commonly required for the accurate localization of loose bodies and, in addition, demonstrates the joint surfaces of the trochlea and ulna more satisfactorily than plain radiography.

WRIST ARTHROGRAPHY

Indications

The cause of persistent pain or limitation of movement in the wrist following trauma may often be elucidated by arthrography. In particular, suspected damage to the triangular cartilage is best confirmed or excluded by this technique.

Technique

The hand is placed palm downwards on the radiographic table, with the wrist flexed to approximately 40° over the radiolucent pad. A skin mark is made during fluoroscopy directly above the wrist joint, between the lunate and the radius. A 22 gauge needle is passed vertically into the joint following infiltration of the skin with local anaesthetic. Between 2 and 4 ml of contrast medium is sufficient to fill the joint and a

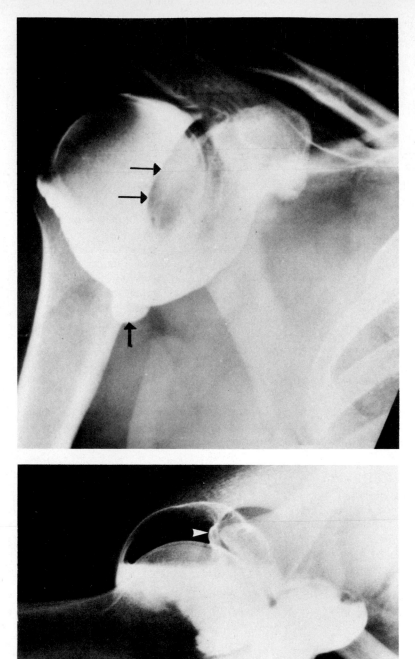

Fig. 21.5 Shoulder arthrogram. (Courtesy of Dr. B. J. Preston)
(a) Arm in internal rotation, showing glenoid labrum and bicipital tendon sheath.
(b) Prone axial view, showing posterior part of the glenoid labrum and bicipital tendon sheath.

single contrast technique is adequate for satisfactory demonstration.

Radiographic technique

Radiographs are taken in the postero–anterior projection, in the neutral position and with radial and ulnar deviation, together with lateral and both oblique projections. Tomograms or stress views are usually unnecessary.

REFERENCES

Butt W. P. & McIntyre J. L. (1969) Double contrast arthrography of the knee. *Radiology*, **92**, 487–99.

Frieberger R. H. & Kaye J. J. (1979) *Arthrography*. Appleton-Century-Crofts, New York.

Grech P. (1972) *Hip Arthrography*. Chapman and Hall, London.

Hall F. M. (1974) Epinephrine enhanced knee arthrography. *Radiology*, **11**, 215–17.

Kutz J. F. (1968) Arthrography in Legg Calvé Perthes disease. *J. Bone Jt. Surg.*, **50A**, 467–72.

Liljedahl S. O., Lindvall N., & Wetterfors J. (1965) Early diagnosis and treatment of acute ruptures of the anterior cruciate ligament. *Acta Radiol. Diagn.*, **19**, 582–600.

Minford J., Hutson M. & Preston B. J. (1982) Radiological involvement in sports injuries. Joint Radiological Meeting, Nottingham, April, 1982.

Preston B. J. & Jackson J. P. (1977) Investigation of shoulder disability by arthrography. *Clin. Radiol.*, **28**, 259–66.

Ricklin R., Ruttimann A., & del Buono M. S. (1971) *Meniscus Lesions*, Georg Thieme Verlag, Stuttgart.

Roebuck E. J. (1977) Double contrast knee arthrography. Some new points of technique including the use of Dimer X. *Clin. Radiol.*, **28**, 247–57.

Salvatti E. A., Freiberger R. H. & Wilson P. D. (1971) Arthrography for complications of total hip replacement. *J. Bone Jt. Surg.*, **53A**, 467–72.

Stoker D. J. (1980) *Clinical Arthrography*. Chapman and Hall, London.

RECOMMENDED FOR DETAILED READING

Dalinka M. K. (1980) *Arthrography*. Springer Verlag, New York.

Freiberger R. H. & Kay J. J. (1979) *Arthrography*. Appleton-Century-Crofts, New York.

Ricklin P., Ruttimann A. & del Buono M. S. (1971) *Meniscus Lesions*, Georg Thieme Verlag, Stuttgart.

The Breast

E. J. ROEBUCK

The radiological demonstration of the breast differs in many respects from that of other organs. A knowledge of the radiological anatomy and a familiarity with the possible radiographic projections are fundamental prerequisites. Radiologists must consider the risk of inducing carcinoma by irradiation. Since the production of a high quality image is mandatory, radiologists must be familiar with the technical problems involved in order to balance achievable radiographic quality and radiation hazard.

RADIOLOGICAL ANATOMY

The breast is a hemispherical structure, with a concave base applied to the chest wall, and the axillary tail as a supero-lateral prolongation. Each breast is divided into 15–20 lobes by fibrous septa. Between 50 and 80 lobules of glandular tissue, each consisting of terminal lactiferous ducts, join successively so that each lobe is drained by a single duct to the nipple.

In the absence of pregnancy, mammary gland tissue occupies the whole of the breast disc for only a short period after adolescence when it is demonstrated as fairly dense homogenous shadowing. Mammographic evidence of involution coincides with the replacement of interlobular connective tissue by fat, initially giving a granular appearance due to the lactiferous ducts and acini which gradually clears completely with the progression of lobular atrophy. Radiological evidence of involution commences early in the second decade of life, with clearing of glandular tissue opacities from the subcutaneous region. Involution progresses first from the infero-medial quadrant and, subsequently, from the supero-medial and infero-lateral quadrants. Finally, glandular tissue disappears from the supero-lateral quadrant and axillary tail. Radiological involution is usually completed many years before the menopause, and it is not uncommon to have no visible evidence of glandular tissue on mammograms of women in the third decade.

With the onset of pregnancy, glandular tissue reappears throughout the breast disc with rapid re-involution following the cessation of lactation.

Since 80–90% of women show one or more types of *dysplasia* of varying severity on mammography, these changes should be considered as normal radiographic appearances. There are three different mammographic appearances of dysplasia. Each type of dysplasia is variable in severity and extent within the breast. In addition, there is variation in the degree of activity of the dysplastic process.

Dysplasia affecting the ducts

The radiological appearances of prominent ducts may be due to either duct ectasia, or periductal collagenosis. The former is more commonly found close to the areola, whereas the latter tends to extend deeply within the gland.

Dysplasia affecting the glandular lobules

Two types of change may be identified:

1. A mixture of epithelial proliferation, micro-cyst formation and stromal fibrosis are seen on histology. On mammography, there are ill-defined denser areas within the glandular tissue, condensing into bands and then thinner strands of fibrosis with cessation of dysplastic activity and progressive involution.
2. Sclerosing adenosis is shown on mammography as areas of density within the homogenous glandular tissue with superimposed microcalcification. These calcifications are commonly rounded and of relatively low density for their size, but occasionally exactly simulate the microcalcifications seen in intra-ductal carcinoma.

RADIOGRAPHIC PROJECTIONS

The radiographic projections employed depend to some extent on the available apparatus and the status of the patient. Two views of each breast are recommended in symptomatic women, whereas only a single oblique view is often taken on asymptomatic women in the first instance. For details of positioning for the projections summarized below, the reader is referred to one of the standard works on radiography.

The oblique projection has been popularized by Lundgren as the sole projection in a screening

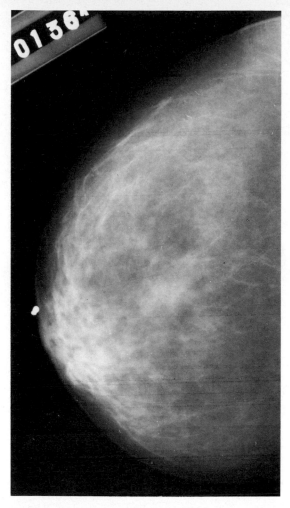

Fig. 22.1 Normal breast, oblique projection.

programme (Lundgren & Jackobsson, 1976), but it is now used as one of the projections in a standard two view technique. The gland tissue is positioned perpendicular to the X-ray beam by angulating the tube approximately 45° to both the patient's sagittal and transverse planes, the exact angulation depending upon individual breast configuration. Superimposition of intramammary structures is thereby minimized, the posterior aspect of the disc of glandular tissue being relatively easily demonstrated and the axillary tail of the breast, with the lower-most axillary glands, usually being well shown (Fig. 22.1).

The erect lateral projection   may be taken with either a medio–lateral, or latero–medial technique. The former is more likely to demonstrate posterior breast structures and laterally placed lesions, whereas the latter more clearly demonstrates medially placed abnormalities.

The supine lateral projection   When a suitable 'over-couch' X-ray tube is available, a lateral view of the breast may be taken with the patient supine. It has the advantage of demonstrating the retro-mammary space more consistently than any other projection. This projection is useful for patients with large breasts, when a large radiograph is required, and is the lateral projection of choice in xeromammography.

The supero–inferior projection   is the standard second radiograph in any two view technique. Since the two projections are taken at right angles to each other, it provides accurate localization of intra-mammary abnormalities when combined with a lateral view. In circumstances where a supine lateral film is not practicable, it is better used in combination with an oblique view to demonstrate the maximum amount of breast tissue.

Rotated supero–inferior projections   The standard supero–inferior view projects the nipple on the midline axis of the radiograph. Since the posterior aspect of the breast is curved, corresponding to the thoracic wall, this standard projection fails to demonstrate the postero-medial and postero-lateral extremities of the breast. In order to overcome this deficiency, it is necessary to rotate the patient laterally to demonstrate any medial lesions or medially to show lateral lesions. Since glandular tissue disappears from the medial half of the breast at a relatively early stage during normal involution, it is recommended that a degree of medial rotation of the patient is employed as a routine instead of the standard projection, in order to show the maximum amount of glandular tissue on the radiograph (Fig. 22.2).

RADIATION-INDUCED BREAST CANCER

Although every effort must be made to reduce the radiation dose to the breast, this factor is relatively less important in women with breast symptoms. The radiation dose assumes great importance when screening women by mammography. It is well-established that there is an increased incidence of breast cancer associated with radiation (Fig. 22.3). Studies of women receiving relatively high doses of radiation have been compared to non-irradiated women (Feig, 1979).

Because the cancer induction rate from mammography is extremely low, it is impossible to estimate

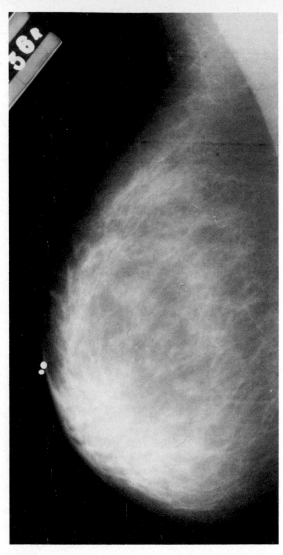

Fig. 22.2 Normal breast, cranio-caudal projection.

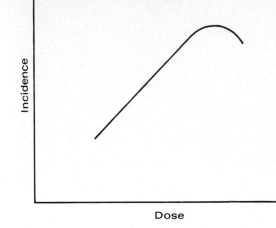

Fig. 22.3 Dose-incidence relationship for radiation induced carcinoma.

suggests that there is a latent period of approximately 15–17 years before the onset of breast cancer, except in the case of the atomic bomb survivors where the latent period was between 5 and 9 years. This variation may be due to the neutron component of the atom bomb irradiation, to the fact that a whole body dose was received, or it may be an expression of a variation in susceptibility between Japanese and Caucasian women. The duration of the radiation effect is uncertain but the population studies indicate this is at least 30 years. One factor of importance to be considered regarding the induction of breast cancer is the increased sensitivity to radiation of younger women; the cancer induction rate in women more than 50 years being approximately 20% of that in women aged between 20 and 34 years. No age relationship was identified in the post-partum mastitis study, suggesting that glandular tissue is the radiation sensitive element, whether it is present as a normal physiological state in the younger women or follows reactivation associated with pregnancy.

THE BASIC IMAGING SYSTEM

A mammographic image is required to have excellent resolution and good contrast between adjacent structures. The image must be easily reproducible to facilitate comparison between present, previous and future films. From these requirements arise a series of technical possibilities which are constrained by two factors:

1. A low kilo-voltage is mandatory because the breast

accurately the low dose risk relationship by epidemiological means without studying groups of irradiated and controlled populations which each number several millions.

The radiation risk of mammography may be calculated from the assumption that there is no threshold below which radiation has no effect and that the dose/response curve remains linear for low doses. However, these basic assumptions result in an overestimate of risk. The validity of assuming linearity is not confirmed by animal experiments in which there is an exponential decrease of the low dose risk (Fig. 22.4).

Study of the data on the groups of irradiated women

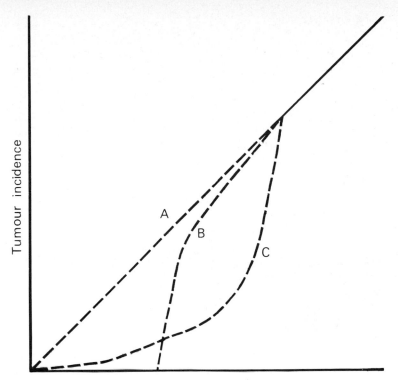

Fig. 22.4 Possible induced cancer incidence for humans at low levels of irradiation:
Solid line—Known linear relationship.
Curve A—Straight line extrapolation.
Curve B—Extrapolation assuming a threshold dose.
Curve C—Relationship as found in animals.

Tumour incidence

Dose (Rads)

consists of soft tissues and the detection of very small calcium deposits in the breast is of extreme importance.

2. It is essential to employ the lowest possible dose of radiation because the breast is an organ liable to develop radiation-induced carcinoma.

The radiologist must decide the 'trade off' point where a further reduction of dose is intolerable because the resultant degradation of image would cause the loss of important diagnostic detail.

Two main modalities are currently used for mammographic images: film mammography using an X-ray tube with a molybdenum target, and xeromammography using a tungsten target.

Film mammography

Non-screen 'industrial', X-ray film was used exclusively until recent years. This gave ideal results in terms of low noise, high resolution and good contrast in the higher film density areas. However, non-screen techniques have the important disadvantage of requiring a radiation dose which is 10–30 times that of film-screen combinations. A long exposure time with an increased risk of movement blurring is also

necessary and there is poorer contrast in the low density areas of the film. Moreover, a manual or dedicated automatic processor is a requirement.

The development of vacuum sealed packs containing a single emulsion film and a single intensifying screen has resulted in lower radiation dosage, shorter exposure times, better contrast at lower film densities, and the ability to use conventional 90 second automatic processing facilities. However, film screen combinations have the disadvantage of lower resolution, higher noise, and the risk of artefacts produced by screen faults or dust.

Xeromammography

The production of the xeroradiographic image results from the partial discharge of an electrostatically charged selenium plate by the emergent X-ray beam. A powder of charged blue particles is then dusted over the plate and adheres to various areas on the plate surface proportional to the residual charge. The image so produced is then transferred on to paper and fixed.

The advantages of xeromammography include a very wide latitude, the chest wall and retro-mammary space being as well demonstrated as the skin and subcutaneous fat. Very high contrast is achieved

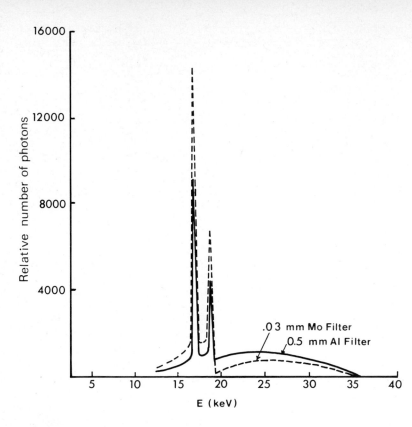

Fig. 22.5 Energy spectrum from a molybdenum anode with molybdenum and aluminium filtration.

within a small area of the xeroradiographic image as a result of the edge enhancement effect, while the overall contrast is low and gives the effect of good penetration of dense glandular breasts.

X-ray beam quality

It is now generally accepted that a narrow spectral band is desirable in order to optimize the mammographic image within the low kilo-voltage range essential for breast examination, the quality of the beam being chosen to give maximal response from the preferred recording system (Hanss *et al.*, 1976).

Molybdenum is a technically convenient material for anode target construction, emitting a very narrow spectral band with characteristic radiation at 17.9 and 19.5 keV. There is, however, in addition to the double peak of characteristic radiation, a significant emission of higher energy radiation, and the use of a 0.03 mm molybdenum filter to suppress strongly the spectrum above 20 keV is recommended to give a higher subject contrast (Fig. 22.5). Energy of this quality gives good contrast in film mammography, but requires a rather high dose level for thick breasts. Target materials with higher atomic numbers would give a lower dose but

inferior contrast. Operating voltages for X-ray tubes with molybdenum targets are usually in the 26–30 kVp range.

After the introduction of xeroradiography in 1971, the use of a tungsten target with low kVp and minimal beam filtration was recommended and the xeroradiographic image was produced in the positive mode. More recently, it has been realized that it is possible to reduce the radiation dose by 20–30% without any significant loss of image content by using the negative mode and a tungsten target with approximately 3 mm of aluminium filtration (van der Riet & Wolfe, 1977). This combination gives a narrow spectral beam at 35 keV, which coincidentally also gives better visualization of dense breasts. There is loss of diagnostic detail if the kVp is raised too high, or if the thickness of the aluminium filtration is increased too much.

It is possible to use a xeroradiographic recording system with a molybdenum X-ray tube target provided there is a 0.5 mm aluminium filter. This reduces the intensity of the characteristic radiation relative to the higher energy portion of the emitted X-ray beam. As more aluminium filtration is added, the beam becomes harder and more closely simulates that emitted by a tungsten target, the resultant reduction in subject contrast being compensated to some extent by the edge enhancement effect characteristic of the xeroradiographic technique. Aluminium filtration also reduces patient radiation dose, the balance between a lower dose and image quality determining the amount of filtration.

The mAs is best determined by automatic exposure control, whatever X-ray beam is utilized, using either an ionization chamber or phototimer, since pre-mammographic assessment of breast density is extremely difficult.

Image quality

Geometric unsharpness is an important factor in image quality and depends upon the size and shape of the tube focal spot, together with the ratio between the focus–object and object–film distances. The development of microfocal spots not only gives the potential for improvement in image quality by reducing geometric unsharpness, but also makes possible the employment of magnification techniques.

Compression of the breast towards the film improves the image quality by:
1. Reducing geometrical unsharpness.
2. Minimizing blurring due to movement.
3. Improving contrast by a reduction of scattered radiation.
4. Giving an equal tissue thickness which results in an homogenous film density with the posterior portion of the breast being as well visualized as the anterior part.
5. Reducing the overlapping projection of image by the spreading apart of intra-mammary structures. It is necessary to compress the average breast to a thickness of about 4 cm in order to achieve these improvements. This degree of compression has the additional benefit of reducing the required exposure and thus the radiation dose to glandular tissue.

Degradation of the final image by scattered radiation can be reduced by a collimating cone, and by the insertion of a 'soft tissue' grid or an air gap between the breast and the film. These last two measures, however, necessitate a higher dose rate and also result in an increase of geometrical unsharpness. The moving slit system, whereby synchronously moving matched grids are inserted proximal and distal to the breast, also reduces scatter without the disadvantages of a higher dose to the breast, although there is some increase in geometrical unsharpness.

It cannot be over-emphasized that while the radiation dose to the breast must be kept to a minimum, it is essential that each step in the production of the final image is calculated to minimize image degradation.

The application of the mathematical concept of Modulation Transfer Functions (MTF) allows accurate assessment of the efficiency of each part of the imaging system (Meredith & Massey, 1979). Since the quality of the final image depends upon the product of the MTF of each constituent part of the imaging system (MTF [whole system] $= \text{MTF}_1 \times \text{MTF}_2 \times \text{MTF}_3 \ldots$ etc.), each individual constituent should be chosen to give the highest possible final image. One poor element in this image production chain does not absolutely determine the final image quality, providing the other constituents have a slightly better MTF than the worst element. The balance between a higher MTF and a lower radiation dose is a subjective choice which depends upon the preference of the individual radiologist.

ULTRASONOGRAPHY

The ability of ultrasound to distinguish cystic from solid lesions has been exploited in the investigation of mass lesions in the breast. Reported accuracy rates for cancer detection when mass lesions are investigated by ultrasonography vary between 70% and 85%.

Ultrasonography is regarded in some centres as a routine step in the investigation of mass lesions. Other investigators prefer to introduce a needle into a lesion; with aspiration if it is cystic in nature, and histological examination following either aspiration cystology, Tru-cut biopsy or excision of a solid mass.

If an impalpable lesion is identified mammographically, and management is in doubt, then contact ultrasound may give sufficient additional information to render biopsy desirable. Alternatively, it may enable the lesion to be ignored with a greater degree of confidence (Fig. 22.6).

Substitution of X-ray mammography by non-ionizing ultrasonography is keenly anticipated, but the resolution obtained by early apparatus has been inadequate for use as the sole modality for whole breast examination. Recent technological advances suggest that poor resolution may not be a barrier in the future. Automation of scanning, and computer processing of the resultant images are fields in which improved technology gives promise of systems adequate for breast screening.

Patients are examined lying prone with each breast being successively immersed in a water bath. Transducers in the base of the bath give a succession of 'B' scan images at 0.5 cm intervals through the breast in transverse or sagittal planes. Areas of interest may be examined in greater detail.

Using this technique sensitivities of over 90% have

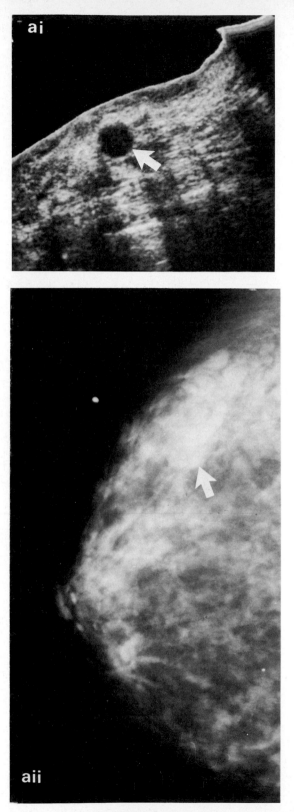

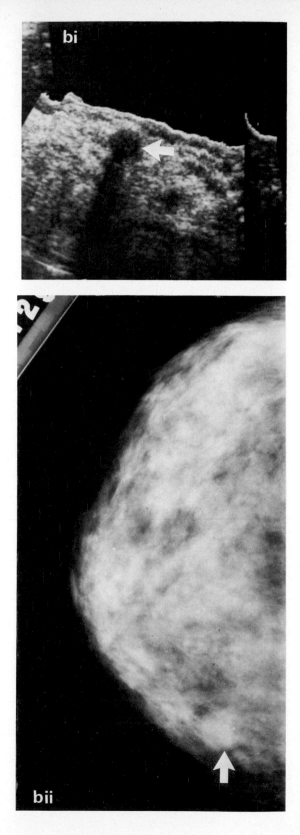

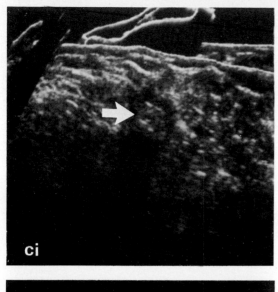

ci

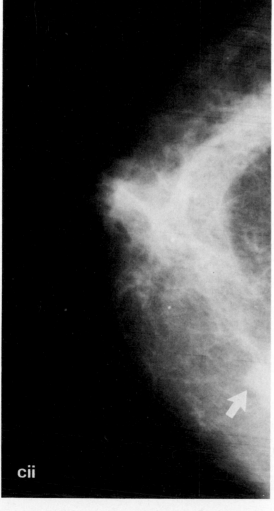

cii

Fig. 22.6 Ultrasonography of (a) Cyst, (b) Fibroadenoma, and (c) Carcinoma, with corresponding mammograms.

been obtained by ultrasonography for lesions greater than 2 cm in diameter, results which are approaching the accuracy of X-ray mammography. However, the sensitivity falls to 60–70% for lesions smaller than 2 cm in diameter, indicating that ultrasonography is not yet sufficiently accurate to be relied upon as the sole image modality.

THERMOGRAPHY

A localized increase in skin temperature may be detected overlying both inflammatory and cancerous breast lesions. These changes may be observed and pictorially recorded by making multiple simultaneous temperature measurements, or by estimations of infrared irradiation from the region.

Telethermography is the technique whereby the patient is positioned in front of an infra-red camera, with the facility of estimating localized temperatures and displaying the overall pattern of temperature variation. Most machines can also produce isotherms and thermal profiles of selected regions.

The examination is performed in the frontal and both oblique positions. The environment temperature must be accurately controlled (21°C ± 1°C) and there must be no draughts or localized heat sources. It is essential that the patient is adapted to this environment by exposure for about 10 minutes prior to recording.

Contact plate thermography employs reusable liquid cholesterol crystal plates directly applied to the breasts.

High false positive and high false negative results are reported when using either technique on a single occasion, although accuracy rates are improved by the classification of results according to the combination of signs present (Gautheric & Gros, 1976). A high reproducibility of pattern is obtained if an individual has successive thermograms. A change from this personal baseline is highly significant and may precede other evidence of disease. Analysis of successive thermograms using computer techniques may prove to be of value in population screening of the sub-group with a 'high risk' pattern on baseline mammography.

DIAPHANOGRAPHY

Translumination is a time-honoured clinical method of examining mass lesions. The technique has recently been considerably refined and apparatus incorporating a very high yellow light source has been specifically designed for breast investigation. The examiner, fully dark adapted, views the breast (diaphanoscopy) and takes photographs (diaphanography) of suspect areas with a highly sensitive infra-red film.

Breast tissue absorbs yellow light more readily than red and infra-red. Dysplastic tissues transmit more red/infra-red than do malignant tissues which have a higher nitrogen content. Thus benign conditions produce a red image and malignant appear brownblack.

Early experience with the improved apparatus suggests that diaphanography has a complementary role to play in the examination of the breast (Gros *et al.*, 1972; Ohlsson *et al.*, 1980). The method may prove to be a sufficiently reliable and relatively economic technique, possibly obviating the necessity for mammography in at least a proportion of cases.

PNEUMO-CYSTOGRAPHY

Indications

Although cysts are common, dogmatic mammographic differentiation from other lesions can sometimes be difficult. The commonest indication for cystography is a lesion within a dense region or with adjacent changes, such as microcalcification, which raise doubts regarding its benign nature.

The lesion is simple to locate if it is palpable, but localization by cranio–caudal and lateral mammographic views may be necessary. Ultrasonographic location can be of assistance.

Technique

As in all techniques of breast examination, a full explanation of the procedure relieves patient anxiety and ensures maximum cooperation. The skin is cleaned with an antiseptic solution and a small injection of local anaesthetic is given into the skin overlying the lesion. A 19 gauge hypodermic needle is then advanced to the lesion. The cyst wall may be so thin as to be scarcely apparent, but it is often surprisingly difficult to penetrate. A reduction in resistance indicates entrance of the cyst.

A variety of aspirate may be obtained, ranging from clear fluid to thick caseous material, while the presence of blood is of particular note. The aspirate should be sent for cytological examination in all cases. The volume of the aspirate is noted and a similar volume

of air is then injected through the needle without a change in position. For a double contrast technique, 0.25 ml of water-soluble contrast medium is injected. The needle is then withdrawn, the puncture site sealed with Nobecutane, and radiographs are taken in cranio–caudal and lateral projections.

ASPIRATION FOR CYTOLOGY

Indications

The technique for cytological examination of breast lesions is similar to that for cytography, but uses a thin needle (0.17 mm). The method is employed if a lesion suspected of being a cyst proves to be solid or as a definitive investigation.

Technique

A 20 ml syringe is applied to the needle and a vacuum is produced by forced manual aspiration or by a special instrument (Cameco, Sweden). The needle is then moved through the lesion five or six times to ensure an adequate aspiration of cells into the syringe lumen. The vacuum is then released, the needle withdrawn, and the aspirate is then ejected on to a microscope slide. The specimen is stained immediately and may be examined at once. Accuracy rates of approximately 90% with very low false positive rates are reported, but it is stressed that a negative result does not exclude the presence of a carcinoma.

LOCALIZATION OF A LESION FOR BIOPSY

Indications

It is often necessary to obtain a histological diagnosis of impalpable lesions which are demonstrated by mammography. On these occasions, the suspicious area must be accurately located to ensure that the correct specimen is submitted for histological examination.

The position of a suspected lesion or area is estimated from lateral and cranio-caudal radiographs with reasonable accuracy. Removal of the correct region is ensured by the insertion of a marker, the relationship of the marker and lesion being demonstrated by repeat mammography. Marking may be achieved either by the injection of contrast medium and a coloured dye (Preece *et al.*, 1977) or by the insertion of a metallic marker (Frank *et al.*, 1976) (Fig. 22.7).

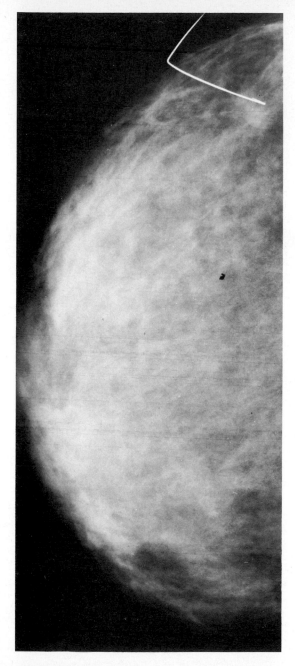

Fig. 22.7 Marker *in situ*.

Technique

The surface marking of the lesion is identified by estimating the distance from, and the angular relationship to, the nipple. The angular relationship is often expressed with reference to a clock face (2 o'clock, 8 o'clock etc.). The depth of the suspect area to the surface marking is then estimated.

Following sterilization of the skin, a small injection of local anaesthetic is given at the surface marking point. The puncture site is then enlarged by the insertion of a 19 gauge needle, to the estimated lesion depth. At this stage, some investigators insert a second hypodermic needle at a slightly different angle and rely upon identification of the relative positions of the needles and the lesion for accurate localization.

If the contrast medium/dye technique is being employed, a mixture of 0.5 ml of Conray 420 and Patent Blue is injected through the needle, which is then withdrawn, and the puncture site sealed with Nobecutane. Cranio–caudal and lateral radiographs are taken to check the position of the needle or injected contrast medium relative to the suspect lesion.

If a specially designed marker needle is being used, it is substituted for the 19 gauge hypodermic needle and is inserted to the required depth with any necessary change in angulation. The barbed stilette is then passed through the marker needle, which is then removed. Migration of the stilette should be prevented by bending the protruding segment through 90° and taping it to the skin, or by using a Denis Browne collar clip.

Various types of on-lay grids have been designed to make accurate positioning of the markers more easily achieved and are advocated by some investigators.

DUCTOGRAPHY

Indications

Demonstration of the lactiferous ducts (galactography) is indicated in patients with persistent single duct discharge of any type, and particularly if the discharge contains blood. It may also help to determine the diagnosis of mammographically demonstrated lesions which are considered to involve a duct.

Technique

Following antiseptic cleansing of the nipple, the suspected duct is gently dilated by a Nettleship dilator. Between 0.5 and 1.0 ml of water-soluble contrast medium is then slowly injected via a fine sialography or dacro-cystography cannula. The injection is terminated when the patient experiences a feeling of intra-mammary pressure or pain, whereupon the cannula is removed. The duct is then immediately blocked by the external application of Collodian or Nobecutane. Cranio-caudal and lateral films are then

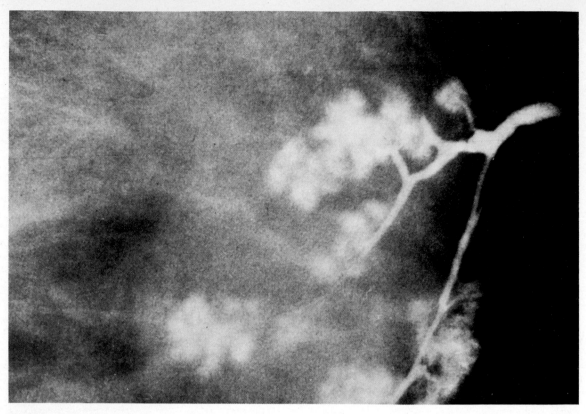

Fig. 22.8 Normal ductogram.

obtained and inspected (Fig. 22.8), supplementary oblique films occasionally demonstrating a particular segment of duct more clearly than the standard projections.

REFERENCES

Feig S. A. (1979) Epidemiology of radiation related breast cancer. *Reduced Dose Mammography*. (Eds. Logan W. W. & Muntz E. P.) pp. 9–19. Masson Publishing Inc., USA.

Frank H. A., Hall F. M. & Steer M. L. (1976) Pre-operative localization of non-palpable breast lesions demonstrated by mammography. *New Engl. J. Med.*, **295**, 259–60.

Gautheric M. & Gros M. (1976) Contribution of infra-red thermography to early diagnosis, pre-therapeutic prognosis and post-irradiation follow-up of breast carcinomas; *Medicamundi*, **21**, 135–49.

Gros C. M., Quenneville Y. & Hammel Y. (1972) *Journal Radiologie Electrolique Medecine Nucléaire*, **53**, 297.

Hans A. G., Metz C. E., Chiles J. T. & Rossman K. (1976) The effect of X-ray spectra from molybdenum and tungsten target tubes on image quality in mammography. *Radiology*, **118**, 705–9.

Lundgren B. & Jackobsson S. (1976) Single view mammography: a simple and efficient approach to breast screening. *Cancer*, **38**, 1124–9.

Meredith W. J. & Massey J. B. (1979) *Fundamental Physics of Radiology*, pp. 674–83. John Wright & Sons.

Ohlsson B., Quenneville Y. & Hammel Y. (1972) *World J. Surg.*, **4**, 701–7.

Preece P. E., Gravelle I. H., Hughes L. E., Baum M., Fortt R. W. & Leopold J. G. (1977) The operative management of sub-clinical breast cancer. *Clin. Oncol.*, **3**, 165–9.

Van de Riet W. G. & Wolfe J. N. (1977) Dose reduction in xeroradiography of the breast. *Amer. J. Roentgenol.*, **128**, 821–3.

R. K. LEVICK

GENERAL PRINCIPLES

Heat loss Neonates and infants lose body heat rapidly, the risk of hypothermia being greatest in the premature baby with little subcutaneous fat. Local warmth may be obtained by special table-top heating cradles, but the most convenient way of avoiding heat loss is to maintain a room temperature of about 80°F in the X-ray room. A room thermometer is an important piece of equipment. Enhanced humidity is not normally required for the duration of an X-ray examination.

Radiation dosage It is good practice to limit the dose of ionizing radiation to the patient as much as possible. Gonad protection is important. Image intensification and dynamic recording on video-tape must be available for screening procedures. A very important principle, which may reduce the radiation dose by as much as 50%, is gridless screening. Infants under one year of age are always examined with the explorator grid removed, there being little scatter and no appreciable loss of detail. When fine detail such as a mucosal pattern is not required, gridless screening may be used in children up to five years of age.

Special X-ray equipment Screening equipment is available which is designed specifically for the examination of infants and children. It is not always possible to accommodate older children on such apparatus. Cradle holding devices are provided which enable the infant to be rotated in relation to the table top. When this type of equipment is not available, views such as the prone 'shoot-through' swallow for tracheo-oesophageal fistula may be obtained by using a device such as the Charteris baby holder inverted on the step of an upright adult screening table.

UPPER GASTROINTESTINAL TRACT

Contrast study for tracheo-oesophageal fistula

Indications To define a suspected fistula without oesophageal atresia, or a recurrent or second fistula after operation. Recurrent chest infections and air distension of the stomach and bowel may have raised the possibility of tracheo-oesophageal fistula.

Technique Contrast medium is injected into the oesophagus with the baby positioned face down (Fig. 23.1). Screening, spot films and video-recording are

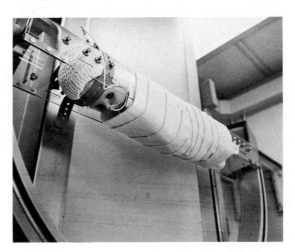

Fig. 23.1 Barium examination for tracheo-bronchial fistula, cradle method. The screening table is erect and the child is held face-down in the cradle after the passage of a naso-gastric tube.

carried out in a prone 'shoot-through' position. A naso-gastric tube such as a No.6F tube or umbilical cannula is passed to the fundus of the stomach. A one in three aqueous dilution of a non high-density barium is prepared and warmed to body temperature. Water-soluble contrast should not be used as aspiration produces pulmonary oedema. A rapid injection of 5 ml barium is made whilst the catheter is withdrawn to the lower cervical region (Fig. 23.2). Screening, video-recording, and possibly spot films, are carried out during withdrawal. Most fistulae are in the upper dorsal (D3 or 4) or lower cervical region, rarely at both levels. The procedure may be repeated if the trachea remains free of aspirated barium.

Complications Barium may be aspirated through the larynx or a fistula. Suction equipment must be available and expert resuscitation at hand. Cardiac arrest is known to have occurred during oesophageal filling and may be prevented by warming the contrast medium.

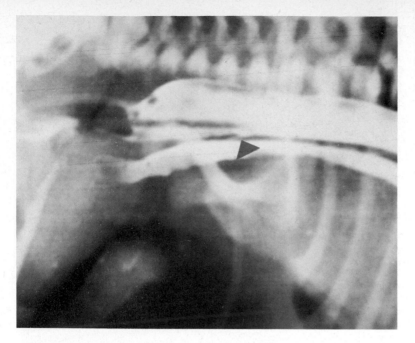

Fig. 23.2 A shoot-through spot film taken during the injection of barium through a tube into the baby's oesophagus. A hair-line fistula (arrow) runs upwards and anteriorly from the oesophagus to the lower cervical trachea.

Barium swallow for reflux and hiatus hernia

Indications Recurrent blood-stained vomiting suggests a serious oesophagitis with a risk of stricture formation.

Technique A one in three aqueous dilution of non high-density barium, sweetened with sucrose, is given from a normal feeding bottle and teat. The sucking and swallowing mechanisms are observed. If the feed is not taken, a No.8F umbilical cannula is threaded through a flanged teat with about 1 cm catheter tip projecting (Fig. 23.3), and barium is injected slowly through the catheter. Not more than 10 ml barium is given. Oesophageal peristalsis is observed and the manner of closure at the cardia after each bolus is recorded. The baby is then turned prone oblique, left side up, and gastric emptying observed before the stomach is too full to see the pylorus through the empty fundus. If emptying is normal, the baby is turned to the opposite prone oblique position in order to pool barium in the fundus. Evidence of gastro-oesophageal reflux and/or hiatus hernia is sought during episodes of crying (Fig. 23.4), which may be produced by gentle plantar tickling, and during further swallowing of barium. Video-recording is of great help for the later slow-motion analysis and reduces screening time.

Complications Suction must be available in case of aspiration.

Alternative examinations While oesophagitis is assessed by endoscopy, the barium swallow is necessary to show reflux and hiatus hernia. Isotope studies are used to show that aspiration of gastric contents is a cause of recurrent pneumonia.

Barium meal for pyloric obstruction

Indications Barium examination is reserved for infants with a typical clinical presentation of pyloric obstruction but without a palpable tumour.

Technique The examination is commenced as described for reflux and hiatus hernia. It may be found that emptying of the stomach is slow, especially if the baby is upset when feeding is stopped. The use of a 'dummy' will often hasten pyloric relaxation. Glucagon, 1 µg/kg body weight intravenously, may be employed to overcome pylorospasm. The pylorus must be seen to open widely to exclude functional stenosis.

Complications Water-soluble contrast should not be used because of the risk of aspiration.

Alternative examination Ultrasonography in either the B-scope or real-time modes may demonstrate the hypertrophied pyloric muscle.

Malrotation is a possible cause of high small bowel obstruction. It is important to record the position of

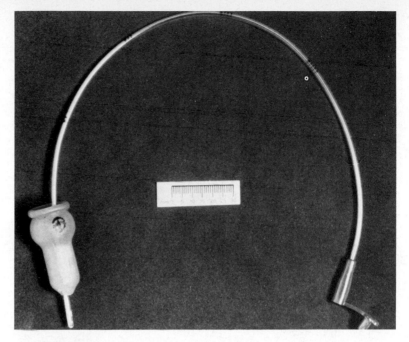

Fig. 23.3 A simple teat and catheter system for barium swallow examinations in babies. The catheter should be cemented to the teat or a wide flanged teat used to prevent the possibility of accidental swallowing of the teat.

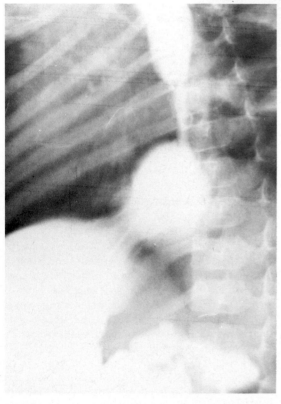

Fig. 23.4 The infant's stomach has been filled with barium. Whilst lying prone-oblique, crying produces an intermittent hiatus hernia. There is gastro-oesophageal reflux and lower oesophageal spasm due to oesophagitis.

the duodeno-jejunal flexure on all barium examinations carried out for vomiting and probable obstruction. On an A–P film the flexure should lie to the left of the spine and at about the same level as the pylorus.

LOWER GASTRO INTESTINAL TRACT

Contrast enema for distal bowel obstruction

Indications Distal bowel obstruction which is not due to ano-rectal anomalies.

General considerations It is important to choose the correct type of contrast medium. When there is no definite diagnosis and the level of obstruction is uncertain, a diagnostic enema may be carried out using a nearly isotonic water-soluble contrast medium such as 25% sodium diatrizoate or, alternatively, a non-ionic water-soluble contrast agent. When meconium ileus obstruction is to be relieved, a hypertonic contrast medium such as Gastrografin is needed. Finally, if Hirschprung's disease is probable, barium is used so that delayed films may be obtained at up to 24 hours.

Technique A soft rubber catheter of about 5 mm outside diameter is passed into the rectum and retained with strapping or by a suitably protected assistant holding the buttocks together. In a diagnostic situation, a pressure head of about 1 foot (30.5 cm) is

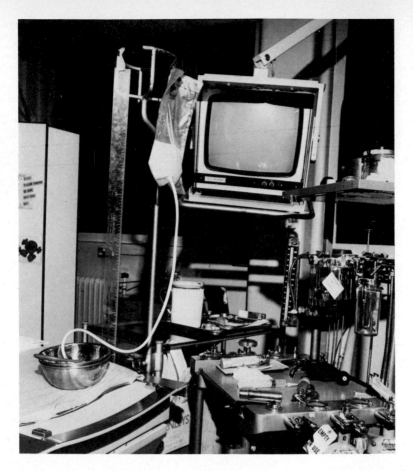

Fig. 23.5 The screening room prepared for attempted enema reduction of an intussusception. The level of barium in the reservoir is about 80 cm above the table top. The infant has a general anaesthetic for the attempt.

employed in case compromised bowel is present. If a firm diagnosis of meconium ileus is then reached, a hypertonic contrast medium is substituted with a pressure head of up to 3 feet (1 metre). Similarly, if a corkscrew or narrow segment is seen, barium is then used for presumed Hirschprung's disease.

Complications Bowel perforation is always possible, so isotonic contrast and low hydrostatic pressure are used if this risk is thought to exist and an examination is still necessary. The use of hypertonic contrast medium in the relief of meconium ileus and milk inspissation is known to produce a considerable shift of tissue fluid into the bowel with a risk of serious dehydration. This type of enema should only be carried out when fluid is already being given intravenously.

Diagnostic and therapeutic barium enema for intussusception

Indications Clinical findings and plain film confirmation of intussusception. The length of history and the passage of blood per rectum are not contra-indications provided the child's condition is satisfactory.

Contra-indications Shock, peritoneal rebound tenderness, plain film findings of perforation or of small bowel obstruction.

General considerations The high success rate of reduction and low incidence of complication noted in various centres is mainly due to proper selection of patients. No infant who is shocked, has signs of peritoneal irritation or plain film evidence of small bowel obstruction, should have an attempted enema reduction. Selection should be made by the paediatric surgeon together with the radiologist.

Technique (Figs. 23.5 & 23.6)   Relaxation is the key to good results. If it is possible to transfer the child directly to the operating theatre should the enema reduction fail, a general anaesthetic should be induced before the enema. Heavy sedation is often less effective, but relaxation may be improved by i.v.

Fig. 23.6 (a) The intussusception has been reduced to the caecum, where the mass and 'coil spring' appearance is visible. (b) A few seconds later reduction is complete and barium has entered the appendix and terminal ileum.

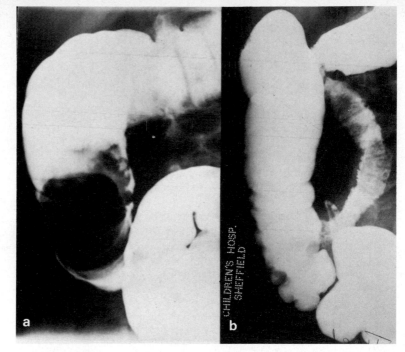

glucagon 1 μg/k body weight. The enema of a one in three aqueous dilution of barium is warmed to body temperature and run in through a soft non-lubricated catheter of 5–10 mm diameter. The catheter is retained in the rectum by manual compression of the buttocks by an assistant working over a lead-rubber sheet, who may also steady the infants legs with his other hand. The diagnosis is confirmed with a pressure head of not more than one foot (30.5 cm). Reduction is then attempted with a pressure of not more than three feet (1 metre). Pressure is maintained for up to five minutes and the attempt may be repeated once or twice, provided there is no deterioration of the child's condition. Ideally, barium should be seen to enter the small bowel. It is important to obtain a post-evacuation film at about ten minutes as a recurrence is occasionally found.

Distal colonogram in ano-rectal atresia

Technique The distal opening is identified and isotonic water-soluble contrast medium run in through a soft catheter. Lateral screening of the pelvis with a marker on the anal dimple will demonstrate the lowest point of the rectal pouch, although a distal plug of meconium may produce a temporary false higher level. Lateral and oblique views are needed to show a fistula present in nearly all high lesions. If barium is

used, it must be washed out to avoid subsequent concretions.

REFERENCES

Levick R. K. (1970) Intussusception—conservative versus surgical management. *Clin. Paediat.*, **9**, 457–62.
Levick R. K. (1972) The choice of contrast medium in neonatal obstruction. *Ann. Radiol.*, **15**, 231–6.
Sauvegrain J. (1969) The technique of upper gastro-intestinal investigation in infants and children. In *Progress in Paediatric Radiology*, Vol. 2, pp. 26–51. S. Karger, Basel.

CONTRAST STUDIES OF THE CENTRAL NERVOUS SYSTEM

Ventriculography in infants

Indications Ventriculography is no longer carried out to determine ventricular size, having been replaced by CT scanning and ultrasonography. However, the ventricles can be outlined by air or positive contrast when a ventricular tap must be carried out to obtain a CSF sample or to measure directly ventricular pressure. Injection of the third ventricle may be the only way to demonstrate lesions of the aqueduct.

Contra-indications A history of previous convulsions make a similar reaction to contrast medium more likely. The risk of upward brain-stem herniation should be considered when a posterior fossa lesion presents with clinical evidence of raised intra-cranial pressure.

Technique In infants of less than six months of age, the anterior fontanelle is usually large enough to allow a parasagittal approach to the lateral or third ventricles. The baby is sedated and placed supine on the screening table in an immobilizing cradle (Fig. 23.7). The vertex must be easily accessible. The

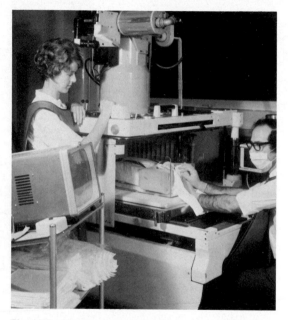

Fig. 23.7 Third ventricular puncture in a hydrocephalic baby. The baby is held in a movable plastic cradle. Puncture is made under screen control. Vertical beam films are taken on the explorator. The 'overcouch' tube is set up for horizontal beam films. (Courtesy of the Editor, Clinical Radiology.)

fontanelle region is shaved and prepared with iodine in spirit. With the usual aseptic precautions, a 21 gauge lumbar puncture needle of $3\frac{1}{2}$ in (9 cm) length is introduced about $\frac{3}{4}$ in (2 cm) lateral to the mid-line at the widest point of the fontanelle. The needle is directed towards the base at an angle of 30° inwards toward the line of the falx. A 'give' may be felt as the tip enters the lateral ventricle, otherwise the stylet is withdrawn after advancing the needle 1 in (2.5 cm) and an attempt made to aspirate CSF. Further advancement may be required. When the lateral

ventricle is reached, the pressure is measured and 5–10 ml of CSF withdrawn. Up to 20 ml of sterile air may then be injected from a 20 ml syringe which has been sterilized with the plunger drawn back. Six standard views are then obtained: erect A–P and lateral, lateral brow-up and brow-down (Fig. 23.8),

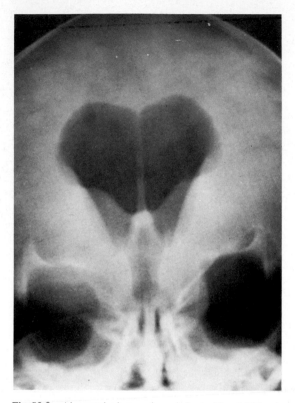

Fig. 23.8 Air ventriculogram in an infant with mild (Grade 1) hydrocephalus. The brow-up film shows the wide lateral and third ventricles.

inverted A–P and lateral after a somersault. Alternatively, a water-soluble contrast medium, suitable for ventriculography, is injected and allowed to diffuse. Good detail of the third ventricle aqueduct and fourth ventricle is not usually obtained, especially when there is dilatation of the lateral ventricles. Direct injection into the third ventricle may be achieved under screen control. The needle is advanced through a lateral ventricle to a point about $\frac{1}{2}$ in (1.3 cm) above the sphenoid body in the mid-line. The tip should lie just anterior to a line joining the external auditory meati. Backflow of CSF is confirmed, or the needle is repositioned, followed by the injection of 2–4 ml of water-soluble contrast medium. An immediate lateral 'shoot-through' is taken with the baby still lying brow-up after the injection, followed by an A–P view. The

Fig. 23.9 Infant myelogram. The anaesthetized baby is placed face-down over a pillow or large pad so that the lumbar spine is well-flexed. Screening may be used to ensure a mid-line approach.

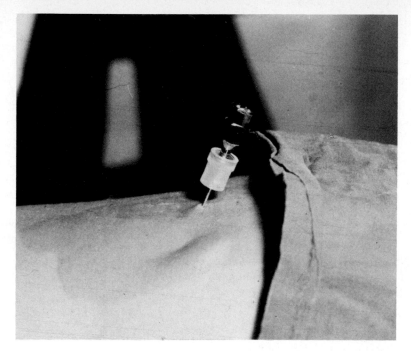

contrast medium is rapidly dispersed unless there is an aqueduct obstruction.

Complications

If convulsions or twitching occur, i.v. diazepam in a body-weight related dose is usually adequate for control.

Myelography in infants

Technique General anaesthesia is advisable as the examination can be alarming. The prone approach is advised for infants under two years of age. The patient is laid face-down with the lumbar spine flexed over a pad (Fig. 23.9). It is important not to use too fine a needle, otherwise the dural 'give' will not be felt. A $1\frac{1}{2}$ in (3.8 cm) 21 guage spinal needle is suitable. The needle is screened into the spine at the 2/3 or 3/4 lumbar level and advanced until dural resistance is felt. The stylet is then withdrawn and a 2 ml syringe attached to the needle. If an attempt to aspirate CSF is unsuccessful, the needle is further advanced very slowly with aspiration until CSF is withdrawn. Dural venous blood will appear if the needle is advanced too far. It is better to postpone contrast injection for a few days if this occurs, as there will almost always be a leakage of contrast medium outside the subarachnoid space. Having achieved a good puncture, the examination proceeds in a conventional manner. Five to

eight millilitres of Niopam 200 (Iopamidol, 200 mg iodine per ml) are introduced, the exact amount depending on the appearances while screening.

Lumbar puncture and myelography in the older child are carried out in the same way as in the adult.

Cerebral angiography in infants

Indications Cerebro-vascular malformations may require arteriography either prior to surgery or to attempted embolization. It should be noted that large lesions, such as vein of Galen 'aneurysms', can be clearly shown on contrast enhanced CT scans.

Technique Direct puncture of the carotid or vertebral arteries is possible. A $1\frac{1}{2}$ in (3.8 cm) 21 gauge lumbar puncture needle with a modified short bevel may be used, proprietary needles being available. However, most examinations are carried out via selective arterial catheterization. As in the adult, a straight catheter advanced from a femoral artery puncture into the dorsal aorta usually enters the left vertebral artery via the left subclavian artery. Special catheters are available in infant sizes for carotid studies. Clean femoral artery puncture is aided by a needle and stylet without an external cannula and by extending the thigh with a pad under the buttocks to fix the rather mobile artery. Saline or local anaesthetic injected around the artery also helps to fix it in position.

REFERENCES

Harwood-Nash D. C. F. & Fitz C. R. (1976) Neurological techniques and indications in infancy and childhood. In *Progress in Paediatric Radiology*, Vol. 5, pp. 49–52. S. Karger, Basel.

Steiner G. M. (1974) Positive contrast ventriculography with Dimer X in hydrocephalus. *Clin. Radiol.*, **25**, 517–23.

ARTHROGRAPHY

This investigation is usually requested for hip dysplasia in the infant. In older children, examination of the knee or shoulder is carried out in the same way as in adults.

Hip arthrography in the infant

Indications Congenital hip dislocation which does not respond to splinting, prior to operative reduction. Doubtful hip dislocations, as in infants with limited abduction, is a further indication. There is some prognostic value in Perthe's disease, but arthrography is rarely used in this condition.

Contra-indications The only major complication is septic arthritis, so that puncture should not be carried out through inflamed or infected skin. Inter-current infections in the chest or urinary tracts may increase the risk of blood-borne infection following joint puncture. Allergic reactions to contrast injection are very rare.

Technique The examination is carried out under general anaesthesia. Adequate asepsis is essential to avoid septic arthritis. The skin is cleaned with an aqueous preparation, such as Cetavalon, and the puncture site further cleansed with iodine in spirit. The infant lies supine on the screening table with the thigh slightly abducted, flexed and externally rotated, about 10° in each direction. A short bevel needle of 22 gauge and 1½ in (3.8 cm) length, with stylette, is used. Of the four different approach routes which have been described, the inferior and lateral routes have the advantage that an initial extra-articular trial injection does not obscure joint detail. However, an initial trial injection of about 3 ml normal saline, after introducing the needle by any route, produces distension of the joint capsule and fluid is pushed back into the syringe

when there is correct placement of the needle. The *inferior* approach is made posterior to the adductor tendon, with the needle advanced parallel to the table top. The *lateral* approach is made anterior to the greater trochanter and the needle is passed superiorly along the femoral neck. The *anterior* approach is screened directly down to the lateral border of the femoral head ossification centre. The *superior* approach is made inward and downward at 45° screening to the same point as the anterior method. The final approach is made under screen control in all methods. Correct placement within the synovial cavity is checked with either the saline method or a small injection of contrast medium. Not more than 2 ml of water-soluble contrast medium is normally needed, the contrast agent being spread by joint movement (Fig. 23.10). Four standard 'spot films' are taken: in the neutral position, 45° abduction in both internal and external rotation, and a 'frog view' lateral. To these may be added a hyper-adducted cross-over view and a 'frog view' with downward pressure on the

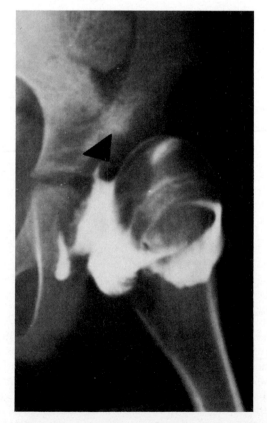

Fig. 23.10 Hip arthrogram. Unsuccessful treatment for a congenital hip dislocation. The capital epiphysis does not return to the shallow acetabulum due to the limbus (arrow).

Fig. 23.11 Equipment for cystourethrography: warmed aqueous contrast medium is held in the bottle and giving set. A trolley with sterile packs is ready for the catheterization. A sterile specimen bottle is available for a urine sample.

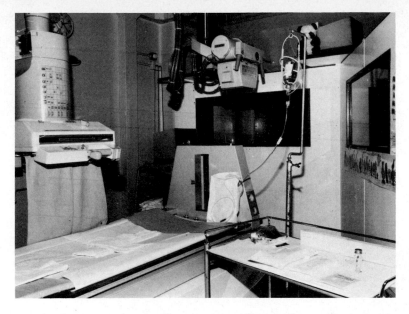

knee. Video-recording of joint movement is of great help.

REFERENCE

Grech P. (1977) *Hip Arthrography*. pp. 15–27. Chapman and Hall, London.

GENITO-URINARY TRACT

Inferior veno-cavography

Indications In the urographic examination of any intra-abdominal mass, it is good practice to combine this with an inferior veno-cavogram. Opinions vary as to the value of this as a diagnostic procedure, but the small addition to normal urographic procedure is worthwhile.

Contra-indications and complications The risk of contrast injection are the same as those for urography, and require the usual precautions. Femoral vein puncture is not advised in infants due to the risk of septic hip arthritis.

Technique This is usually carried out as part of the contrast injection for i.v. urography. A 21 gauge needle with flexible tube extension is inserted into a suitable ankle or foot vein and strapped in position. The system is kept open with a slow injection of normal saline. The explorator of the screening table is positioned over the pelvis and abdomen with spot films in readiness. The contra-lateral femoral vein is compressed manually and a rapid contrast injection is made. The contrast medium is observed in the pelvic veins and inferior vena cava and spot films are then obtained. If the child is old enough, a Valsalva manoeuvre may be applied at the same time.

Cysto-urethrography by urethral catheterization

Indications These include recurrent urinary tract infection and developmental abnormalities such as ectopic ureter.

Contra-indications This examination should be avoided during an acute urinary infection as reflux may occur only during a cystitis.

Technique Sedation is rarely needed. A local policy is needed in regard to antibiotic cover. The operator is 'scrubbed-up' and gloved. The perineum and peri-urethral area is cleaned with a suitable aqueous antiseptic solution. A No.6 or 8F umbilical feeding tube with a closed end and a side hole is a very suitable catheter for babies. The sterile catheter is lubricated with an anaesthetic jelly prior to its introduction. Resistance due to external sphincter in boys is gently overcome, while occasionally it may be necessary to inject normal saline from a syringe whilst advancing the catheter. When the bladder has been entered, the catheter is secured with external strapping. It is good practice to obtain a urine specimen and to measure the volume of residual urine at this stage. A suitable water-soluble contrast medium is then dripped in from a container about one metre above the table top, using a standard i.v. giving set (Fig. 23.11). Filling is

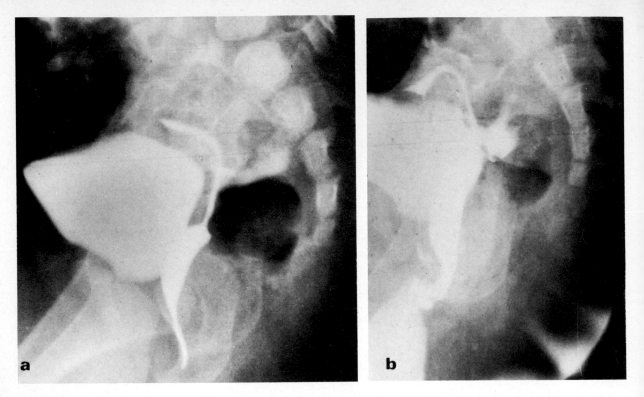

Fig. 23.12 Catheter study of a urogenital sinus in a baby with an intersex problem. (a) Filling of the urethra and bladder anteriorly. The wide vagina and narrower uterine cavity are filled with the uterus curving forward over the back of the bladder. (b) The uterine cornua are shown on a slightly oblique projection. Filling of the fallopian tubes is sometimes obtained.

continued until contrast medium begins to be passed alongside the catheter into the bladder neck and upper urethra. If the catheter is removed at this stage in infants, voiding may continue and save a long wait for spontaneous micturition. In older children, protestations of fullness may be checked by observing extension of the great toes! Spot radiographs record the bladder shape and size, vesico-ureteric reflux if seen, and the bladder outlet and residue on voiding. In children with neurogenic bladders, the residue is recorded after expression. Emptying may have to be achieved by expression if cysto-urethrography is combined with an examination under anaesthesia.

Alternative examination Bladder residue may be found by ultrasonography. Ureteric reflux is demonstrable by gamma camera isotope imaging.

Cysto-urethrography by supra-pubic puncture

Indications This method is used when a urethral obstruction is suspected in an infant. Posterior urethral

valves are usually sought in this way because urethral catheterization may temporarily fold back the membranous valve and make it difficult to visualize.

Contra-indications

Puncture should not be made through infected skin.

The presence of a full bladder may be confirmed by ultrasonography before examination. Skin preparation with a suitable water soluble antiseptic is carried out over the lower abdomen. A syringe is attached to a 21 or 23 short bevel needle which is introduced in the midline about 1 cm above the symphysis. The needle is advanced perpendicularly, or at a slight upward angle, until urine is aspirated. When in position, a urine sample is obtained and the needle is connected to a 'drip-set' for contrast filling. The needle may be steadied by a swab held by strapping. The examination then proceeds as previously described for the per urethral study. If pressure measurements are to be obtained, or if catheter drainage is required for some length of time, a flexible open-end catheter may be introduced by the Seldinger technique.

Complications Normal asepsis should prevent infection. Puncture of other organs, such as bowel or injection of contrast medium into peri-vesical tissues is avoided if the bladder is full, which may be checked by ultrasonography.

Genitography for intersex problems

Indications Ambiguous external genitalia.

Contra-indications Local infection in the perineum.

As contrast medium may spill through the Fallopian tubes into the peritoneal cavity, aseptic techniques are necessary to avoid infection.

Perineal examination shows whether there is either a wide cloacal type opening or one or more small orifices. In the latter case, a catheter examination is made in the same way as a cystogram. A single large opening may be examined by the 'flush' method described by Schopfner (1964). A 10 ml syringe is filled with a water-soluble contrast medium as used for cystography. A soft rubber acorn, similar to that used in the clamp for adult urethrography, is fitted to the syringe nozzle and the acorn applied with gentle pressure to the opening. An injection of 3–4 ml is made under screen control and spot films obtained in A–P and lateral planes (Fig. 23.12) The process may be repeated several times if necessary.

REFERENCES

Chiswick M. L. (1978) *Neonatal Medicine*. p. 80 (supra-pubic puncture).
Shopfner C. F. (1964) Genitography in intersex problems. *Radiology*, **82**, 664–74.

SINOGRAPHY

This term is used to denote the radiological examination of a cutaneous opening.

There are two problems in regard to sinuses and fistulae:

1. Where there is a cutaneous opening, the extent and direction of the track must be delineated and any communication with an abscess cavity or the bowel demonstrated. The track is examined by sinography.
2. Where there is the possibility of an internal fistula, a more complex series of investigations is required depending on the site of the fistula.

The track may be probed to determine its direction and to give an estimate of its size, which helps in the selection of a catheter. Probing must be very gentle to avoid damage to underlying tissues or the formation of a false passage. A red rubber catheter (Jacques 10 French gauge) is suitable in most cases. Finer Portex catheters are required for very narrow sinuses, but they are stiff and must be inserted with care.

No special sterile precautions are necessary, apart from sterilizing the instruments and catheters. The catheter is held with forceps and inserted into the cutaneous opening in the direction of the track, as determined by the probe, until firm resistance is felt. Water-soluble contrast medium is then injected fairly rapidly from a 20 ml syringe under screening control, in order to appreciate the ramifications of the tracks and their communications. Two spot radiographs should be taken at right angles to each other. Usually a supine and lateral view are all that is required (Fig. 24.1).

Complications are rare. Trauma to the track may cause slight bleeding, but the greatest danger is forceful probing and insertion of the catheter. If there is free spillage into the peritoneal cavity, the injection should be stopped because interperitoneal contrast medium may cause a profound ileus.

The timing of sinography in relation to other investigations is important. Plain films and ultrasonography should be performed first. Sinography may be performed during computed tomography, using water-soluble contrast of low density. Sinography should precede any barium study.

Internal fistulae

Not all fistulae can be demonstrated by radiological means. For example, only about 40% of colo-vesicular fistulae due to diverticular disease are shown on barium enema or by the presence of air in the bladder.

Although a fistula connects two hollow viscera, it may fill from only one side. The higher the applied pressure, the more likely the fistula will be shown. A high pressure examination is performed first. For instance, a barium enema or small bowel enema rather than a small bowel meal, or a cystogram in preference to an IVU.

The alternative investigation is used if the first does not show the fistula.

The choice of contrast medium depends on the site of the fistula and should be safe, wherever the fistula might take it. Gastrografin must never be used if there is the possibility of a fistula between the oesophagus and the bronchial tree, because of the risk of severe pulmonary oedema. In this situation aqueous Dionosil is recommended, although barium is generally adequate.

The progress of the contrast medium through the viscus is monitored, in order not to miss early filling of the other viscus from the fistula. This applies particularly to ileo-sigmoid fistula when early filling of the distal large bowel, before the proximal part contains barium, is diagnostic of a fistula but may be missed if the films are delayed until filling of the entire colon (Fig. 24.2).

Fig. 24.1 Following a road traffic accident, which involved damage to the pelvis, this patient developed an intermittent discharge from a sinus opening situated posteriorly in the mid-thigh. A catheter was introduced via the opening and could be inserted for a considerable distance. Contrast medium outlined a broad track extending up to the pelvis (a). A lateral view (b) shows that the track entered the pelvic cavity via the obturator foramen and ended in several branches within the ischiorectal fossa.

Fig. 24.2 Ileo-colic fistula due to Crohn's disease. A small bowel film (a) shows barium in the sigmoid, but not the rest of the colon. The caecum has filled and diseased terminal ileum is noted. Early filling of the rectum suggested a fistula, which was confirmed by a barium enema (b) showing barium filling the ileum from the sigmoid colon.

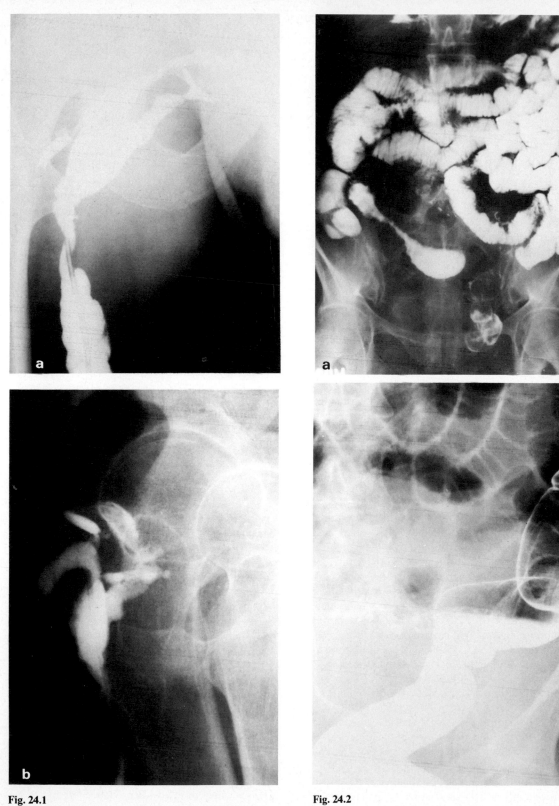

Fig. 24.1

Fig. 24.2

THE EARLY DEVELOPMENT OF WATER-SOLUBLE CONTRAST MEDIA FOR UROGRAPHY AND ANGIOGRAPHY

In 1923, Berberich and Hirsch used strontium bromide for the opacification of blood vessels in the extremities. Brooks employed sodium iodide solution for this purpose in the following year, but both of these agents caused pain and damage to the vascular walls. Moniz, in 1927, used sodium iodide for carotid arteriography but switched to colloidal thorium dioxide for this purpose in 1931 (Moniz, 1940).

Thorium dioxide had the advantage of being highly radio-opaque, at a time when radiographic film and equipment was much less efficient than it is nowadays, and of not causing pain on intravascular injection. Unfortunately, thorium is radioactive—being an emitter of α particles and having a half life of 1.4×10^{10} years. Thorium dioxide is permanently retained by the body within the reticulo-endothelial system, particularly the liver and spleen (Fig. 25.1). Indeed, large doses of the substance were injected intravenously to delineate these organs on abdominal radiography. The first recorded neoplasm in man attributed to thorium was an endothelial sarcoma of the liver (MacMahon et al., 1947), almost 20 years after colloidal thorium dioxide was introduced as a contrast agent. Other tumours have also been related to thorium; including hepatomas, biliary adenocarcinomas and myelogenous leukaemia. Retention of thorium by the urothelium following retrograde pyelography has been associated with subsequent transitional cell carcinomas (Wenz, 1967), while local injections into the breast and the maxillary sinuses have been followed by carcinomas at these sites (Swarm, 1971). The perivascular extravasation of thorium dioxide caused local granuloma formation.

Osborne et al., (1923) noted that the urine in the bladder often became radio-opaque in patients who received i.v. sodium iodide for syphilis. While this established that iodine could cause radiographic opacification of urine, delineation of the urinary tract was generally poor and sodium iodide was too toxic for use in urography.

In the late 1920s when Moniz's pioneering work was underway in Portugal, other developments in radiographic contrast media were being made in Germany. Binz and Räth, in Berlin, synthesized a large number of pyridine compounds, some of which contained iodine, with a view to treating syphilis and other infections. Swick, under the aegis of first Lichtwitz and then von Lichtenberg, investigated one of these compounds, Selectan, in regard to intravenous urography. Selectan (Fig. 25.2) was found to be of low solubility and unsuitable for this purpose. However, the sodium salt of one of the iodinated pyridines synthesized in 1927 by Binz and Räth—5-iodo-2-pyridone-N-acetic acid—was named Uroselectan (Fig. 25.3) and was used by Swick to produce the first successful intravenous urograms (Swick, 1929). The history of the development and recognition of Uroselectan has been elegantly and fully described by Grainger (1982).

Binz and Räth formulated two improved pyridine derivatives, iodopyracet (Diodone) (Fig. 25.4), and iodoxyl (Uroselectan B) (Fig. 25.5), each containing two iodine atoms per molecule, which soon replaced Uroselectan and remained the water-soluble contrast agents of choice until the early 1950s, some 20 years later.

THE SUBSTITUTED TRI-IODOBENZOIC ACID COMPOUNDS

Swick, while working in America in the 1930s, proposed the use of the benzene ring as an alternative iodine carrier to the pyridine ring. On this basis, sodium iodohippurate was developed as a potential contrast medium, but was discarded because of its high toxicity. Wallingford, who had extensively investigated iodinated benzoic acids as intermediates in the synthesis of iodohippurates, found that the introduction of an amine ($-NH_2$) group to the benzene ring resulted in a reduction in toxicity. The most soluble and least toxic of a large series of substituted amino tri-iodinated benzoic acids synthesized by Wallingford was 3-acetyl-amino-2,4,6,-tri-iodo-benzoic acid, the sodium salt of which was introduced as sodium acetrizoate (Urokon, Diaginol) in 1952 (Fig. 25.6).

Hoppe and his co-workers (Larsen et al., 1956)

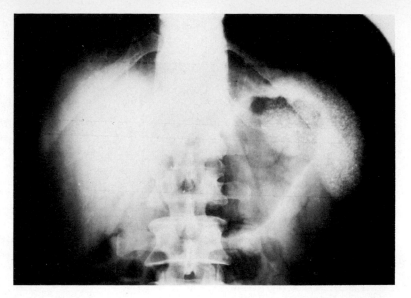

Fig. 25.1 Speckled opacification of the spleen due to accumulation of thorium, which was injected at arteriography more than ten years previously.

found that the insertion of a second acetamino group at the 5 position reduced toxicity and increased solubility still further; resulting in diatrizoic acid (Fig. 25.7), the sodium salt of which is marketed as

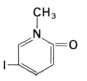

Fig. 25.2 Selectan: N-methyl-5-iodo-2-pyridone

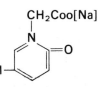

Fig. 25.3 Uroselectan: 5-iodo-2-pyridone-N-acetate-sodium

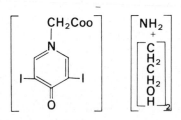

Fig. 25.4 Iodopyracet (Diodone)

Hypaque. Urografin (Schering) consists of a mixture of the sodium and methylglucamine salts of diatrizoic acid, available in various concentrations, in an attempt

to balance the high viscosity of methylglucamine salts against the higher toxicity of sodium salts.

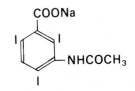

Fig. 25.5 Iodoxyl (Uroselectan B)

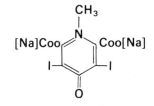

Fig. 25.6 Sodium acetrizoate (Urokon, Diaginal)

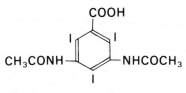

Fig. 25.7 Diatrizoic acid

Iothalamic acid (Fig. 25.8), which has given rise to the Conray range of contrast media, is an isomer of diatrizoic acid, the —NHCOCH₃ grouping at position 5 being changed to —CONHCH₃. Metrizoic acid (Fig. 25.9) differs from diatrizoic acid in having a methyl group (—CH₃) added to one acetamido side

Water-soluble Contrast Media   339

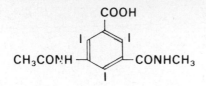

Fig. 25.8 Iothalamic acid

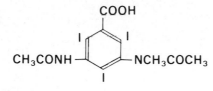

Fig. 25.9 Metrizoic acid

chain. The sodium salts of iothalamic acid and metrizoic acid are much more soluble than sodium diatrizoate, allowing high iodine concentrations to be achieved without higher viscosity. In the Triosil range of metrizoate compounds, calcium and magnesium ions are used, in balance with the methylglucamine salt, as an alternative to some of the sodium ions, as an attempt to reduce the toxicity incurred by high concentrations of sodium.

In general, sodium salts are more toxic to the brain and myocardium than the corresponding methylglucamine salts.

DISADVANTAGES OF HYPEROSMOLAR CONTRAST MEDIA

The majority of adverse effects from water-soluble contrast media are due to their high osmolarity (Grainger, 1980). The osmolarity of conventional contrast media is five to eight times that of plasma; an imbalance which becomes especially significant when large amounts of contrast medium are injected rapidly into the circulation, when contrast studies are performed in infants and small children, and when high concentrations are injected into end arteries which supply sensitive structures such as the heart and brain. The effects of hyperosmolarity occur at various sites:

Erythrocytes (Asperlin, 1979)

A rise in plasma osmolarity, due to the injection of contrast medium, causes water to leave the erythrocytes and to enter the plasma. The erythrocytes then become shrunken and deformed, loosing the pliability which normally allows them to traverse capillaries of

smaller diameters than themselves. This impairment of capillary transit and sludging of red blood cells results is tissue anoxia and an increase in the peripheral vascular resistance.

Endothelium (Almen et al, 1973)

Exposure of endothelial cells to hyperosmolar contrast media results in their damage, the degree of which is proportional to the concentration of the contrast medium. At capillary level, this endothelial compromise results not only in cellular damage but also an increased permeability of the capillary wall. This effect is of particular significance in relation to the blood–brain barrier, there being extensive experimental work demonstrating the increased permeability and the ensuing damage which results from direct contact between the contrast medium and brain cells (Gonsette, 1978).

Haemodynamic effects

The intra-arterial injection of any solution which is hyperosmolar to blood results in vasodilatation. In arteriography, this vasodilatation is manifested by pain and a sensation of heat in the limbs whose arteries are being delineated by contrast medium. The intra-aortic injection of contrast medium results in a transient fall in both systolic and diastolic blood pressure, indicating that the contrast medium has both vasodilator and cardiotoxic effects (Snowdon & Whitehouse, 1981), and often a rise in pulse rate. An increase in blood flow occurs within the legs (Delius & Erikson, 1969). These haemodynamic changes may be of clinical significance in patients who have cardiovascular disease. The i.v. injection of contrast medium, while often resulting in warmth and other symptoms attributable to vasodilation, rarely causes any appreciable alteration to blood pressure and pulse (Eyes et al., 1981). Transient hypervolaemia is another result of the intravascular injection of a large volume of hyperosmolar contrast medium. Water is rapidly transported from the extravascular compartment to the circulation and causes a marked fall in the haemocrit.

NON-IONIC CONTRAST MEDIA

All conventional water-soluble contrast media, being substituted tri-iodobenzoic acid derivatives, are salts of strong acids. As such, they all completely dissociate in solution, forming one cation (sodium or methylglucamine) and one anion (the tri-iodinated benzoate radical). Only the iodine-containing anion serves a useful purpose by providing opacification, the radiographically useless cation exerting the same osmotic effect as the anion. A natural development would therefore be a contrast medium which did not ionize in solution, thereby having approximately half the osmolarity of a conventional contrast medium of equal iodine concentration. The adverse effects due to hyperosmolarity should also be reduced by half.

The practical application of this proposition was made by Almén, a Swedish radiologist, in 1968. He suggested that the ionizing carboxyl group of conventional contrast media could be transformed into a non-dissociating group, such as an amide ($-CONH_2$). Further research led to the development of metrizamide (Amipaque, Nyegaard), a substituted amide of metrizoic acid, in which one of the hydrogen atoms in the amide radical is replaced by a simple grouping (Fig. 25.10). Metrizamide has the disadvantage of not

Table 25.1 Comparison of osmolality and viscosity of various contrast media.

Contrast medium	Concentration mgI/ml	Viscosity (m Pa.s)		Osmolality (mol/kg H₂O)
		20°	370	
Urografin 370	370	18.9	8.5	2.07
Hypaque 50%	299	3.3	2.5	1.52
Triosil 350	350	6.0	3.4	1.97
Metrizamide	280	9.7	5.0	0.43
Iopamidol	280	7.5	3.8	0.57
	370	18.0	9.5	0.80
Iohexol	280	8.8	4.8	0.62
	370	29.6	13.5	0.98
Hexabrix	320	15.7	7.5	0.58

oped by Bracco in Italy, is stable, may be autoclaved in solution and is cheaper than metrizamide (Fig. 25.11). Iopamidol is now used in myelography (Smaltino *et al.,* 1980), arteriography (Whitehouse & Snowdon, 1982) and in cardiac angiography (Cucchini

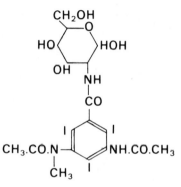

Fig. 25.10 Metrizamide (Amipaque)

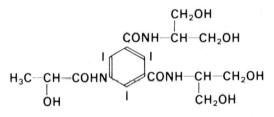

Fig. 25.11 Iopamidol

being sterilized by autoclaving, therefore having to be presented in freeze-dried lyophilized form, having a high viscosity (Table 25.1) and being much more expensive than conventional contrast media. Despite these shortcomings, metrizamide has revolutionized myelographic procedures (Lindgren, 1977). The lower osmolarity than previous contrast agents has also meant that metrizamide is well-tolerated in arteriography, in which it causes much less haemodynamic effects (Almén *et al.,* 1977; Snowdon & Whitehouse, 1981), and in peripheral venography where there is less local venous damage than with conventional contrast media. (Albrechtsson, 1979). The good toleration of metrizamide is shown in the specific instances of coronary arteriography (Enge *et al.,* 1977) and carotid arteriography (Enge *et al.,* 1977) and carotid arteriography (Wilmink, 1979).

A second generation of non-ionic contrast media has developed since metrizamide. Iopamidol, devel-

et al., 1979). The cardiovascular effects of iopamidol are less than with conventional contrast media, but are not quite as small as the changes from metrizamide (Whitehouse & Snowdon, 1982) although patient toleration is good.

Iohexol (Nyegaard) (Fig. 25.12) is a newer non-ionic contrast medium which is undergoing clinical evaluation but which shows promise (Lindgren, 1980).

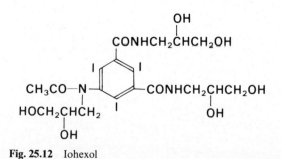

Fig. 25.12 Iohexol

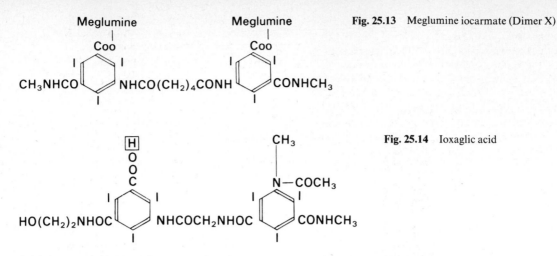

Meglumine   Meglumine

Fig. 25.13   Meglumine iocarmate (Dimer X)

Fig. 25.14   Ioxaglic acid

It may be that non-ionic contrast media are less allergenic than conventional media, but this is still a speculative and unproven consideration.

MONO-ACID DIMERS

It is possible to link two molecules of monomeric salts of substituted tri-iodobenzoic acids, by a side chain bridge, to produce a dimeric dicarboxylic acid. A dimeric acid produced from iothalamic acid is known as iocarmic acid, the methylglucamine salt of which (meglumine iocarmate) was introduced as Dimer X in 1970. Each molecule of Dimer X contains six atoms of iodine and dissociates in solution into two meglumine cations and one large iodinated anion (Fig. 25.13). The ratio of iodine atoms to ions is therefore 6 : 3, which is an improvement on the 3 : 2 ratio of conventional monomeric salts.

Subsequently, one of the carboxyl groups of a dimeric dicarboxylic acid has been converted into a non-ionizing radical, the other carboxyl group being linked to a cation to produce a salt. This compound is then a monomeric salt of a monoacid dimer, one molecule of which dissociates in solution into one large dimeric anion containing six atoms of iodine, and one cation. The iodine atom : ion ratio is then 6 : 2. Ioxaglate is such a compound, being commercially available as Hexabrix (Fig. 25.14), with a two to one mixture of meglumine and sodium salts of ioxaglic acid at an iodine concentration of 320 mg/ml. Hexabrix, like the non-ionic contrast media, is well tolerated in angiography, being of value in respect to carotid arteriography (Grainger, 1982), femoral arteriography (Holm & Praestholm, 1979) and angiocardiography (Cumberland, 1980). The small blood pressure changes and slight alteration in heart rate on aortography are comparable with metrizamide (Whitehouse & Snowdon, 1982).

A totally non-ionic dimer, the next logical step, is a current development. Iotasul is an example of a non-ionic dimer (Fig. 25.15), having less than half the osmolarity of metrizamide and the same osmolarity as plasma in the high concentration of 400 mg iodine/ml. The intradermal injection of Iotasul has been found to give a high quality lymphogram (Siefert *et al.,* 1980).

Theoretically, solutions of the non-ionic contrast media and Hexabrix should have an osmolarity of exactly half that of solutions of conventional monomeric salts, for the same iodine content (Table 25.1).

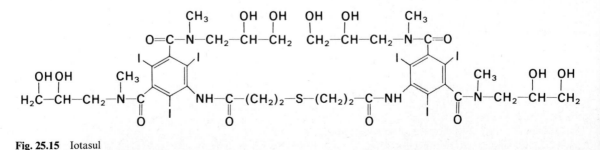

Fig. 25.15   Iotasul

In practice, the osmolarity of solutions of these agents is a third, instead of the anticipated half, because some of the molecules of the newer agents aggregate in solution with a resultant reduction in the number of particles.

The treatment of allergic reactions to water-soluble contrast media is discussed in the section on Intravenous Urography (p. 222).

REFERENCES

Albrechtsson U. (1979) Side effects at phlebography with ionized and non-ionized contrast media. *Diagnostic Imaging*, **48**, 236–40.

Almén T., Hartel M., Nylander G. & Olivecrona N. (1973) Effects of metrizamide on silver staining of aortic endothelium. *Acta Radiol*. Supplementum **335**, 233–8.

Almén T., Boijsen E. & Lindell S. E. (1977) Metrizamide in angiography I femoral arteriography. *Acta Radiol. Diagn.*, **18**, 33–8.

Aspelin P. (1978) Effect of ionic and non-ionic contrast media on red cell deformity *in vitro*. *Acta Radiol.*, **20**, 1–12.

Berberich J. & Hirsch S. (1923) Die röntgenographische Darstellung der Arterien und am lebenden. *Klin. Wschr.*, **9**, 2226–8.

Brooks B. (1924) Intra-arterial injection of sodium iodide. *J. Amer. med. Ass.*, **82**, 1016–19.

Cucchini F., Didonato M., Baldi G., Effendy F. N., Bongrani S., Colla B. & Visioli O. (1979) Left ventriculography and selective coronary arteriography with a new non-ionic contrast medium. *G. ital. Cardiol.*, **9**, 744–52.

Cumberland D. C. (1980) Hexabrix—a new contrast medium in angiocardiography. *Brit. Heart J.*, **45**, 698–702.

Delius W. & Erikson U. (1969) Effect of contrast medium on blood flow and blood pressure in the lower extremities. *Amer. J. Roentgenol.*, **107**, 869–76.

Enge I., Nitter-Hauge S., Andrew E. & Levorstad K. (1977) Amipaque: a new contrast medium in coronary angiography. *Radiology*, **125**, 317–22.

Eyes B. E., Evans A. F. & Whitehouse G. H. (1981) A comparative trial of two urographic contrast media—Conray 420 and Urografin 370. *Aust. Radiol.*, **25**, 150–6.

Gonsette R. E. (1978) Animal experiments and clinical experience in cerebral angiography with a new contrast agent (ioxaglic acid) with a low hyperosmolality. *Ann. Radiol.*, **21**, 271–3.

Grainger R. G. (1980) Osmolality of intravascular radiological contrast media. *Brit. J. Radiol.*, **53**, 739–46.

Grainger R. G. (1982) Intravascular contrast media—the past, the present and the future. *Brit. J. Radiol.*, **55**, 1–18.

Holm M. & Praestholm J. (1979) Ioxaglate, a new low osmolality contrast medium used in femoral angiography. *Brit. J. Radiol.*, **52**, 169–72.

Larsen A. A., Moore C., Sprague B., Clok J., Moss J. & Hoppe J. O. (1956) Iodinated 3,5-diamino benzoic acid derivatives. *J. Amer. chem. Soc.*, **78**, 3210–16.

Lindgren E. (1977) Metrizamide—Amipaque. The non-ionic water-soluble contrast medium. Further clinical experiences in neuroradiology. *Acta Radiol*. Suppl. 355.

Lindgren E. (1980) Iohexol. A non-ionic contrast medium. *Acta Radiol*. Suppl. 362.

MacMahon H. E., Murphy A. S. & Bates M. I. (1947) Endothelial cell sarcoma of the liver following thorotrast injection. *Amer. J. Path.*, **23**, 585–611.

Moniz E. (1940) *Die cerebrale Arteriographie und Phlebographie*. Springer Verlag, Berlin.

Osborne E. D., Sutherland C. G., Scholl A. J. & Rowntree L. G. (1923) Roentgenography of the urinary tract during excretion of sodium iodide. *J. Amer. Med. Ass.*, **80**, 368–73.

Siefert H. M., Mutzel W., Schobel C., Weinman H. J., Wenzerl-Hora B. I. & Speck V. (1980) Iotasul, a water soluble contrast agent for direct and indirect lymphography. *Lymphology*, **13**, 150–7.

Snowdon S. L. & Whitehouse G. H. (1981) Blood pressure changes resulting from aortography. *J. roy. Soc. Med.*, **74**, 419–21.

Shaltino F., Ciccarelli R., Cirillo S., Corrado A., D'Auria T., Gambardella R., Rotondo A. & Santor S. (1980) Myelography with B15000, a new non-ionic water-soluble contrast medium: technical aspects and early clinical experience. *Radiol. med.*, **66**, 210–14.

Swarm R. L. (1971) Colloidal thorium dioxide. In *Interventional Encyclopaedia of Pharmacology and Therapeutics*. Radiocontrast Agents, Vol. 2, Pergamon Press, Oxford.

Swick M. (1929) Darstellung der Nieren und Harnweg in Roentgenbild durch intravenöse Einbringung eines neuen Kontraststoffes: des Uroselectans. *Klin. Wshr.*, **8**, 2087–9.

Wallingford V. H. (1952) Iodinated acylaminobenzoic acids as X-ray contrast media. *J. Amer. pharm. Ass.*, **42**, 721–8.

Wenz W. (1967) Tumours of the kidney following retrograde pyelography with colloidal thorium dioxide. *Ann. N. Y. Acad. Sci.*, **145**, 806–10.

Whitehouse G. H. & Snowdon S. L. (1982) An assessment of iopamidol, a non-ionic contrast medium, in aorto-femoral angiography. *Clin. Radiol.*, **33**, 271–4.

Whitehouse G. H. & Snowdon S. L. (1982) An assessment of Hexabrix, a low osmolality contrast medium, in aortofemoral angiography (in press).

Wilmink J. T. (1979) Patient reactions in angiography of the head and neck using an ionic and non-ionic contrast medium. *Diagn. Imag.*, **48**, 196–8.

Anaesthesia in Diagnostic Radiology

S. L. SNOWDON

ANAESTHESIA IN DIAGNOSTIC RADIOLOGY

Although a large number of procedures undertaken in the X-ray Department require some form of anaesthesia or analgesia, this subject has been surprisingly neglected in the past.

There is evidence that the results of a significant number of invasive radiological procedures do not influence patient management (Bell *et al.*, 1980). The patient may therefore be subjected unnecessarily to the hazards of anaesthesia in the radiology department.

Anaesthesia in radiological cases is often delegated to a junior member of the anaesthesic staff and there are frequently limited and outdated anaesthetic facilities provided in radiology departments. Few standard texts advise on the problems that are likely to be encountered, despite the unfavourable circumstances for anaesthesia on what are often poor risk patients (Barnes & Havill, 1980). Such investigations are not uncommonly followed by operative intervention which requires further anaesthesia. It is, therefore, essential that a high standard of anaesthetic care is employed in the first instance. An experienced anaesthetist may also be useful in the Radiology Department, not only for administering a general anaesthetic, but also in advising on suitable analgesia, sedation, resuscitative procedures, regional blocks and clinical measurement.

Facilities required for general anaesthesia in the X-ray department

Because the hazards encountered in anaesthetizing a patient in the X-ray department may be as great as those encountered in the main operating theatre, the facilities should be of comparable standard. There should be a separate room for induction of anaesthesia and subsequent recovery. A fully equipped anaesthetic trolley must be available and should include ventilators and a comprehensive monitoring system. Careful monitoring is important during anaesthesia in the X-ray Department, but may be especially difficult because of the darkened conditions as well as the position and the need to move the patient during some procedures. The table provided for anaesthetizing a patient should be capable of being tipped and there should be facilities for obtaining a sitting position. A full range of anaesthetic drugs is required, including 'DDAs' and those drugs which are needed for resuscitation.

A patient who is anaesthetized is, of course, unable to respond or move away from a source of electrical shock and fatal electrocution has occurred in these circumstances. All equipment should therefore be rigorously checked, especially the earth leakage current in monitoring apparatus and in radiological equipment.

An operating department assistant is useful in moving and repositioning the patient. He is also required to check carefully all the anaesthetic and monitoring equipment which is often neglected, outdated and within an isolated X-ray department.

A fully qualified nurse should also be available during the administration and recovery from anaesthesia. She may have to manage a patient who is only semi-conscious, and who may have suffered an anaphylactic attack or other complication such as laryngospasm.

Preparation for anaesthesia

Adequate consultation between clinician, radiologist and anaesthetist is required to avoid confusion on the ward concerning the necessity for anaesthesia when a patient is about to undergo a radiological investigation. An appreciation of the likelihood for general anaesthesia is required so that the patient should receive appropriate preparation. The patient should have a full general examination and the routine investigations.

For patients over 60 years of age, an electrocardiograph (ECG), chest radiograph, haemoglobin level, blood count and serum electrolytes are recommended on a routine basis. In younger patients, investigations may also be required where there is a specific indication, for instance a chronic cough necessitates a chest radiograph. The primary disease requiring radiological investigation may well be linked with other disorders, for instance the association of diabetes and arteriopathy, which require appropriate investigation and treatment prior to anaesthesia.

Sedation may be needed prior to the procedure and is especially important when the investigation is performed under local anaesthesia rather than general anaesthesia.

Type of anaesthesia for procedure

The decision as to whether a patient should receive general anaesthesia or local anaesthesia seems to be arbitrary in many cases. This is exemplified by the wide variety of anaesthetic 'techniques' used for the same radiological procedure in different centres. There are definite risks associated with general anaesthesia which should be borne in mind when considering procedures which are diagnostic and seldom therapeutic, making it difficult to set any direct benefit to the patient against any potential hazard. Having established the real need of the procedure and its influence on the subsequent management of the patient, it is then necessary to examine the indications and relative contra-indications for general anaesthesia.

INDICATIONS FOR GENERAL ANAESTHESIA

1. When the procedure is painful, either because of the technique or the nature of the injected contrast medium.
2. Where severe anxiety is anticipated (Finby & Kanick, 1970).
3. When the radiological procedure may produce complications which require control of the ventilation or circulation.
4. If subsequent general anaesthesia is required immediately following the procedure.
5. If general anaesthesia makes the performances of the radiological procedure easier and improves the quality of a particular investigation.

RELATIVE CONTRA-INDICATIONS

1. Pre-existing diseases; for example, coronary thrombosis, diabetes and severe respiratory embarrassment.
2. Technical anaesthetic problems; for instance, an unstable neck and limited neck or jaw movement.
3. Recent ingestion of food or fluid.
4. Inadequate patient preparation for general anaesthesia, when there has not been an examination or insufficient investigation.

5. A history of allergy, particularly with a previous general anaesthetic or contrast medium examination.
6. Acute or active chronic respiratory infection.
7. The coexistence of other disorders of greater importance with a higher priority for treatment than the disease about to be investigated by the radiologist.

If, on balance, general anaesthesia is contra-indicated, consideration should be given to local anaesthesia or neurolept-anaesthesia. Whilst neurolept-anaesthesia has gained popularity in many parts of the world, the patient often feels disorientated during the procedure and unable to fully express his fears (Moor et al., 1971). Patients occasionally obstruct their airway during neurolept-anaesthesia, necessitating emergency intubation and controlled ventilation.

Careful preparation is also required if the radiological investigation is performed with local anaesthesia. The confidence of the patient should be gained and the procedure carefully explained to him well in advance. Suitable pre-operative sedation may do much to relax the patient and facilitate the examination. The patient should be engaged in conversation and encouraged throughout the investigation. Local anaesthesia occasionally proves inadequate either because of discomfort experienced by the patient or because of radiological technical difficulties. General anaesthesia may then be required and the patient should be prepared for such an eventuality.

ANAESTHETIC PROBLEMS ASSOCIATED WITH SPECIFIC TECHNIQUES OF X-RAY EXAMINATION

Aortography

Patients presenting for aortography frequently have generalized cardiovascular disease. There is often a history of smoking and patients may have multisystem disease, including respiratory problems which require careful pre-operative preparation. Investigations should include a chest radiograph, pulmonary function tests, electrocardiogram, a full blood count including platelets, and serum electrolytes.

The two commonest approaches to aortography are the translumbar route and the Seldinger technique from a femoral artery. General anaesthesia is usually required for translumbar aortography. Intubation and controlled ventilation are then indicated because of the prone position of the patient. Special care should be taken to ensure the secure fixation of the endotra-

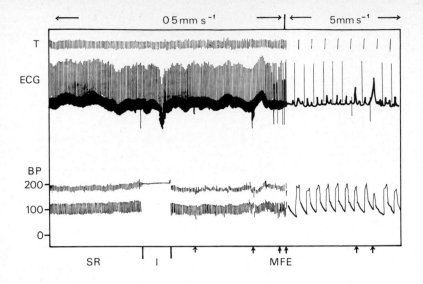

Fig. 26.1 Tracing of ECG and arterial pressure (BP) recorded during and following the injection of contrast media (I) demonstrating the subsequent appearance of multifocal ectopic complexes (MFE) and fall in arterial pressure. The patient showed a stable sinus rythm (SR) prior to injection and, as is commonly noted in patients presenting for aortography, hypertension.

cheal tube. A patient may be moved more than a metre during the radiological exposure, so that excessive tension may develop on the tubing attached to the anaesthetic machine. Sudden extubation in the prone position, especially in a darkened room, is serious because re-intubation is difficult in this position. Careful positioning is also important during translumbar aortography because of the movement of the X-ray table, care being taken to secure the arms and legs. The pelvis and chest must be raised to enable free movement of the abdomen during controlled ventilation, otherwise excessively high inflation pressures are required to ventilate the patient in this position. The patient should never be moved without first informing the anaesthetist. A ventilation alarm is of great help to the anaesthetist in ensuring satisfactory respiration and maintaining the anaesthetic circuit connection attaching the patient to the anaesthetic machine.

Routine monitoring of the ECG is very important because of the common occurrence of pre-existing cardiovascular disease and also because of the cardiovascular side-effects resulting from the injection of the contrast medium. The frequency of the latter has not been fully appreciated in the past and blood pressure monitoring is advisable. It is possible to monitor continuously the blood pressure, by connecting the angiographic catheter to a pressure transducer. Many of the contrast media employed for aortography produce a significant fall in the blood pressure immediately following their injection (Moss & Johnson, 1981; Snowdon & Whitehouse, 1981), and sometimes cardiac dysrhythmias (Fig. 26.1). This uncontrolled hypotension is especially undesirable in patients with cardiovascular disease. Post-operative

laryngospasm is another largely unrecognized complication associated with translumbar aortography. The laryngospasm may not be immediately apparent following extubation, and the first signs may only appear several minutes later. If severe, this complication is life threatening and may require urgent re-intubation of the patient. It is, therefore, advisable that the patient remains in the recovery area under careful observation for twenty minutes. Milder forms of laryngospasm may be managed by intravenous sedation and oxygen therapy. A vicious circle may develop with the patient becoming increasingly anxious and agitated with resultant worsening of the laryngospasm. The cause of the laryngospasm is uncertain but is probably related to intubation in the prone position causing irritation of the vocal cords. Inhalation of secretions, which accumulate especially in the nasopharynx in the prone position, may trigger the spasm. An allergic reaction to the contrast media with laryngeal oedema has also been implicated as a cause.

Pulmonary oedema has complicated translumbar aortography, the first signs appearing after reversal of anaesthesia (Aps, 1975).

A poor cardiac reserve, the change from positive pressure ventilation to spontaneous respiration, and an increased circulatory blood volume due to hyperosmolar contrast media, are precipitating factors in these cases. The femoral Seldinger approach using local anaesthesia should, therefore, be adopted whenever possible. Until recently, general anaesthesia was even required for the femoral Seldinger approach because of the severe pain with followed injection of the contrast medium. The newer contrast media with low osmolality have the advantages of causing considerably less pain as well as producing less significant hypotension (Snowdon & Whitehouse, 1981).

Epidural anaesthesia has been used to facilitate aortography. There is a small but definite incidence of spinal cord and nerve damage following epidural anaesthesia (Miskin *et al.*, 1973). Spinal cord damage may also be encountered following aortography due to high concentrations of contrast media reaching the spinal cord via the lumbar arteries. The skills of the anaesthetist in clinical measurement and monitoring are useful in the assessment of functional improvement achieved by transluminal angioplasty.

Carotid angiography

Patients referred for carotid angiography from a vascular surgical unit are often managed in a similar manner to that described for aortography. Those patients presenting in a neuroradiological unit may, however, cause different problems for the anaesthetist. A raised intracranial pressure, and associated vomiting with its consequent electrolyte disturbance, are features which must be recognized and dealt with by the anaesthetist. It is particularly important to correct sodium and potassium disturbances which may lead to potentiation of muscle relaxants and prolonged muscle relaxation.

The anaesthetic technique may considerably affect the intra-cranial pressure (Samuel *et al.*, 1968; Jennet *et al.*, 1969; McDowell, 1975). Intra-cranial pressure is related to changes in blood gases, including oxygen and carbon dioxide tensions (Fig. 26.2), which the anaesthetist may do much to control, normally aiming to keep the arterial carbon dioxide within the normal range. Control of arterial blood gas tensions may be used to alter blood vessel calibre, with significant improvement of the radiographic demonstration of the cerebral vasculature (Dallas & Moxon, 1969). It should be remembered that the neurosurgical patient may proceed directly to further surgery.

There is some evidence that volatile agents, especially halothane, cause a significant rise in the intra-cranial pressure of patients with cerebral tumours (McDowell *et al.*, 1963). Spontaneous ventilation whilst using a volatile anaesthetic agent is, therefore, contra-indicated and a technique employing intubation and controlled ventilation is used in preference. A smooth induction is desirable, avoiding coughing and straining, yet permitting maintenance of the blood pressure which facilitates palpation and cannulation of the carotid artery. A technique using muscle relaxants causes relaxation of the sternocle-

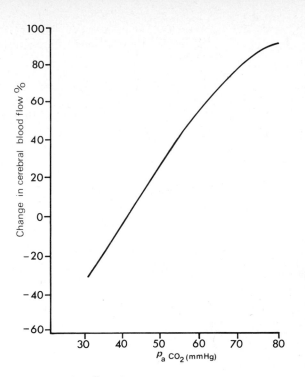

Fig. 26.2 The effect of arterial carbon dioxide tension on cerebral blood flow. Hypercarbia is frequently associated with spontaneous respiration during anaesthesia and the resulting increased cerebral blood flow may raise the intracranial pressure.

idomastoid muscle, allowing it to be displaced, and an easier fixation of the artery. However, the cannulation of the intracranial vessels by a catheter from the femoral artery is replacing direct carotid artery puncture. It is clearly more difficult to assess the neurological state of the patient during general anaesthesia compared to local anaesthesia. For this reason, some anaesthetists routinely employ electroencephalographic monitoring in addition to careful monitoring of the ECG and of the blood pressure. If carotid angiography has been performed under general anaesthesia, a neurological examination should be undertaken during the recovery period to ensure that there has been no cerebral damage. An intense burning sensation and severe retrobulbar pain occasionally makes if difficult for patients to remain motionless if only local anaesthesia has been used, resulting in an unsatisfactory study. The advent of low osmolality contrast media has made this less of a problem. Unexpected cardiovascular collapse may also occur during the investigation (Campkin *et al.*, 1977). The presence of an anaesthetist is therefore useful during local anaesthesia, if only to assist with resuscitation and to intercede if the patient finds the procedure unbearable. Prolonged apnoea has been observed following vertebral angiography (Davis & Statham, 1962), providing a further reason for using controlled ventilation during general anaesthesia.

A sudden rise in blood pressure has been noted following carotid angiography and may be a complication of the contrast media (Campkin *et al.*, 1977), especially in patients having a subarachnoid haemorrhage, and the reversal of narcotics with nalaxone (Cottrell & Estilo, 1981). Narcotics may, of course be used with either local or general anaesthesia. Cottrell and Estilo (1981) have described a case where a sudden rise of arterial blood pressure to 260/140 was associated with the rupture of a cerebral aneurysm, 5 minutes after nalaxone reversal of fentanyl, and a resultant right hemiplegia.

Pneumoencephalography

While many of the difficulties associated with carotid arteriography are seen, there are some specific problems associated with general anaesthesia in pneumoencephalography. Development in computed tomography, however, have led to a progressive decline in the use of this procedure although it is still used occasionally in many centres. A considerable rise in intracranial pressure has followed the injection of air as the contrast agent when nitrous oxide has been used in general anaesthesia (Saidman & Eger, 1965; Artrue *et al.*, 1978). Nitrous oxide is highly soluble in water and in blood while air, particularly nitrogen, is relatively insoluble. Following induction of anaesthesia with nitrous oxide, the concentration of nitrous oxide rapidly increases in the blood with simultaneous clearance of nitrogen. Air injected into the ventricle is, however, only slowly taken up into the blood stream because of its poor solubility. Following the initially low partial pressure of nitrous oxide within the ventricle into which air has been injected, nitrous oxide will rapidly cross the capillary membrane until there is equilibrium between the partial pressures of the liquid and gaseous phases. The volume of nitrous oxide entering the ventricle, whilst coming into equilibrium for a given partial pressure, is considerably larger than the volume of nitrogen leaving the ventricle. Nitrogen, being relatively insoluble, achieves an equivalent partial pressure in solution for a much smaller dissolved volume. Volume expansion, due to the unequal transfer of nitrous oxide and nitrogen inside the ventricle, results in a considerable rise of intracranial pressure. The injection of nitrous oxide is a more satisfactory alternative to injecting air

in pneumoencephalography (Betts, 1977). The same is true when this procedure is performed under local anaesthetic or neuroleptanalgesia (Edwards and Flowerdrew, 1980; Wolfson *et al.*, 1968). Air embolism has occurred following pneumoencephalography (Jacoby *et al.*, 1959), the risk of embolism also being minimized by the use of a soluble gas such as nitrous oxide.

Hypotension is another complication of air encephalography. Many anaesthetic agents diminish the autonomic control of the peripheral vascular system, resulting in postural hypotension. Careful monitoring of the blood pressure is essential whilst changing the patient from the supine to erect position during air encephalography. A peripheral vasocontrictor may be used to overcome the postural hypotension, but positioning the patient supine is the most effective management.

Cardiac angiography

Cardiac angiography has separate considerations in the adult and paediatric age groups.

In the adult, cardiac angiography is usually performed under local anaesthesia with the assistance of sedation. Dysrythmias are not uncommon as a result of the direct stimulation of the heart by the catheter and following injection of the contrast medium, although this has been considerably reduced by the introduction of non-ionic contrast agents. Electrocardiographic monitoring should always be undertaken. Left heart failure, myocardial infarction and 'crescendo angina' have all been noted to occur during coronary angiography. Sedation or anaesthesia must, therefore, disturb the cardiovascular system as little as possible. Diazepam is most commonly used for sedation (Hendrix & Malory, 1971). It is preferable to use a lipid-based emulsion such as Diazemuls because of the high incidence of pain on injection and of thrombophlebitis following the injection of plain diazepam. Diazepam has a significant depressant effect on respiration. This is particularly evident if a narcotic or opiate is also given, whereupon profound respiratory depression may occur and require intubation and controlled ventilation. Hypotension occasionally follows the intravenous injection of diazepam, which should therefore be given carefully while observing the patient's response in terms of respiratory changes and of blood pressure. A suitable level of sedation may be achieved by giving 5–30 mg intravenously in increments of 1–2 mg until the onset of ptosis.

Two particular considerations decide the form of anaesthesia for paediatric cardiopulmonary investigation. Firstly, the infant is usually uncooperative and hence general anaesthesia may well be required regardless of any other consideration. Secondly, it is most important to maintain cardiovascular stability. While heavy sedation is employed in some centres (Nicholson & Graham, 1969), it may well be associated with marked respiratory depression and a resultant considerable disturbance of the normal physiological state. Sudden cardio-respiratory failure may also occur during cardiac catheterization. If the child is already anaesthetized, he will almost certainly have been intubated and an intravenous line established—two vital steps in resuscitation.

The aim of the anaesthetist is to present the child for investigation with a stable circulatory state. This requires careful preoperative preparation. Some children present in cardiac failure as potential surgical emergencies. A muscle relaxant technique with controlled ventilation has been used to provide stable conditions. Great care must be taken to avoid hypoxaemia. It is especially important in the smaller child to maintain body temperature. Continuing therapeutic support of the cardiovascular system may be required throughout anaesthesia, with corrections to the arterial blood gas status. Ideally, these infants require the skills of a paediatric anaesthetist in specialized centres.

Bronchography

Bronchography is usually undertaken with local anaesthesia to the pharynx and sedation of the patient, but may also be performed under general anaesthesia with more comfort for the patient. Special endotracheal tubes have recently been developed to enable bronchography to be undertaken during general anaesthesia.

Venography

Intraosseous venograms are rarely performed nowadays but require general anaesthesia because of the discomfort to the patient. Patients with multiple pulmonary emboli may have a poor cardiopulmonary reserve and should be assessed by means of chest radiographs, isotope studies, pulmonary function tests and, most importantly, blood gas analysis following clinical assessment. The normal hypoxaemia may be found on blood gas analysis. The normal homeostatic mechanisms which maintain the distribution of blood flow and ventilation are disturbed during anaesthesia, with marked increase in the physiological shunt. This leads to an increase in hypoxaemia unless there is a high inspired oxygen tension, controlled ventilation and, possibly a continuous positive airway pressure (CPAP).

CT scanning

It is occasionally necessary, even with the short scan times now available, to use some form of sedation and occasionally general anaesthesia in infants and patients who are unable to cooperate.

Orthopaedic radiology

The radiological investigation of a joint under mechanical stress sometimes requires general anaesthesia. Caution is required in the manipulation of joints, especially if muscle relaxants are used, because considerable damage may occur to the joint which is no longer protected by the normal muscle tone.

Injection of contrast medium into the nucleus pulposus is sometimes employed in the investigation of 'prolapsed disc' prior to chemonucleolysis by chymopapain. Precise positioning of the needle before injection is required, and may cause considerable discomfort to the patient. Cooperation of the patient is very important during the contrast injection to determine if pain has been provoked and to ensure that no damage is caused to the nervous system. Light anaesthesia and neurolept-anaesthesia allows the patient to be awakened at appropriate times, questioned as to any discomfort, and requested to move his legs. The anaesthetist must anticipate well in advance when anaesthesia is to be lightened in order that the patient may communicate coherently with the operator.

POST-OPERATIVE COMPLICATIONS AND CARE

Because the radiology departments are frequently isolated from the other medical units in the hospital, special care is required during the recovery from anaesthesia. An experienced nurse must be available to tend to the patient. Facilities should be provided for the patient to stay long enough to recover fully prior to his return to the ward. An inexperienced nurse should not escort the patient back to the ward, because of the potential risk of serious and life-endangering complications.

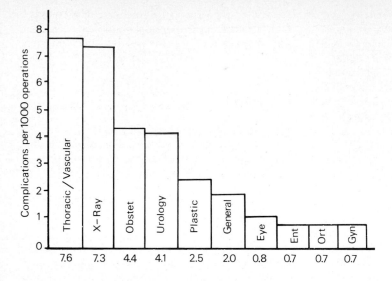

Fig. 26.3 Incidence of complications per thousand procedures requiring admission to an intensive therapy unit in various surgical groups. (Courtesy P. J. Barnes & J. M. Havill, *Anaesthesia and Intensive Care,* **8**, No. 4, November 1980).

A recent investigation showed a surprisingly high morbidity following anaesthesia for radiological procedures (Barnes & Havill, 1980). On comparing the morbidity rate per thousand procedures requiring admission to an intensive care unit after a variety of surgical procedures (Fig. 26.3), anaesthesia for radiological investigations had a morbidity second only to cardiothoracic surgery. The combination of factors responsible for this relatively high morbidity included ignorance of the hazards which may arise within the radiology department and the delegation of anaesthesia to junior and inexperienced staff.

The facilities provided in the recovery room should include an adequate suction and oxygen supply. Endotracheal tubes, laryngoscopes and suitable drugs for resuscitation must be immediately available. The trolley on which the patient is recovering must allow the patient to be tilted head down in case of vomiting or hypotension. An ECG and defibrillator must be available, together with intravenous fluids and infusion sets. Whilst much of the X-ray department may be darkened, the recovery room should be well lit. The anaesthetist is frequently hampered in assessing his patient during periods of reduced illumination in the X-ray room. He therefore loses the valuable sign of skin colour which gives him information about the patient's circulation and peripheral perfusion, the adequacy of oxygenation, and hence the normal and proper functioning of the anaesthetic apparatus.

CONCLUSION

A greater mutual understanding of the problems involved at the interface between Anaesthesia and Radiology will result in improved standards of safety and should also lead to a safer conduct of radiological investigations and an improvement in the quality of the results. The diagnostic radiologist now also undertakes therapeutic procedures, for example transluminal angioplasty. The skills of the anaesthetist in clinical measurement and monitoring are useful in the assessment of functional improvement achieved by these procedures.

REFERENCES

Alps C. (1975) Pulmonary oedema following translumbar aortography. *Proc. roy. Soc. Med.,* **68**, 966.

Artru A., Sohn Y. J. & Eger E. T. (1978) Increased intracranial pressure from nitrous oxide—five days after pneumoencephalography. *Anaesthesiology,* **49**, 126–37.

Barnes P. J. & Havill J. A. (1980) Anaesthetic complications requiring intensive care—a five year review. *Anaesth. Intens. Care,* **8**, 404.

Betts K. (1977) (Correspondence) Nitrous oxide encephalography. *Anaesth. Analg.,* **56**, (3), 469.

Campkin T. V., Hurchings G. M. & Phillips G. (1977) Arterial pressure studies during carotid angiography. *Brit. J. Anaesth.,* **49**, 163–7.

Cottrell J. E. & Estilo A. E. (1981) Naloxone, hypertension and ruptured cerebral aneurysm. *Anaesthesiol.,* **54**, 352.

Dallas S. H. & Moxon C. P. (1969) Controlled ventilation for cerebral angiography. *Brit. J. Anaesth.,* **41**, 597–602.

Davis S. & Statham C. (1962) Prolonged apnoea following vertebral angiography. *Brit. J. Anaesth.,* **34**, 119–20.

Edwards J. C. & Flowerdrew G. D. (1970) Diazepam and local analgesia for lumbar air encephalography. *Brit. J. Anaesth.,* **42**, 999–1104.

Finby N. & Kanick V. (1970) Radiological special procedures and the difficult patient. *Radiology,* **94**, 101–3.

Hendrix G. & Malory W. (1971) Intravenous diazepam in coronary arteriography. *J. S. Carol. Med. Ass.,* **67**, 5–6.

Hopkin D. A. Buxton (1980) *Hazards and Errors in Anaesthesia in Radiological Departments.* Springer, Berlin, New York.

Jacoby J., Jones T. R., Ziegler J., Clanen L. & Garvin J. P. (1959) Pneumoencephalography and air embolism: simulated anaesthetic death. *Anaesthesiol.,* **20**, 336–40.

Macpherson D. S., James D. C. & Bell P. R. F. (1980) Is aortography abused in lower-limb ischaemia? *Lancet,* **ii**, 80–82.

Manners J. M. (1971) Anaesthesia for diagnostic procedures in cardiac disease. *Brit. J. Anaesth.,* **43**, 276–87.

McDowall D. G., Harper A. M. & Jacobson I. (1963) Cerebral blood flow during halothane anaesthesia. *Brit. J. Anaesth.,* **35**, 394–402.

McDowall D. G., Barker W. B. J. & Fitch J. (1969) Effect of anaesthesia on intracranial pressure in patients with space occupying lesions. *Lancet,* **i**, 61–4.

McDowall D. G. (1975) Anaesthesia for neuroradiology. *Proc. roy. Soc. Med.,* **68**, 765.

Miskin M. M., Baum S. & Di Chiro G. (1973) Emergency treatment of angiography induced paraplegia and tetraplegia. *New Engl. J. Med.,* **288**, 1184–5.

Moore P. H., Morgan M. & Loh L. (1971) Ketamine as the sole anaesthetic agent for minor surgical procedures. *Anaesthesia,* **26**, No. 2.

Moss P. J. & Johnson R. C. (1981) Case report—temporary blindness following anaesthesia after translumbar aortography. *Anaesthesia,* **36**, 954–5.

Nicholson J. R. & Graham G. R. (1969) Management of infants under six months of age undergoing cardiac investigation. *Brit. J. Anaesth.,* **41**, 417–25.

Saidman L. J. & Eger E. (1965) Change in cerebrospinal pressure during pneumoencephalography under nitrous oxide anaesthesia. *Anaesthesiol.,* **26**, (1), 67–72.

Samuel J. R., Grange R. A. & Hawkins T. D. (1968) Anaesthetic technique for carotid angiography. *Anaesthesia,* **23**, (4), 543–51.

Snowdon S. L. & Whitehouse G. H. (1981) Blood pressure changes resulting from aortography. *J. roy. Soc. Med.,* **74**, 419–21.

Wolfson B., Siker E. G., Wible L. R. & Dubansky J. (1968) Pneumoencephalography using neuroleptanalgesia. *Anaesth. Analg.,* **47**, (1), 14–17.

Index